THE U.S. HEALTH SYSTEM
Origins and Functions
4th Edition

THE U.S. HEALTH SYSTEM
Origins and Functions

FOURTH EDITION

Marshall W. Raffel, Ph.D.

Professor of Health Policy and Administration
The Pennsylvania State University
University Park, Pennsylvania

Norma K. Raffel, Ph.D.

Health Services Research
State College, Pennsylvania

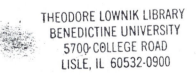
Delmar Publishers Inc.™

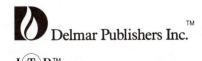
I(T)P™

NOTICE TO THE READER

Publisher does not warrant or guarantee any of the products described herein or perform any independent analysis in connection with any of the product information contained herein. Publisher does not assume, and expressly disclaims, any obligation to obtain and include information other than that provided to it by the manufacturer.

The reader is expressly warned to consider and adopt all safety precautions that might be indicated by the activities described herein and to avoid all potential hazards. By following the instructions contained herein, the reader willingly assumes all risks in connection with such instructions.

The publisher makes no representations or warranties of any kind, including but not limited to, the warranties of fitness for particular purpose or merchantability, nor are any such representations implied with respect to the material set forth herein, and the publisher takes no responsibility with respect to such material. The publisher shall not be liable for any special, consequential or exemplary damages resulting, in whole or in part, from the readers' use of, or reliance upon, this material.

Cover design by: Timothy Conners

Delmar Staff
Senior Acquisitions Editor: Bill Burgower
Assistant Editor: Debra Flis
Project Editor: Carol Micheli
Production Coordinator: Jennifer Gaines
Art and Design Coordinator: Michael Traylor

For information, address Delmar Publishers Inc.
3 Columbia Circle, Box 15-015
Albany, New York 12212

Copyright © 1994 by Delmar Publishers Inc.
The trademark ITP is used under license

Delmar Publishers' Online Services
To access Delmar on the World Wide Web, point your browser to:
http://www.delmar.com/delmar.html
To access through Gopher: gopher://gopher.delmar.com
(Delmar Online is part of "thomson.com", an Internet site with information on more than 30 publishers of the International Thomson Publishing organization.)
For information on our products and services:
email: info@delmar.com
or call 800-347-7707

Printed in the United States of America
Published simultaneously in Canada
By Nelson Canada,
A Division of The Thompson Corporation

 4 5 6 7 8 9 10 XXX 00 99 98 97 96

Library of Congress Cataloging-in-Publication Data

Raffel, Marshall W.
   The U.S. health system : origins and functions / Marshall W.
Raffel, Norma K. Raffel. -- 4th ed.
      p.   cm.
   Includes bibliographical references and index.
   ISBN 0-8273-5408-8
   1. Medical care--United States. 2. Public health--United States.
I. Raffel, Norma K. II. Title. III. Title: US health system.
   [DNLM: 1. Delivery of Health Care--United States. 2. Delivery of
Health Care--history--United States. 3. Public Health--United
States. 4. Public Health--history--United States. 5. United
States.   W 84 AA1 R2u 1994]
RA395.A3R33 1994
362.1'0973--dc20
DNLM/DLC
for Library of Congress   93-11931
                                                              CIP

Contents

To Robert, Dorothy, and Timothy

Preface

A growing number of colleges and universities are offering an introductory course on the health services in the United States to enable students in health, business, and public administration, as well as those in public health, nursing, and other health professional programs, to learn more about our system for providing health services—how the system developed, how it works today, why it costs so much, and what its problems are. *The U.S. Health System: Origins and Functions* was written for such a course. The fourth edition has undergone extensive revisions to take account of the many changes that have occurred in the last few years, not the least of which is that over 35 million Americans are now without health insurance protection against the costs of health care. Costs continue to rise at an ever faster pace despite the increased competition among physicians, hospitals, and health insurance companies. During this same period there has been an explosion in new knowledge and technology that enables physicians to treat old and new medical problems more effectively.

In late 1992 the need for health care reform was on the minds of most Americans, and political candidates all had their prescriptions to bring about needed changes—to control costs but at the same time to assure access for all to the highest quality health care. Meaningful health care reform requires, however, an understanding of not only the historical developments of our health system but also how and why its current problems arose. It is only in this way that we can assess the economic, clinical, and political constraints that will determine what kind of reforms are possible.

With these factors in mind, the fourth edition has been prepared. Our debt to a host of national organizations for data and permission to reprint material is considerable. Their contributions are evident throughout the text. They are not responsible, however, for the interpretations as they appear in the text or for any errors; for these, the authors are responsible.

As important as all those organizations are, a very special debt is owed to the students of HPA 101. They may not know or fully appreciate it, but they were all the motivating force for the development of this text in all of its editions.

Marshall W. Raffel
Norma K. Raffel

Chapter 1

History of Medical Education and Medical Practice in America

Medical practice and education in the United States evolved from the democratic, egalitarian, and individualistic character of early America. Although strongly influenced by Europe, the education of physicians and the practice of medicine are largely the result of historical developments within the country and have been shaped by a free enterprise philosophy. Until recently the medical profession fashioned the training and practice of medicine with little interference from government.

The physician today is a person vastly different from the practitioner in seventeenth and eighteenth century America. Today's medical practitioner pursues a rigorous course of study and clinical practice under the close supervision of faculty who are typically at the forefront of the health professions. Not only must today's medical practitioner pass courses in a premedical curriculum at a college or university and those offered by the medical school, but he or she must also pass the licensing exam. Nearly all practitioners, moreover, now undertake at least three years of additional supervised specialty training in a nationally accredited residency training program on completion of medical school. In most states, physicians must also participate in approved continuing medical education programs. The end result is a person licensed by the state government to practice medicine, a physician who is competent to diagnose and treat most illnesses and to know when to refer the patient for specialist care.

This is not to suggest that every physician is excellent, that all are competent, that all provide the best possible medical care, or that diagnostic and treatment errors are not made. It is to say, rather, that the physician who is consulted is probably a competent physician and that the patient has reasonable grounds for believing this.

Medical Practice and Training in Colonial America

In colonial times most of the sick were treated at home by women in the family. They used medicinal herbs, relied on family and friends for advice,

1

and later used medical guides that were specifically published for lay people. During that period, people with little or no training could also treat the sick and be regarded as physicians. Most "physicians" were trained under an apprenticeship system, and there was no organized method for testing the competence of those practitioners or their students, nor were there effective licensing bodies that could attest, by the granting of a license, to the physician's competence. Packard quotes from William Smith's 1758 *History of New York* (1, p. 284):

A few physicians among us are eminent for their skill. Quacks abound like locusts in Egypt, and too many have been recommended to a full practice and profitable subsistence; this is less to be wondered at, as the profession is under no kind of regulation. Loud as the call is, to our shame be it remembered, we have no law to protect the lives of the King's subjects from the malpractice of pretenders. Any man, at his pleasure, sets up for physician, apothecary, and chirurgeon. No candidates are either examined, licensed, or sworn to fair practice.

Smith's reference to "physician, apothecary, and chirurgeon" reflects the then British categorization of practitioners. The physicians typically held university medical degrees and practiced what we would call internal medicine. The apothecary was not a physician nor university trained. He was trained as an apprentice and was concerned with the dispensing of drugs. People frequently sought medical advice from the apothecary as they do from today's pharmacist, and the apothecary became, in Britain, the equivalent of a general practitioner. The chirurgeon, or surgeon, was also apprentice trained.

These distinctions became blurred in colonial America, for very few physicians came to the New World, and there were, at Smith's time, no medical schools in America to train them. Furthermore, at Smith's writing, there was only one hospital in all the colonies, the Philadelphia Hospital, and it had

been open for only a few years.* The first medical school was established in 1756 at the College of Philadelphia (later, University of Pennsylvania). The second school was at King's College (later, Columbia University), founded in 1768. By the time of the Revolutionary War, neither school had made significant medical manpower contributions to the total number of medical practitioners in the colonies. Accurate figures are hard to obtain, but it would appear that the Philadelphia school graduated fewer than ten students a year from 1768 to 1773; the first class at King's College in 1769 consisted of two.

Shryock notes that on the eve of the Revolutionary War, "it has been estimated that . . . there were about 3,500 established practitioners in the colonies and that not more than 400 of these had received any formal training. Of the latter, only about half—or barely more than 5 per cent of the total—held degrees" (2, p. 9). Most of the 200 degree holders in medicine were from European, and mainly British, medical schools.

Some of the early nonmedical degree practitioners were simply learned men†— ministers, planters, lawyers, teachers—who could gather a smattering of knowledge from books they read and could apply that knowledge. As Shryock puts it (2, p. 16):

A man who had graduated from an arts college, read in medicine, and acquired some experience was the near-

---

*Today, the physician and surgeon are both graduates of accredited medical schools and hold either the degree of Doctor of Medicine (MD) or Doctor of Osteopathy (DO). In American terms today, the physician is any MD or DO whereas in Britain the physician is still the equivalent of our specialist in internal medicine. The surgeon in America is thus a physician, with the added specialty qualifications in surgery. The apothecary has, in America, become the pharmacist and is the graduate of a university pharmacy program.

†At this point, the use of the word *men* is appropriate, for medicine was a male domain. Female involvement in "medical" matters was confined to midwifery, and to the extent that some of them received formal training, it was frequently provided by medical practitioners. The first female medical-school graduate was from the Geneva Medical College around 1850. See Shryock, R.H.: Women in American Medicine, *J Am Med Women's Assoc*, Vol. 5; No. 9, September 1950 (reprinted in Shryock, R.H.: *Medicine in America*. Baltimore, Johns Hopkins Press, 1966).

est thing to a formally trained practitioner that the colonial environment produced before the 1760s. As late as about 1830, it may be added, the University of Virginia still provided instruction in medicine for all its undergraduate students.

Most who aspired to medical practice apprenticed themselves for a number of years to established physicians. Upon completion of the training period, during which time the apprentice would watch and assist his preceptor and read his books, the physician would give the apprentice a signed testimonial that would constitute the certificate of proficiency. The real competence of the "graduate" from apprentice training would be as good or as bad as the preceptor, as the books available, and as the conscientiousness of the apprentice.

Samuel Treat, for example, was apprenticed to Dr. John Redman in Philadelphia and received his medical certificate in 1765 after nearly four years' service. Treat was fortunate in being able to learn from more than just one teacher: the Pennsylvania Hospital opened in 1752, and Treat was afforded the opportunity to attend there during his apprentice period. He was also fortunate to be in Philadelphia when some learned physicians began to offer lectures in various subjects. Treat attended the anatomical lectures offered by Dr. William Shippen, Jr. Treat's medical certificate was thus signed by many, as quoted in Packard (1, p. 278):

MEDICAL CERTIFICATE TO MR. SAMUEL TREAT, 1765, PHILADELPHIA.

This is to certify to all whom it may concern that Mr. Samuel Treat hath served as an Apprentice to me for nearly four years, during which he was constantly employed in the practice of Physic and Surgery under my care, not only in my private business, but in the Pennsylvania Hospital, in which character he always behaved with great Fidelity and Industry. In Testimony of which, I have thereunto set my hand this first day of September, One Thousand Seven hundred and Sixty-five.

(Signed)   John Redman

We whose names are under written do Certify that Mr. Samuel Treat hath diligently attended the practice of Physic and Surgery in the Pennsylvania Hospital for several years.

(Signed)   Thos. Cadwalader,
Phineas Bond,
Th. Bond,
Wm. Shippen,
C. Evans.

This is to certify that Samuel Treat hath attended a course of Anatomical Lectures with the greatest diligence and assiduity.

(Signed)   William Shippen, Jr.

More commonly in the colonial period, the medical certificate was signed by only one physician. Still others, as Corner notes (3, p. 3), "probably had no other qualifications beyond an interest in the sick and assurance enough to hang out a shingle."

Apprenticeship to a single physician was the more common approach to training for a long time because there was, until 1752 in Philadelphia and 1791 in New York, no institution that could rightly be called a hospital.* With the opening of the Pennsylvania Hospital, however, a significant new pattern of training began to develop. Physicians not only began to take their apprentices with them to the hospital to assist (as Dr. John Redman did with Samuel Treat), but also they began to allow other students to follow them as they examined and treated their hospital patients. So many students sought this privilege that the hospital resolved in 1763: "It is the unanimous opinion of the Board that such of them at least who are not apprentices to the Physicians of the House, should pay a proper Gratuity for the Benefit of the Hospital for their privilege" (1, p. 323).

By 1773, the hospital decided to regulate this

---

*The New York Hospital apparently served briefly during the Revolutionary War as an American military hospital until the British occupied New York, at which time it became for seven years a barracks, and possibly also a military hospital, for British and Hessian soldiers. It was not until 1791 that the hospital admitted its first civilian patient. See *Hospital Care in the United States,* Commission on Hospital Care. New York, the Commonwealth Fund, 1947, p. 439.

system so that an aspiring physician could pay a fee to the hospital and be formally apprenticed to the institution for five years, upon completion of which the institution would grant a certificate. With the establishment in 1765 of the medical department at the University of Pennsylvania, the hospital apprentices attended lectures there. Packard states that this practice continued until 1824, when the hospital required that future residents had to be regular graduates from the medical college before taking up their hospital appointment (1, p. 327). Packard also provides us with a sample Pennsylvania Hospital certificate (1, p. 281):

This is to Certify that . . . , son of . . . , West Jersey, entered regularly as a pupil of the Pennsylvania Hospital . . . , 1763, and continued his attendance with Diligence and Application to . . . , 1764, during which time we hope and have reason to believe he has made considerable Progress in the Knowledge of Anatomy and the Practice of Physick and Surgery, therefore wishing Happiness and success we give from under our hands and the seal of the Corporation, this Testimonial of our Esteem and Approbation.

Lecture series on various medical subjects were sometimes provided by the better trained physicians in the larger cities long before the founding of medical schools. The lecturers were mostly physicians trained abroad, some of whom were products of colonial apprentice training who went overseas subsequently for the additional training, chiefly to Scotland and England. Typically, fees were collected for their lectures, and even after the founding of medical schools, professors were paid by the students for the privilege of attending their lectures.

Many of these early practices continue today in a somewhat modified form. Aspiring physicians are now apprenticed not to individual physicians or to hospitals, but to an entire faculty, and the assisting process in the treatment of patients continues as an important part of clinical training in all med ical schools. Students also pay fees for lectures and for apprenticing, but instead of paying individuals—the preceptor, the lecturer, or the hos-

pital—the fee is now given as tuition to the medical school.

Nineteenth Century Medical Education

Only four medical schools—Harvard University (1783), Dartmouth College (1797), and the schools in Pennsylvania and New York that were already mentioned—were established by 1800. We should not think of these schools as being like those today. Three or four faculty members were sometimes all that were available, but not always. Corner tells us that Dartmouth "appointed the formidable Harvard graduate Nathan Smith to be a one-man medical faculty. For ten or 12 years he alone ably taught all the courses" (3, p. 57). The science and art of medicine were extremely limited in what they could offer in the way of cure, and one can appreciate, therefore, the great appeal in the nineteenth century of cultists and quacks. However weak the first schools were, they marked an important forward step. Stevens notes that "the foundation of the medical school in Philadelphia . . . was a part of the movement by university trained physicians to organize and rationalize medicine on a European model and to institute recognizable educational standards" (4, p. 17). The early medical faculties at Pennsylvania, Harvard, and Columbia, and even at Dartmouth, were dominated by men with European medical training. As the number of medical schools grew, and as more and more American medical graduates went abroad to Edinburgh, London, Paris, and other cities of Europe, many returned and gravitated to the medical school faculties, and they championed reform.

It is typical of most endeavors that those who are most expert seek to raise standards, to elevate the level of practice. So it was in medicine. It was evident in the founding of university medical schools, the early establishment of medical societies, and the initiation of medical journals—all designed to share knowledge, to communicate, to improve the quality of practice, and to establish a profession in which standards and esteem were comparable to those of their European colleagues.

Medical licensure was rarely effective in the colonial and postcolonial periods, in large measure because there was an insufficient number of well-trained practitioners. Early attempts at licensure included the establishment of state licensing boards, the granting of authority to the medical society, and recognition of the university (Doctor of Medicine, MD) degree both as entitlement to a license and as an alternative to licensure by the medical society or state licensing board. Georgia was the first state to restrict medical licenses to graduates of medical schools (1821). However, opposition to licensure was strong from the apprentice trained physicians, to whom licensure loomed as a threat; from other kinds of quasi-health practitioners, whose practices were threatened; as well as from many segments of the lay population that resented medical elitism. Resentment against the profession is illustrated in the matter of vital statistics registration: "In Georgia . . . the legislature 'fairly hooted' when a registration bill was introduced in 1849, and the whole matter was viewed as just another 'trick of the doctors' " (5). By the middle of the nineteenth century, many licensure acts had been either repealed or so drastically altered that they were rendered ineffective (4, pp. 26–28).

But the trend toward formalized medical education was firmly established. As the decades advanced in the nineteenth century, more and more medical practitioners came from medical schools; a decreasing percentage came from the apprenticeship system. In the absence of a strong licensing mechanism, the measure of a physician's competence came to rest on the standard of whether or not the physician had graduated from a medical school with an MD degree.

This encouraged development of a large number of new medical schools, some at universities that were ill-equipped to support and nourish them, and a great many freestanding schools with no university ties. Sometimes a school consisted of two rooms, one for lectures and one for dissections. There were few, if any, laboratories, and very limited libraries. Many schools were located in rural areas with no hospital or other clinical facilities.

The notion of university based medical education, it should be remembered, came to this country primarily from Scotland; University of Edinburgh trained physicians strongly influenced the structuring of the schools at Pennsylvania and Columbia. University based medical education was also dictated by the absence of strong hospitals in colonial America that could provide the milieu for excellence. In England, however, a number of medical schools grew up around such long established hospitals as St. Thomas' and Guy's, from which came the acceptable model of freestanding and hospital based schools in nineteenth century America. By then, hospitals were more common in the states than they were in the later part of the eighteenth century, though not all of the new medical schools could claim meaningful hospital affiliation.

Some of the new nonuniversity schools were good and had reputable faculties. Some of the schools were weak and were allegedly set up to make money, because the professors in most of the schools (good and bad) were paid directly by each student for attendance at lectures. Stevens cites the first of the proprietary schools, which was established by three local physicians in Castleton, Vermont, in 1818 (4, p. 25). Whether it was an improvement over apprenticeship to a single physician we can only guess, but the school did survive until 1862. Norwood, moreover, tells us that for some time the school was, in form, the medical department of Middlebury College and that in some of its faculty were people of considerable ability (6, pp. 204–208). In Boston, among the better private schools, Packard cites the Tremont Street School, established in 1838 by four physicians, including Oliver Wendell Holmes, and the Boylston Medical School (1, pp. 446–447).

The Tremont Street School flourished and offered lectures in embryology and anatomy, surgical pathology, chemistry, auscultation and percussion, and microscopic anatomy. The faculty was mostly moonlighting Harvard faculty, something we should not be surprised at, since rarely did a faculty member in those days rely solely on medical school income. The school thus had a close relationship with Harvard and eventually became Harvard's summer program.

The Boylston Street School opened in 1849. Despite opposition from Harvard, it received authority to grant degrees in 1854. It had a good faculty, illustrated by the fact that soon after receiving degree-granting authority, Harvard recruited the best of them, and the school "faded out of existence" (1, p. 447).

But even the quality of education at the "better" schools left much to be desired. Burrow tells us (7, p. 9):

When Charles Eliot became president of Harvard in 1869 (the year that the institution provided its first microscope for medical students), his early effort to institute written examinations for medical degrees met opposition from the director of the medical school who asserted with little exaggeration that a majority of the students could hardly write.

Under such conditions, one can sympathize with those in the population who relied on quacks of various sorts or who cherished their apprentice trained doctors as being as good as any coming out of a university medical school. Medical science was rather primitive, with a very limited understanding of the causes or options in the treatment of disease.

During the next decade, Harvard increased its length of training from two to three years, instituted written exams, and then required a college degree or the passing of a qualifying exam for admission. In 1892, the training was lengthened to four years. In 1893, Johns Hopkins University launched its pioneering effort in medical education with a four-year curriculum. This curriculum became, as we shall see, the model used to reform all medical education.

It was noted previously that a great many of the early leaders in American medical education received training in Britain and France. In the later part of the nineteenth century, the development of scientific medicine reached its height in Germany and Austria. Bonner has estimated that some 15,000 Americans undertook serious medical studies in German-speaking universities, 10,000 of these drawn to Vienna. Many others (over 10,000 more in Vienna), he estimates, familiarized themselves with the medical scene from short visits and vacation tours, and the medical faculties at Johns Hopkins, Harvard, Yale, and Michigan were dominated by professors who had spent time at German-speaking universities (8, pp. 39, 60–64, 69). How many others received training during this period in France, Britain, and other centers of European excellence is not known. But the German influence at this stage was critical. Shryock states (9, p. 30):

German-trained leaders in the better schools (Hopkins, Harvard, Michigan) found the continued mediocrity of medical education intolerable. Medical professors in this country still retained private practice, although incomes from apprentices vanished when this practice declined, after 1870, with the lengthening of the curriculum. Hence, professors were able to infiltrate the medical societies as practitioners, and appealed to the AMA (American Medical Association) to reform the schools. The latter [schools], because of their power to license, were primarily responsible for the low state of both training and practice; and the reformers—consciously or unconsciously—returned to an earlier program in appealing for control by medical societies. The latter, in turn, succeeded in persuading most states to re-establish the examining and licensing boards which had earlier been abandoned; and such bodies (1875–1900) were able to exert some pressure for better educational standards. By 1900, moreover, liberals in the AMA secured its reorganization, and in 1904 set up a Council on [Medical] Education which began to rate the various schools.

The American Medical Association and the Association of American Medical Colleges

The American Medical Association (AMA) was founded in 1847, and its primary goal was to improve medical education. At the organizational meeting in Philadelphia (Fig. 1–1), a Committee on Medical Education was established. The first

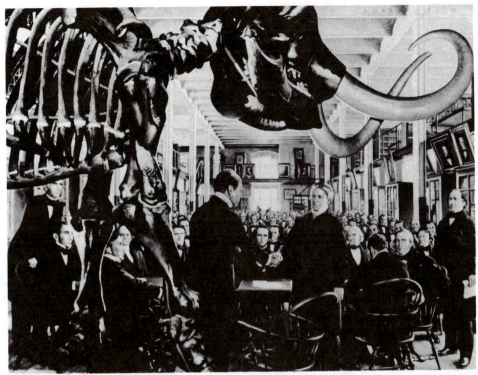

Figure 1–1. First meeting of the American Medical Association, in Philadelphia, 1847. (Courtesy, Parke-Davis, Division of Warner-Lambert Company, Morris Plains, NJ.)

pronouncement of the committee was to decry "medical instruction which does not rest on the basis of practical demonstration and clinical teaching; . . . it is . . . the duty of the medical schools to resort to every honorable means to obtain access for their students to the wards of a well-regulated hospital" (10, p. 888).

Although the AMA at its founding had as a primary goal the reform of medical education, its efforts were diluted for many years because so many of its members had an interest of one sort or another in the continuation of the weaker schools. One can surmise that this vested interest was not only financial investment and return but also included a desire to buy time so that the improvements could be made. Some practitioners did not want to see their schools put out of business, and there was a certain skepticism about what reform

would accomplish, because the discoveries of Lister on antiseptic surgery and Pasteur on germs were not to come until the 1860s, and anesthetic was introduced into surgery only in 1846. One can also speculate a resistance resulting from impolitic expressions from medical school faculty whose words seemed arrogant and condescending to the more traditionally trained physician.

In its 1872 report, the Committee on Medical Education observed that "it seems much easier to show the defects in our present system than to advise a suitable and practical remedy" (10, p. 890). The influence of the medical school professors "has always been so great in the Association as to prevent its doing what it should have done long ago, viz., establishing a national standard for medical teaching and demanding that colleges shall accept it or not be recognized" (10, p. 890).

A similar problem arose in 1876 when 22 medical schools organized the Association of American Medical Colleges (AAMC) as part of the effort to improve the quality of medical education. Coggeshall notes that "the embryo organization soon foundered over an issue involving its principal concern for higher standards. The question was whether graduation requirements should be extended to three years rather than two" (11, p. 49).

Both the AMA and the AAMC thus encountered the problem that besets all representative bodies: to continue to exist, the organization, like the elected politician, must retain the support of its constituency; get too far ahead and the effort will founder because it will not enjoy support from the majority of the membership. Standards thus tend to be minimal, so that most of the present members can meet them. Progress is still made, as it was by the AMA and the AAMC, but with incremental steps by which the constituency is persuaded that it is in the constituency's interests to support whatever is being proposed.

Sometimes an organization can make little progress on an issue. Individual members may charge ahead, but there may simply not be enough support for the entire group to do so. The reluctance of the entire group to move may be based on any number of reasons, such as not being convinced that the proposed course of action is merited or wise, fear that the course of action may produce undesirable outcomes, fear that the action will harm or destroy the efforts of individual members, as well as satisfaction with the way things are at present. In such instances, an organization may simply have to tread water until some other body is able to make the necessary breakthrough, on the assumption that a breakthrough is appropriate. Reform of medical education is a good illustration of this.

Despite the fact that Harvard lengthened its curriculum to three years in the early 1870s, it and others could not move the AAMC on this matter in 1876. Not until 1891 did the AAMC support a three-year training period, only to have Harvard a year later again go its own way and lengthen its

curriculum to four years. Hopkins, as we have noted, introduced its four-year curriculum after Harvard, in 1893. The AAMC was persuaded in 1894 also to support a four-year curriculum. The organization played an important role, increasingly so from the 1890s on, but clearly it did not have enough clout to bring about the necessary reform by itself. It was at this point that the AMA played a significant role.

In 1901, the AMA was restructured to become a more representative body, with business transactions conducted by a House of Delegates consisting largely of elected representatives from the states but also including a representative from each of the scientific sections of the association and from each of the federal government health services (Army, Navy, and Public Health). This reorganization made the association a more representative national body, lessening the domination by those close to the city in which the annual meeting was being held; the reorganization also lessened the influence of medical educators in the governing House of Delegates. In 1904, the House of Delegates acted on a report of the Committee on Medical Education and created a new Council on Medical Education whose functions were, as quoted by Johnson (10, p. 892):

1. To make an annual report to the House of Delegates on the existing conditions of medical education in the United States
2. To make suggestions as to the means and methods by which the American Medical Association may best influence favorably medical education
3. To act as the agent of the American Medical Association (under instructions from the House of Delegates) in its efforts to elevate medical education

The first council consisted of four medical school professors and one dean, from what might fairly be cited as the more reputable schools, that is Rush, Harvard, Pennsylvania, Michigan, and Vanderbilt. The council still exists, and its annual report, published each year in the *Journal of the American Medical Association (JAMA)*, offers, agreeably surprised not only at the efforts being made to correct conditions surrounding medical education but at the enormous amount of important data collected.

He agreed with the opinion previously expressed by the members of the Council that while the Foundation would be guided very largely by the Council's investigation, to avoid the usual claims of partiality no more mention should be made in the report of the Council than any other source of information. The report would therefore be, and have the weight of an independent report of a disinterested body, which would then be published far and wide. It would do much to develop public opinion.

It was considered wise to withhold publication of the list of satisfactory colleges until the Carnegie report comes out . . . [so that] that report would make the Council's report at a later date more effective.

The Flexner Report and Reform

The study was begun almost immediately. In January 1909, Flexner, who was not a physician but an educator, the holder of a baccalaureate degree from The Johns Hopkins University and a master's degree from Harvard, began the first of his medical school visits. On most, if not all, of his visits, he was accompanied by Dr. N.P. Colwell, who was the secretary of the AMA's Council on Medical Education. In his autobiography, Flexner tells us how he carried out his survey (12, pp. 120–122). He notes that it was essentially an educational survey, not a medical one. He identified five factors that would provide him with conclusive data as to the quality of a school:

First, the entrance requirements. What were they? Were they enforced?

Second, the size and training of the faculty.

Third, the sum available from endowment and fees for the support of the institution, and what became of it.

Fourth, the quality and adequacy of the laboratories provided for the instruction of the first two years and the qualifications and training of the teachers of the so-called preclinical branches.

Fifth and finally, the relations between medical school and hospitals, including, in particular, freedom of access to beds and freedom in the appointment by the school of the hospital physicians and surgeons who automatically should become clinical teachers.

Much of the data he sought was secured through interviews with the dean and a few of the faculty. A "stroll through the laboratories" revealed to him much about the availability of equipment and specimens, and a "whiff" revealed something about the teaching of anatomy. He goes on to say:

In the course of a few hours a reliable estimate could be made respecting the possibilities of teaching modern medicine in almost any one of the 155 schools I visited in the United States and Canada. Having visited perhaps half a dozen schools, sometimes more, I would return to New York and set my facts in order—never the same facts respecting any two of them. These brief summaries I returned to the dean of the school by mail with the request that he correct any misstatements. I had the feeling during the whole time that the faculties were more than candid with me, because though I endeavored to disabuse them of the idea, they were convinced that Mr. Carnegie, having once made a gift to a medical school in Atlanta, contemplated further activities of the same kind.

His autobiography vividly describes the conduct of his study and is rewarding to read. Flexner's formal report, *Medical Education in the United States and Canada,* was published by the Carnegie Foundation in 1910 (13). Though more controlled in language than the accounts given in his autobiography, it nonetheless provided a candid, searing critique of medical education in both the United States and Canada. It named schools, their assets, and their liabilities, and it offered a prescription for each school, for each state and region, and for the country as a whole. Where the schools were no more than business ventures (such as the Jenner Medical College in Illinois and Still College of Osteopathy in Iowa), he said so. Regarding the California Medical College, he stated that "the school is a disgrace to the state whose laws permit its existence." The Los Angeles College of Osteopathy had all the aspects of a "thriving business." Chicago was described as "the plague spot of the without question, the most definitive account of the current state of medical education.

But even before the council's work began, leadership in the AMA was making progress. Beginning in 1902, *JAMA* published medical school failure statistics on state board licensing examinations, a form of exposure that could not help but embarrass and lead to institutional reform. In 1907, the assessment of schools were made even easier by grouping the schools into four classes. Class 1 had fewer than 10 percent failure; class 2 had 10–20 percent failure; class 3 had more than 20 percent failure; class 4 consisted of a miscellaneous grouping of smaller schools (fewer than 10 graduates) and not otherwise classifiable institutions (10, p. 895).

The council subsequently decided to rate each school based not only on the state board exam performance but also on such factors as entrance requirements, medical curriculum, laboratory facilities, hospital facilities, faculty quality, library, and research. The resulting scores would place each school in one of three categories: class A (acceptable, with a point score above 70); class B (doubtful, with a score of 50–70); and class C (unacceptable, with a score of less than 50). Each school was visited; in 1907, the findings were reported.

The council chairman noted that "the Council was very lenient in its markings," and of the 160 schools, 82 were in class A, 46 in class B, and 32 in class C. The classifications were not published, though each school was notified of its standing. The council chairman, some years later, stated (10, p. 897):

As a result of the report of this first inspection a great wave of improvement in medical education swept over the country. Fifty schools agreed to require by 1910, or before, at least one year of university physics, chemistry and biology and one modern language as a preliminary education before matriculating in medicine. Immediately a number of consolidations were arranged in many cities having several schools. A number of schools, as a result of state boards refusing examinations to their graduates, went out of business and it became evident that the 160 schools would be reduced within a short time to probably less than a hundred.

The improved situation was evident. The AMA's work was clearly facilitated by effective leadership in the organization as well as by medical educators from some of the better schools who were also working within the AAMC. The AAMC began to inspect the schools and put pressure on the poorer schools to improve or else get out of the association. There was, however, a clear political constraint on the AMA classification of schools. The ratings were made leniently perhaps in recognition of the fact that it had to take one step at a time if it was to be effective and that to be successful in this, a clear majority of schools had to be acceptable; and so it was: 51 percent of the schools (82) fell into the acceptable class; only 20 percent (32) were unacceptable; the remainder, while doubtful, could pass muster if they improved. This, then, was perhaps as far as the AMA could go by itself. Johnson notes that there was considerable resentment over these reports by many of the colleges, and as a result of this, he quotes the council chairman, who said years later (10, p. 897): "It occurred to some of the members of the Council that, if we could obtain the publication and approval of our work by the Carnegie Foundation for the Advancement of Teaching, it would assist materially in securing the results we were attempting to bring about."

Johnson then quotes from the minutes of the council meeting held in New York in December 1905 (10, p. 897):

At one o'clock an informal conference was held with President Pritchett and Mr. Abraham Flexner of the Carnegie Foundation. Mr. Pritchett had already expressed, by correspondence, the willingness of the Foundation to cooperate with the Council in investigating the medical schools. He now explained that the Foundation was to investigate all the professions, law, medicine and theology. He had found no efforts being made by law to better the conditions in legal education and had met with some slight opposition in the efforts he was making. He had then received the letters from the Council on Medical Education and expressed himself as most country" in terms of medical education, and the provisions of the Illinois state law "are, and have long been, flagrantly violated" with the "indubitable connivance of the state board."

Small wonder Flexner's life was threatened and a libel suit filed and other suits promised. But not all was so negative. With regard to Dartmouth, he noted difficulties that the institution had in attracting a sufficient number of medical cases for teaching purposes because of its remoteness and expressed doubt about a compulsory fifth-year internship in a large hospital. The college's preclinical training in the basic sciences was excellent. He concluded (13, pp. 264–265):

That the school cannot much longer continue in its present stage is clear; for with the requirement of two years of college work for entrance in 1910, it asks a student to spend six years to get a degree in medicine, in attaining which he can enjoy only a very limited opportunity to learn internal medicine. It is safe to predict that on that basis the present facilities will not hold the student body together during the third and fourth years.

Subsequently, Dartmouth took Flexner's observations to heart and abandoned clinical instruction, retaining only the two years of preclinical instruction in what is known as a *school of basic medical sciences,* with the students transferring to other schools for the third and fourth years of clinical instruction. Many other schools could expand their clinical classes on two accounts: (1) the big blockages in medical education are the very expensive preclinical labs and (2) clinical training is easily expandable in big cities because of the large population base, a plentiful range of medical and surgical cases for teaching purposes, and plentiful hospital beds. Because of population growth and improved transportation, Dartmouth went back to a four-year curriculum in the 1960s.

Other schools that showed both weaknesses and promise received constructive criticism from Flexner. At Yale, for example, the teaching staff was cited for being "overworked and without a proper force of assistants." At New Haven Hospital the

available beds were well used, but criticism was registered. "The obstetrical and gynecological wards . . . are not used for teaching; nor is there a contagious disease pavilion. Post-mortems are scarce" (13, p. 200). At Columbia, the criticism was also constructive: there was no real medical library and endowments were insufficient (but, he felt, readily correctable). More serious was a problem regarding "rights" in the hospitals in which the teaching was carried out.

Some institutions received high praise, particularly Harvard, Western Reserve, McGill, Toronto, and Johns Hopkins. It was Johns Hopkins School of Medicine, launched only 17 years earlier (1893), that was singled out and became his preferred model for medical education. In addition to the school's requiring a bachelor's degree for admission, Flexner states (13, p. 12):

This was the first medical school in America of genuine university type, with something approaching adequate endowment, well-equipped laboratories conducted by modern teachers, devoting themselves unreservedly to medical investigation and instruction, and with its own hospital, in which the training of physicians and the healing of the sick harmoniously combine to the infinite advantage of both. The influence of this new foundation can hardly be overstated. It has finally cleared up the problem of standards and ideals; and its graduates have gone forth in small bands to found new establishments or to reconstruct old ones.

The Flexner report caused some schools to close and some to consolidate. Some allegedly closed before the report's publication in order to escape the criticism. In Chicago, where there had been 15 schools, Flexner tells us that the number was reduced to three (12, p. 31). In all, Flexner recommended that the number of schools be reduced from 155 to 31. By 1920, the number of schools was down to 85. By that time, however, the need for more than 31 was apparent because of population increases and new knowledge that permitted more to be done for patients.

The report, coming from an independent body, strengthened the hand of medical reformers in the

AMA, AAMC, state medical societies, and, importantly, state licensing boards. Licensing legislation in the states mandated more rigorous control. The council, moreover, leaned on people in the state societies, even before the Flexner study, to see to it that reform-minded people got appointed to state licensing boards. Many boards began to set new requirements, which included increasing the length of medical training and providing students with modern laboratories, libraries, and clinical facilities. Stevens notes (4, p. 68):

In 1905 only five schools had required any college preparation for admission. Ten years later eighty-five schools prescribed a minimum of one or two years' college preparation; by 1932, every recognized medical school and most of the state licensing boards required at least two years' college work, many required three, and several a college degree . . . . By 1925, forty-nine boards required candidates for their examinations to be graduates of a medical college, and forty-six states refused to recognize low-grade schools as a preparation for the license. Since the only national rating of colleges continued to be that of the AMA Council on Medical Education, the profession by then held effective monopoly control of educational regulation.

The increased leverage provided by the work of the AMA and the AAMC was evident in their increased coordinated efforts, leading, in 1942, to the establishment of a Liaison Committee on Medical Education (LCMC), which developed educational program guidelines, inspected schools, and became the official accrediting body for medical schools. Their efforts were supported by the growing number of medical graduates from the better schools who, in their own ways, were persuasive within their state societies, before legislative bodies, and with the public.

But the final lever for reform came from the foundations and from individuals whom the foundations could persuade. Flexner's influence here was a critical factor. Shortly after his report, he joined the General Education Board, a Rockefeller charity, which poured enormous sums into medical education. Flexner estimated that the General Education Board's $50 million for medical education had been successful in getting other contributors to come up with half a billion dollars or more from 1919 to 1928, a period when the dollar bought much more than it does today. His role in the allocation of these funds and in persuading others to complement the board's contributions is described in his autobiography, *I Remember*. The monies, of course, went to the better schools and to those that showed promise of moving in the direction laid out in his report. University medical schools usually had a better academic reputation and a more solid financial base than proprietary schools, and therefore acquired the new money that became available for medical education. Because of this influx of money, universities gained control of medical education (14). The monies were also strategically allocated where they would do the most good in terms of influencing reform at nearby institutions: the grant to the University of Rochester, for example, was designed to stimulate the reform of all New York schools; the grant to the University of Iowa was meant to do the same in the Midwest (12, p. 296).

Our story of medical schools might appropriately end here. We now backtrack to look at the development of medical specialties. We will return to medical schools in a later chapter.

The Development of Medical Specialties

Most physicians in the colonial and postcolonial periods were general practitioners; this was the great need at the time. Moreover, it was made necessary because the state of medical science was rather primitive, hardly justifying a specialist, and because surgical practice was limited, until 1846, by the absence of anesthesia. Where physicians did develop special skills or interests and became known for them, they primarily remained general physicians and practiced their specialties (such as obstetrics or surgery) only on occasion. As to the state of medical science, Shryock reminds us that this was the age of bleeding and purging (the former carried on as late as the 1870s), when illness was attributed to some generalized problem such as "impurities of the blood or the existence of excessive tension or laxity in the nervous and vascular systems" (15). Under such a philosophy, there was little need for specialists. Surgery inside body cavities would be pointless as well as painful, and surgery was thus limited largely to trauma cases. Benjamin Rush, besides being a signer of the Declaration of Independence and a prominent Philadelphia physician, was a great advocate of both bleeding and purging. A contemporary critic of Rush (William Cobbett) described his mode of practice as "one of those great discoveries, which are made from time to time for the depopulation of the earth" (2, p. 70). The unpleasantries of such treatment and the risks they entailed made the milder treatments offered by quacks and cultists appealing.

During the first half of the nineteenth century, a growing number of American physicians went to France for advanced study. It was during this period that French investigators were effectively proving the errors of bleeding and purging, as well as the ineffectiveness of many drugs then in common use. Their investigations pointed to specific pathology in different locations and systems of the body, there being no single, let alone simple, explanation for disease. These findings, of course, made the whole notion of specialization appealing to those physicians whose interest was excited by special health problems.

But old ideas die hard, and it was not until the 1860s that specialties began to make headway on the medical scene. Resistance to specialties was, at times, vigorous, and the issues were complex. Fishbein, in his history of the AMA, summarizes the issues pertaining to specialization in a report at the association's 1866 meeting in Baltimore (16, pp. 74–75):

This year was notable for the majority and minority reports of the Committee on Medical Ethics dealing with specialization. The majority report listed the advantages of specialization as including minuteness in observation, acuteness in study, wideness of observation, skill in diagnosis, multiplicity of invention and superior skill in manipulation. The disadvantages were a narrowness of view, a tendency to magnify unduly the diseases which the specialty covers, a tendency to undervalue the treatment of special diseases by general practitioners, some temptation to the employment of undue measures for gaining a popular reputation and a tendency to increased fees. The advantages far outweighed the disadvantages from the point of view of the patient and of the advancement of the specialty. The committee felt that these disadvantages could be overcome if the specialist would begin as a general practitioner and gradually grow into his specialty.

The committee was especially concerned with the means by which the specialist made himself known to the community. They felt that there should be no advertising either in newspapers or medical journals.

The minority report was signed by Dr. Henry I. Bowditch. He considered that the whole tendency of modern science was toward specialism but he felt that the Association had no business passing on the question of the advertisements unless they were evidently of a mountebank character. It was his opinion that "any Association would be better occupied in the hearing of able papers and in discussions on all subjects connected with medicine than in any movements for the mere discipline of erring members."

To some of these issues and related ones there are no easy or hard-and-fast answers. Many of the same issues persist to this day. Should a patient go first to the general practitioner or directly to the specialist? Will the specialist treat the whole patient? Should a specialist be permitted to advertise, and how? Will the surgeon operate because that is what a surgeon is taught to do? Does specialty practice lead to unnecessary procedures? Will the higher fees accorded specialists lead people into medicine and the specialty for the sake of money? But don't we want the best medical care, and isn't the specialist the best?

It was only six years earlier (1859) that the scientific sections of the AMA began to be set up. Initially, they focused on what were then well-defined areas of scientific interest as the AMA delegates saw them: anatomy and physiology, chemistry and materia medica, practical medicine and obstetrics, and surgery. Obstetrics became part of the new section of Obstetrics and Diseases of Women and Children in 1873. Children were separated to become a section on Diseases of Children in 1879. Ophthalmology, laryngology, and otology sections were formed in 1878, and so on. The AMA's responses to specialty interests were often slow because of the occasional reluctance of AMA membership to recognize the validity of the specialty. Is there such uniqueness in diseases of children, for example, to justify the problems' being spun off from general practice to be treated as a specialty? Will the specialist become so narrowly focused that he or she might miss the critical contributions that can be made by those more generally oriented? Though it is true that the specialist may tend to draw paying patients away from the general practitioner, there is also considerable evidence that a specialist practicing in too isolated an environment runs grave risks of practicing bad medical care because of the tendency to magnify concerns of the specialty and to be insensitive to the contributions and skills of other specialties. The resistance to some specialty development was thus genuinely concerned with quality of patient care as well as the economics of medical practice.

General practitioners' concerns on the economic score were also well founded, for by the mid-twentieth century general practitioners were squeezed out of many hospitals by the specialists in some larger cities. The argument advanced by the specialists was: If you're sick enough to be in the hospital, you're sick enough to need a specialist. This led the general practitioners to fight back, organizing, in 1947, the American Academy of General Practice (AAGP), with state and local chapters, and applying pressure for hospitals to add general practice departments. To prove their worth, members of the academy were required to have 150 hours of approved continuing education credits every three years. In 1969, general practice, now called family practice, became a recognized specialty. The AAGP is now the American Academy of Family Physicians (AAFP).

Because of the slow response by the AMA to specialty interests, the specialists began to form their own societies and associations. These groups, by and large, did not fight the AMA but simply went their own way. Often, some members held leadership positions both in the AMA and in their specialty group. The specialty organization could focus more quickly than the more generally oriented AMA on the problems and concerns of the specialty. Some of the early specialty groups were the American Ophthalmological Society (1864), the American Otological Society (1868), the American Gynecological Society (1876), the American Association of Obstetricians and Gynecologists (1888), and the American Pediatric Society (1888). There were also state and local specialty societies, some established before the national body, some later. Specialty journals followed; in many cities, the specialty was advanced by the presence of specialty hospitals and clinics. Indeed, in most large cities today, one can find specialty hospitals still thriving or only recently merged with other hospitals. Eye and ear hospitals are perhaps the most common example.

These special hospitals and clinics became, in the late nineteenth and early twentieth centuries, the foci for training in those specialties, because, generally speaking, the most outstanding practitioners were affiliated with those institutions. This is not to suggest, however, that some outstanding specialists did not practice and train others in the more generally oriented hospitals.

There was, of course, no standard at the turn of the century for what constituted adequate training in a specialty. Courses were offered by medical societies, hospitals, specially founded schools, and universities. The programs of study lasted anywhere from a few weeks to three years. Flexner described some of these in his report (13, pp. 174–177):

The Postgraduate School

The postgraduate school as developed in the United States may be characterized as a "compensatory adjustment." It is an effort to mend a machine that was predestined to breakdown. Inevitably, the more conscientious and intelligent men trained in most of the medical schools herein described must become aware of their unfitness for the responsibilities of medical practice; the postgraduate school was established to do what the medical school failed to accomplish . . .

The postgraduate school was thus originally an undergraduate repair shop. Its instruction was necessarily at once elementary and practical. There was no time to go back to fundamentals; it was too late to raise the question of preliminary educational competency. Urgency required that in the shortest possible time the young physician already involved in responsibility should acquire the practical technique which the medical school had failed to impart. The courses were made short, frequently covering less than a month; and they aimed preeminently to teach the young doctor what to "do" in the various emergencies of general practice.

The "repair shop" to which Flexner referred was also the rationale in the later part of the nineteenth century for the internship, which over time became standard practice: the requirement of an additional year of supervised training to give the medical graduate (still, in a sense, a student) that extra bit of on-the-job training. The need for some practical on-the-job training was necessitated by the medical schools' adoption of the Harvard practice of not requiring an apprenticeship before medical school. This need for additional training was also, in part, what motivated many other physicians to go abroad. As Stevens notes (4, p. 117), the internship tended to emphasize either medicine or surgery and thus became an introductory phase of specialization.

Early specialty training was thus erratic, and in the absence of accepted standards, the quality of specialty care ran from excellence to complete incompetence. Perhaps the best assessment was made by the United States Army in 1917. Stevens cites army sources and tells us (4, pp. 127–128):

The army acted as a filtering system for quality. No one reached the medical training camps unless they were initially felt to be desirable (thus eliminating the obviously incompetent, the sick, those of bad character, alcoholics, drug addicts, and so on), were from reputable medical colleges, were licensed to practice in the state in which they lived, were already in active practice, and had passed an examination before a local board. At the camps many more were rejected; physical unfitness rather than professional incompetence was used as the reason for rejection wherever possible, to avoid embarrassment.

Specialist qualifications received searching examination. The surgeon general's office card-indexed men whose reputation seemed to warrant their acceptance as specialists, but so many were found to be overrated that the specialists' divisions agreed to make specialist appointments conditional on examination. The results were appalling. Some of the "specialists" examined were found to be unfit to practice any branch of medicine in the service. A study of the examination results at Camp Greenleaf in 1918 revealed only one medical officer in three qualified to do independent surgery, and only about 6 percent were rated as high-class surgeons; there was a similarly small proportion of really high-grade men in internal medicine. Seventy percent of the otolaryngologists, 51 percent of the ophthalmologists, and 38 percent of those who said they were plastic and oral surgeons were rejected. Thus the extent of educational deficiency was glaringly acknowledged—and at the same time directly linked with the potential danger to the public if such practices were to continue.

All these factors were to deepen concern over the preparation and role of the specialist in postwar prosperity, not only in relation to the kinds of intraprofessional questions which had stimulated the surgeons and ophthalmologists to develop separate organizations but also in relation to the provision of high-quality medical care to the public.

But the army's findings described sets of circumstances that were well known by the leaders in many specialty areas. Anyone who wanted to become a specialist did so. There was no mandated course of study or training, nor was a license granted for specialty practice. State licensure acts focused on the basic qualifications for medical practice. A physician, once licensed, had no legal constraints placed on him or her but could legally do all that fell within the definition of medicine and surgery.

To be sure, many, perhaps even most (we have no way of really knowing), of the specialists were conscientious. They sought to learn through special courses, by going abroad, and by reading books and journals. They sought further information and fostered research through local, state, and national specialty societies. When one of their members secured a reputation for special skills, others went to work with that person. Bond, for example, writes of "an enthusiastic pioneer in gynecological surgery, and one of the founders of the Woman's Hospital" who, in the latter half of the nineteenth century, would journey to New York from Baltimore "every year . . . for several weeks to familiarize himself with any new advances in his specialty, in that birthplace of American gynecology, where Marion Sims labored and suffered in his earlier years" (17, p. 73). With the advent of anesthesia, antiseptic techniques, new instrumentation, and new technology learned from the Civil War battle casualties as well as from European research, a new era began to open. Hospitals grew in number, because now people could go to them for general and special surgery with less fear of pain and more assurance that they would survive and improve from the encounter.

But this new era posed new problems. The new opportunities unlocked the specialties, but the advances in most of the specialties entailed surgery. Surgery, which included sewing a laceration, setting a bone, or amputating, used to be the domain of the general practitioner (GP). Now, however, surgery became more complicated, and the better surgeons wanted to restrain not only the GPs but the less qualified surgeons as well.

As noted earlier, this could only mean cutting the volume of paying patients for the GP. It meant that the GP's image to the public might be lowered, that the GP might come to be viewed as a less-than-complete physician. (By 1947, the Council on Medical Education had to issue a special report on the prestige of general practitioners [4, p. 307]). The better surgeons, on the other hand, argued that GPs had no business inside the abdomen. This led, as noted earlier, to the attempt to keep the GP out of the urban hospitals and, in many areas of the country, to restricting the practice of

the GP in the hospital to nonsurgical cases. Today, however, there are still small community hospitals in which the GP does general surgery, because the GP has always done it, because there are no specialists, because some procedures (for example, appendectomy) are relatively simple even though in the abdominal cavity, and because some patients want their doctor to do the operating.

The American College of Surgeons (ACS), which was established in 1912, set specific requirements in an effort to improve the skills of physicians it accepted into fellowship. Stevens notes that "prerequisites included a one-year internship, three years as an assistant, fifty case abstracts, visits to surgical clinics, and for graduates of 1920 and after, two years of college before medical school" (4, p. 92). This suggested a pattern for certifying specialists, the first certifying board being established in 1917. Clearly, the ACS requirements were devices for the employment of peer pressure to improve. Though the college could not license surgeons, it could pass professional judgment and approve of accomplishments and of behavior. As a voluntary group, however, it could only judge those who appeared voluntarily before it. Once accepted into fellowship, it could do little in the beginning to monitor continued excellence; this came much later. All these developments by the ACS were important but not enough. The next step was to inspect the places in which internships were provided, that is, in the general and special hospitals around the nation. Both the AMA and the ACS moved on this front.

The AMA began to pay attention to the internship at the time it established its Council on Medical Education. The council surveyed hospitals that were offering internships and in 1914 published its first list of approved internship hospitals. At about the same time, the ACS began to think about establishing hospital standards for surgical practice; in 1916, it received a Carnegie grant for this purpose. Stevens tells us that at one point the ACS asked the AMA to provide leadership with regard to hospital standardization, but that the cost appeared too much for AMA resources and the ACS was forced to proceed alone (4, p. 119). The first list of hospitals that the ACS felt met its standards was ready in 1919, but the conditions encountered in its survey were so bad that the college suppressed the list. In 1924, the Council on Medical Education began to approve hospitals for residency (specialty) training programs. A key requirement at that time was that the hospital must first have approval for internship programs.

Residency training in one of the recognized specialty fields also posed some problems as it developed. Originally, the residency represented an extra period of clinical training following the internship for a few elite young physicians who wished to become teachers or leaders in medicine. By the mid-1960s, however, nearly all medical school graduates took three or more years of residency (specialty) training after an internship. The growth of the specialties was a direct result of new knowledge and new technology, enabling physicians to do more than ever before to help people in need. As with internships, residency programs proliferated into hospitals of all types and sizes. In some teaching hospitals there was little if any fulltime staff, few of the attending physicians were interested in teaching, and the resident's educational experiences and practice were poorly supervised and coordinated. Some hospitals did not have an adequate number or variety of patients and in some, where there was senior staff, the staff was so involved in research that they often neglected to teach residents.

Another problem was the conflict between the primary purpose of any hospital, that is, patient care, and the requirement for high-quality graduate education. It seemed clear that to a large number of hospitals one of the reasons for expansion of the residency program was to have junior staff to help carry the patient load, as was the case with internships.

Still another problem that affected the quality of residency training was that the programs were typically planned, monitored, and appraised only by members of one individual medical service (medicine, surgery, pathology, etc.), and some-

times only by a single person, the chief of the service.

(Residents, as they train in hospitals, are commonly referred to as the *house staff.* They have, as noted, certain service responsibilities that accompany the educational programs in which they are enrolled. House staff are different from *medical staff* and *hospital medical staff,* which consist of physicians who are not residents and who have full authority and responsibility for treating patients within their hospital-defined areas.)

The need for reform was evident to many medical educators and to leaders of the AMA. The AMA once again assumed a leadership role. It commissioned a Citizens Committee on Graduate Medical Education, chaired by John S. Mills, who was then president of Western Reserve University. The commission consisted of 11 members, only three of whom were physicians.

The Mills Commission

For the second time in its history, the AMA requested an outside examination of the medical education process. (The first one resulted in the Flexner Report.) The mandate this time was to examine graduate medical education—the internship and the residency—and to make recommendations to improve this part of a physician's formal training. The commission's report, *The Graduate Education of Physicians* (18), was issued in 1966.

The report reviewed at some length the origins of both the internship and the residency, and noted strengths and weaknesses in each as they evolved. Among its key recommendations was a call for the elimination of the independent internship, meaning that no internship be approved unless it is linked with and part of an approved residency training program. The first year of each residency program, however, should be one that gives the resident a broad clinical experience. The commission further recommended that this change in the nature of the internship should *not* mean an additional year of residency training.

Another key recommendation related to the role

of the hospital. The commission felt that the existing autonomy of individual hospital departments and the programs they developed was not appropriate, but that the hospital as a whole had to play some role in residency programs in terms of providing resources and facilitating the cooperation of other hospital departments and services. The commission went so far as to recommend that accreditation of residency training programs be given to the institution rather than to the individual services involved. There were many other recommendations, but these are the ones that most concern this discussion.

The Mills report is an excellent example of a health policy plan. Although not completely implemented, it led to considerable discussion within the medical profession and to positive reforms in line with the spirit of the report. In late 1970, the AMA's House of Delegates endorsed the concept that the first year of graduate medical education be in a program approved by the appropriate residency review committee (which each specialty board had) rather than by the AMA's Council on Medical Education. Thus, in effect, the AMA said that it would no longer review and approve internships, that internships would have to be integrated with residency training programs. In fact, since 1975 the AMA has stopped approving internships and has ceased the use of the term in its *Directory of Residency Training Programs*. The AMA's position was reaffirmed and strengthened in 1982 when its House of Delegates adopted a recommendation from its Council of Medical Education that the first year of postdoctoral medical education for all graduates should consist of a broad year of general training.

The Development of Specialty Boards

To become a specialist today in a particular medical area, a physician—following graduation from medical school—must undergo a period of further training in an approved setting and pass a qualifying examination. The physician is then certified as a *diplomate* of that specialty by the appropriate specialty board. The various boards are legitimized by their sponsors—the major specialty society or societies in that area and the appropriate specialty section of the AMA.

The development of the first specialty board by sponsoring groups is interesting, and for this we turn briefly to the field of ophthalmology. Treatment of eye conditions was the domain of many. Optometrists, who were not medically qualified, were active in the field, as were general practitioners. The specialty within medicine only began to emerge during the latter part of the nineteenth century, aided greatly by the developments of the ophthalmoscope and anesthesia.

Over the years, those physicians who developed a special interest in problems of the eye organized specialist organizations. There were three principal organizations. The AMA had within its scientific groups a Section on Ophthalmology. Then there were the American Ophthalmological Society and the American Academy of Ophthalmology and Otolaryngology. There were, in addition, a number of regional and state groups. Concern within each of these groups about the quality of ophthalmologic training and practice and the appropriate role for the nonmedically qualified optometrists led the three national bodies to get together and to recommend to each of their organizations, in 1915, that a single specialty board be sponsored. The board was to consist of three representatives from each of the societies, and "the board would appoint examiners, hold examinations, and determine requirements; that it would grant a certificate or diploma; and that the specialty societies should limit their membership to diplomates" (4, p. 113). The two societies and the AMA Section on Ophthalmology approved the proposal. In 1917, the first specialty board, the American Board for Ophthalmic Examinations, was incorporated; in 1933, it was renamed the American Board of Ophthalmology.

Societies of a closely related group of physicians incorporated the second specialty board in 1924, the American Board of Otolaryngology. They were closely related because many specialists in this area also include ophthalmology in their practices. Younger specialists in these areas today are either ophthalmologists or otolaryngologists, the latter known as ENT (ear, nose, throat) specialists. It is common to find some older physicians who consider themselves EENT (eye, ear, nose, throat) specialists, but they are a dying breed. It was not until the 1930s that other specialty boards were established.

The American Board of Ophthalmology set the pattern for specialty recognition in the nation, that is, the recognition of a national specialty board because of widespread acceptance by societies or groups associated with the specialty. These groups, as noted earlier, consisted in each case of the one or more specialty societies and the appropriate specialty section of the AMA. The logic for legitimacy was simple: any specialist worthy of recognition belonged to one or more of the sponsoring groups. This did not mean that a physician could not be a competent specialist without belonging, but it did say that if that self-styled specialist wanted outside professional recognition of competence, he or she had to belong to one of the societies or to the AMA scientific section. If the specialists belonged, then the society or AMA section, as representative bodies, could legitimately sponsor a specialty board.

Over a span of time, each of the specialty societies modified its requirements for membership. One common element, however, became certification by the appropriate specialty board.

The number of specialty boards in 1991 stood at 23; 20 of those boards are *primary* boards. Three of the boards are *conjoint* boards (see Table 2–4). Two are the American Board of Allergy and Immunology (a conjoint board of the American Board of Pediatrics and of the American Board of Internal Medicine), and the American Board of Nuclear Medicine (a conjoint board of the American Board of Internal Medicine, the American Board of Pathology, and the American Board of Radiology). The third conjoint board (American Board of Emergency Medicine) was established in 1979. Its development is interesting. Initially it was spon-

sored by three groups: the AMA's Section on Emergency Medicine, the American College of Emergency Physicians, and the University Association of Emergency Medical Services. The application by this developing board was submitted to the Liaison Committee for Specialty Boards (LCSB), which body is the joint creation of the AMA's Council on Medical Education and of the American Board of Medical Specialties (ABMS). The ABMS is a coordinative body representing the 23 existing approved specialty boards, with five cooperating or associate members who are there for liaison purposes: the American Hospital Association, the Association of American Medical Colleges, Council of Medical Specialty Societies, the Federation of State Medical Boards of the USA, and the National Board of Medical Examiners. The application of the American Board of Emergency Medicine was somewhat controversial, because some of the existing specialties believed that, at most, it should be a subspecialty of one or more of the existing boards. In 1977 Emergency Medicine was disapproved as a primary specialty, but its sponsors persisted, and in 1979 it received approval as a conjoint board. In addition to the three sponsoring societies, the new board consists of representatives from seven primary specialties boards, including the specialties of family practice, pediatrics, and surgery (which had earlier opposed elevation of Emergency Medicine to specialty status).

Table 2–4 lists the approved boards in the medical specialties and subspecialties as of 1991. Table 2–5 lists the specialties and subspecialties for osteopathic medicine. Both tables can be found in the next chapter.

The American Board of Medical Specialties

When the ABMS was established (as the Advisory Board for Medical Specialties) in 1933, there were only four existing certifying boards: Obstetrics and Gynecology, Ophthalmology, Otolaryngology, and Dermatology and Syphilology (later renamed Dermatology). But the trend toward establishment of specialty certifying boards was clearly established, and to keep some sense of order, the Advisory Board of Medical Specialties was established, with the then four specialty groups as founding members plus the American Hospital Association, the Association of American Medical Colleges, the Federation of State Medical Boards, and the National Board of Medical Examiners. In 1970, the board was reorganized and became the American Board of Medical Specialties with the AHA, AAMC, FSMB, and the NBME as associate members. A fifth associate member, the Council of Medical Specialty Societies, joined in 1973. The regular members consist of representatives from each of the approved primary and conjoint medical specialty boards, and the board now has 23 members plus five associate members who are there for liaison purposes. The major purposes of the ABMS are to act as a spokesperson for approved specialty boards, resolve problems that arise among specialty boards, deal with the approval of new specialty boards and types of certification, and prevent duplication of effort among boards. The ABMS statement on the significance of certification in medical specialties explains that certification is voluntary and warns of the increasing fragmentation of medicine into more specialties and subspecialties in the statement below (19):

Medical specialty certification in the United States, from its inception, has been a voluntary procedure. Since the establishment of the first nationally recognized medical specialty board in 1917, some physicians have elected to seek formal recognition of their qualifications in their chosen specialty fields by presenting themselves for examination before specialty boards comprised of their professional peers. The definitions of each of the specialties and of the educational and other requirements leading to eligibility for board certification have been developed by consensus within the medical profession and, to date, the certification of a medical specialist has remained separate and distinct from licensure by civil authorities of professionals qualified to practice medicine within their jurisdictions.

The voluntary nature of specialty certification is attested to further by the fact that as of December 31, 1973, only 46 percent of the 308,127 physicians not in training included in the national registry of physicians maintained by the American Medical Association are diplomates of one or more of the 22* member Boards of the American Board of Medical Specialties. Yet, as Levit, et al. have recently demonstrated, the trend toward specialty board recognition is accelerating and during the current decade "virtually all United States graduates will undertake residency training and seek specialty certification."

The growth in medical specialty certification must be differentiated from the parallel increasing trend of physicians voluntarily to designate special areas of interest or areas of special practice to which they devote the largest segment of their professional time, whether or not they are diplomates of the 22 member boards of the American Board of Medical Specialties. For such purposes the American Medical Association has expanded its list of specialty designations to 67 categories to assist the individual physician in describing his primary field of medicine for listing in the American Medical Directory. There are no professional or legal requirements for a licensed physician to seek specialty board certification in order to offer his professional services in his specialty.

Many thoughtful observers, both within and outside of the profession, caution that the progressive fragmentation of medicine into more and more medical specialties and subspecialities is contrary to the best interests of the public. Nevertheless, the established specialty boards, as well as the American Board of Medical Specialties itself, are increasingly facing concerted pressures to offer certification in additional specialty or subspecialty categories. This is occurring despite the fact that accredited educational programs and the evaluative examinations on which general certifications are based assign appropriate emphasis to each of the subspecialties or areas of special competence identified with the corresponding primary field. Accordingly, diplomates holding general certification normally acquire, to a greater or lesser degree, all of such special competencies in their educational and specialty practice experience.

Issues in Specialty Development

Some additional issues surfaced in the development of specialties. First, establishment of many

---

*This was adopted in 1975. There are now 23 member boards.

specialty boards inevitably led to conflicts over definition of the specialty. So long as the specialty, however defined, did not pursue a formal legitimizing process, the need for precise definitions was not imperative, but once the boards were established, definitional or domain or "turf" problems arose. Many groups experienced these difficulties. Stevens recounts the controversy as it developed between the optometrists and ophthalmologists, noting, also, that the controversy there still persists. Controversy developed as well among other medical specialists. Stevens notes, for example, that in the area of surgery, a great many of the medical specialties have surgery as an integral part of the specialty. Most of these specialties were incorporated before the American Board of Surgery (1937). Each carved out for itself a piece of the action, leaving little that can be considered unique to general surgery. With the renaming of the Advisory Board of Medical Specialties to the American Board of Medical Specialties in 1970, the umbrella agency's role was strengthened by receiving authority to coordinate the boards.

A second issue to note is that there were a great many organizational conflicts. One can view these conflicts in a negative or positive way. Negatively, they appear as power plays by a body that wishes to dominate. Positively, and we believe more appropriately, they can be viewed as the result of disagreements on how best to do the job. The AMA, for example, at many points sought to bring things under its umbrella, believing that the stronger the AMA was in terms of being *the* voice of American medicine, the more persuasive it could be in bringing about lasting improvements. Others, on the other hand, saw organizational development outside the AMA, but not in opposition to the AMA, as a more effective mechanism. Sometimes the disagreement over strategies was in part a conflict of long-term versus short-term objectives. Clearly, the AMA was not altogether happy that the specialties developed outside its structure, for it wanted a unified medical profession. On the other hand, during the period the specialties were developing, the AMA's principal support came from its rank-

and-file general practitioners, whose anxieties may not have been as great as those of physicians who saw themselves as specialists. One notes in this regard that the AMA's early view of its scientific sections was that the sections should primarily be focal points for the dissemination of knowledge to all physicians and not just serve the needs of the highly trained specialists (16, p. 288); hence, specialty societies and, in time, specialty boards. A major step was taken by the AMA in late 1977 to bring the specialty societies into its policy-making framework. As reported in the AMA's newspaper to its members (20, p. 1):

After nearly three hours of heated debate, the AMA's House of Delegates totally revamped the section council system and set specific criteria for giving specialty societies direct representation in the AMA.

The actions, approved by the house at its interim meeting in Chicago, eliminate delegates to the house from the 28 section councils and instead will enable any specialty society that meets the criteria to request the seating of its own delegate.

The move is a major policy change that can greatly expand specialty society representation in the AMA, and in doing so can provide a stronger, more united voice for American medicine, proponents said.

As one looks at the sweep of history, despite some competitiveness and disagreements, the AMA and most of the organizations sought ways to work together for the good of their profession and of the public. This is evident in the representatives on various committees, set up from time to time by the various organizations. These organizations saw themselves as part of a community in which, to survive, they had to get along with those of standing. The AMA and others felt the fringe areas (such as chiropractic medicine), where there might not even be medical qualifications, could be attacked, for these peripheral groups were not perceived as legitimate parts of the medical community.

The third issue to note relates to specialty terminology. A physician who completed all specialty requirements except the final board examination was, until recently, said to be board *eligible* in that specialty. Some specialties, such as orthopedic surgery, require the person to be a board-eligible practitioner in the specialty area before being permitted to take the examination. In other cases, the board-eligible person practices in the specialty area until the examination is scheduled and results are reported. In some cases, the board-eligible person never bothers to take the examinations. The author of a major textbook on pediatrics who was also professor and head of a university medical school department of pediatrics was, for example, only board eligible. However, this type of case is relatively rare today. Since "board eligible" can cover a multitude of competencies as well as sins (including those who fail the board examinations), there is a move by specialty boards to drop the use of this phrase and, on inquiry, to state precisely what a person's status is in the certifying process. When the physician passes the specialty exam and is awarded a diploma, he or she is then said to be a *diplomate* (holder of a diploma) or *board certified.*

The fourth issue to note is that the time required for training in a specialty varies with the specialty. The training program is known as the *residency* in a particular clinical area. The person being trained is a graduate of a medical school and while in the residency is known as a *resident.* The requirements for each specialty are spelled out in the *Directory of Medical Specialists,* which is published every other year for the ABMS, and they are also published each year by the AMA in its *Directory of Residency Training Programs.*

Federation of State Medical Boards and National Board of Medical Examiners

In the last half of the nineteenth century, licensing boards were established or reestablished in many of the states. But not all states at the turn of the century required passing a state board licensing examination to practice medicine in that state, as illustrated by the following letter to the editor and answer in *JAMA* in 1901 (21, p. 817):

Please let me know where a graduate in medicine could practice without the State Board examination.

Answer. The laws of the following states admit graduates to practice medicine without examination, under varying conditions: Arkansas, Colorado, Kentucky, Michigan, Nevada, Nebraska, Oklahoma, Rhode Island, South Dakota, and Wyoming. In some of the states only diplomas from certain schools are recognized: thus in Michigan the diplomas of some forty or fifty schools only are accepted and in Rhode Island similar scrutiny is exercised. In nearly all, more or less discrimination is made in regard to certain schools, but in these states more particularly than others.

Texas, in 1873, was the first state to establish a state board of medical examiners. By the turn of the century 37 states required credentials of some sort for licensure, and 23 of the states required more than a diploma. Some states also began to recognize the credentials and licenses of certain other states on a reciprocal basis, hence the practice of reciprocity came into being. But, as Womack notes (21, p. 819):

By 1901, 23 states required more than a diploma for licensure, and there were 37 states requiring certain credentials for licensure. By the turn of the century, already a few states had formed groups that could exchange the recognition of credentials, an action that became known as "reciprocity." Such a cooperative venture was at that time not too successful, for the legislation governing the qualification for medical practice differed widely in the various states, as did the effectiveness of the examination. Some examining boards scrutinized a candidate with unusual care. Others did not. Some did not require an examination. Others did. Some examining boards quickly became the pawn of political influence and, too often, could not maintain the type of respect from other boards that would be needed to make reciprocity universal. By 1900, in many areas, the situation was not a happy one.

The need for some kind of national standard was apparent to many, but to bring this about was not easy. As with so many change efforts in all fields, resistance is often encountered. For example, the National Confederation of Medical Examining and Licensing Boards, founded in 1891, had considered the question of a national examining board but had disapproved the idea. Some states still wanted something done in this regard, and Derbyshire states that the Wisconsin board worked out an exchange plan with the Michigan board in 1901 (22, p. 50). The following year, these states met with representatives from Illinois and Indiana, and they established the Confederation of Reciprocating State Medical Examining Boards. Derbyshire states that soon afterward "its membership was increased and its aim broadened to include efforts to improve educational standards and to promote uniform legislation for medical licensure." Merger of the two organizations was achieved in 1912 with the formation of the Federation of State Medical Boards. By 1914, 26 boards were members. Despite many developmental problems over disagreements about the aims of the federation, by 1978, all medical (MD) boards were members; there are, as well, nine member osteopathic examining boards. The Canadian provinces are also among its members.

During the early part of this century, some in the AMA were interested in national licensure, but this never became a strong movement because of constitutional concerns over the question of state rights. This is a nice way of stating two related points of view: concern over federal bureaucratic control of the right to practice and concern by state boards about their rights (self-preservation), and also the belief held by many that the state boards were better able to assess competence to practice medicine. One should not snicker at the defensiveness of some state boards on this issue. Any national system would have to have standards low enough so that most states could qualify. Otherwise, a national system would not be acceptable. Why, then, should a state board with very high standards opt for a system that would lower that state's standards? This is in part why the federation's early successes were limited.

However, reformers wanted to see a raising of standards throughout the nation and, with that, increased reciprocity. In addition, they wanted some

mechanism to assure high-quality physicians in the federal services. The idea, then, of some kind of national examining system as a means for comparing medical graduates from the different schools had a lot going for it, and this led, by 1915, to the formation of the National Board of Medical Examiners (NBME). The initial board included, among others, representatives of the Navy, Army, Public Health Service, the Federation of State Medical Boards, the AAMC, the ACS, and the AMA. The critically important position of secretary was filled by Dr. William L. Rodman, who announced the formation of the NBME (a month after its establishment) during his presidential address at the AMA meeting in San Francisco in June 1915. Rodman labored hard to develop this new organization. He served as professor of surgery at a number of medical schools, was president of the AAMC in 1903 and 1904, was active in AMA clinical affairs and politics, serving in the House of Delegates from 1900 to 1903 and for many years as chairman of its Committee on Reciprocity, and was a founding fellow of the ACS. In 1915 he became the sixty-seventh president of the AMA.

Rodman's career is interesting because it illustrates the pathways through which many medical leaders worked and still work. Such people wear many hats, some of them at the same time. One person is thus able to exert influence in a number of organizations. One can hypothesize, also, that the whole idea of federal representation on the NBME stemmed from a 1902 editorial in JAMA, which has been attributed to Rodman, that called for a national board to examine the qualifications of physicians who serve in the federal services, and this was, in part, prompted by Rodman's previous experiences as an army surgeon. Although early federal government representation later caused some concern in the ranks of medicine, Womack notes that in some of the developmental stages of the NBME, these representatives provided needed consistent support (21, p. 821).

The AMA's endorsement of the NBME came in 1916, and with that endorsement, the NBME was fully legitimized. The AMA noted in its resolution of endorsement that two legal forces, government medical services and state licensing boards, were represented on the NBME and that "finances have been generously provided for its maintenance for a number of years" (21, p. 820). Who provided that generous financial support? None other than the Carnegie Foundation for the Advancement of Teaching.

The NBME quickly began work administering the first examination in late 1916. Thirty-two applicants asked to take the examination, but only 16 were considered sufficiently qualified. Womack reports that only 10 took it, and only five passed. "Between 1916 and 1921, eleven examinations were held. There were, in all, 498 applicants, 427 qualified to take the examination; 325 appeared and 269 passed" (21, p. 820). Initially, eight states indicated that they would accept NBME test results for licensure. Over the years, as testing procedures improved, and as state boards were reassured that the NBME would not usurp their prerogatives and become the licensing agency, more and more states accepted the results. But there were many variations, and some states insisted on setting their own examinations, constructed from the NBME pool of questions, graded by the NBME, but administered by the states under their own names. Some states, moreover, insisted on special basic science examinations, a barrier to licensure that is, Derbyshire states, a matter of increasing exasperation to medical educators and physicians. "In these days of rapid growth of medical knowledge, the burgeoning of medical education, and the increasing mobility of the population, basic science requirements are considered by many to be anachronistic stumbling blocks to medical licensure" (22, p. 118). The original intent of these laws was to deal not so much with physician deficiencies but with chiropractors, cultists, and the like.

Despite the significant advances brought about through the NBME examinations, state structuring of some examinations (from NBME questions) by boards whose personnel were always changing and who generally had no expertise in testing procedures, coupled with state determination of

pass levels, prompted concern. Derbyshire notes, for example, that some states rarely failed applicants. Other states had high failure rates, and one state apparently gave special (favorable) treatment to its native sons. These variations posed very real problems in terms of facilitating reciprocity (endorsement) of licenses among the states. In addition, the NBME examinations were not given to graduates of foreign medical schools (during the late 1940s, a growing number of international medical graduates [IMGs] began to move to the United States).

We should note at this juncture that we do not refer to graduates of Canadian schools as IMGs. Because of the similarities between the educational systems and the medical school accreditation process (which was until recently the same accreditation body), graduates of approved Canadian schools are considered eligible to be examined by all state boards on the same basis as U.S. graduates, and about half of the states grant reciprocity. In recent years, the United States' receptiveness to Canadian graduates has not been viewed sympathetically by the Canadian government because of the talent drain to the south.

The problems that arose, from variations among the states that adapted the NBME tests to their uses, concerned enough of the state boards so that a move began to improve on the situation by creating one national test. The vehicle for this effort was the Federation of State Medical Boards of the United States, which developed the Federation Licensing Examination (FLEX), and FLEX was accepted by all state boards for medical licensure until 1994. The examination is developed nationally by the federation through its FLEX board, from NBME questions. It is administered by each state and graded by the NBME; scores are recorded by the federation for reference purposes and are reported to the appropriate state boards. All states now set the pass level at the FLEX weighted average of 75, although individual states may differ about the number of times FLEX may be taken.

Most licensing boards do not allow graduates to

take the FLEX until they have completed their residency requirements. A few states' boards allow graduates to take the examination before or during residency training, but they do not issue a license until the residency training is completed.

FLEX was taken by graduates who wished to practice in the few states where the NBME was not accepted, by a few medical school graduates who did not have an NBME certificate, and by IMGs. The great majority of medical school graduates took the NBME examinations (the "National Boards") to receive licensure.

The NBME examinations consist of three parts: part I, taken toward the end of the second year of medical school; part II, toward the end of the last year; and part III, during or on completion of the internship or first year of residency training. There is an obvious advantage to the National Boards, in that the candidate takes part I, the basic science portion, when the material is freshest.

Finally, after nearly a century of debate about a national licensing system, the FSMB and the NBME got together and, in 1992, introduced a single, uniform examination for medical licensure called the United States Medical Licensing Examination (USMLE), which replaced the NBME and FLEX. It is expected that all states and some Canadian provinces will use the USMLE because no other national examination will be available after 1994.

The USMLE is an examination program consisting of three parts or "steps" to measure the knowledge and competence of applicants for medical licensure. These "steps" use multiple-choice questions and may be taken at separate times. "Step 1" assesses the understanding and application of basic biomedical skills. "Step 2" assesses the knowledge and understanding of clinical science necessary for patient care under supervision. "Step 3" assesses the knowledge and understanding of biomedical and clinical science necessary for unsupervised practice of medicine. Although states retain the right to set passing grade scores, it is expected that they will all accept the same passing grade.

Controversies in the Development of Medical Practice

The practice of medicine brought neither financial wealth nor social prestige in early America. As mentioned earlier, medicine was practiced by a wide array of individuals, from those who had studied medicine in Europe to persons with little or no medical training. Most families cared for themselves, and many medical practitioners found it difficult to support themselves solely from medical practice and were often forced to resort to a second occupation. Most patients who were treated by physicians remained at home, and their physicians spent many hours traveling to visit them with a horse and buggy for transportation. The hours spent traveling severely limited the number of patients a physician could attend. The number of patients increased as transportation and roads improved, enabling physicians to travel between patients more quickly; patients were also more able to visit the doctors' offices.

Most physicians practiced essentially on their own; they had little need for hospitals. Medical societies were few and tended to draw only the most elite members of the profession, that is, the ones who had more formal training and who were seeking to upgrade the educational process and the overall quality of medical practice.

The practice of medicine began to change significantly as hospital use increased. In the late nineteenth century and early 1900s, the number of hospitals grew rapidly as hospital sanitation improved, hospital infections decreased, and antiseptic surgery was introduced. Urban life that accompanied industrialization (working away from home and having smaller living accommodations) also contributed to the increased use of hospitals, although well-to-do families still preferred treatment in their homes. It was around this time and as a result of these developments that, as Starr notes, "hospitals moved from the periphery to the center of medical practice as well as medical education" (23, p. 146).

As hospitals became a necessary part of medical

practice, medical practitioners increasingly sought access to them, to admit their patients and to continue treatment. They did not become employees of the hospitals, but rather used the hospitals as one of the tools necessary for patient care. Sometimes they established their own hospitals, particularly when they encountered resistance to joining the staffs of existing institutions, which were frequently dominated by the professional elite. Hospitals had no control over the patient's treatment. This was solely the responsibility of the individual physician.

As access to hospitals increased, professional associations, particularly the ACS and AMA, sought ways to tighten the medical control of hospitals, particularly because a number of practices developed that were considered not in the patients' best interests and therefore unethical: ghost surgery, fee splitting, and unnecessary surgery.

Ghost Surgery, Fee Splitting, and Unnecessary Surgery

Ghost surgery is surgery performed by a surgeon other than the one engaged by the patient. If, for example, a patient needed abdominal surgery and the GP was uncomfortable undertaking it, the GP might take it on "to save face" or to satisfy the patient, and when the patient was under anesthesia, a hired surgeon would come in to do the job. The patient would never see the ghost surgeon. This practice is probably nonexistent today.*

Fee splitting is a practice in which the surgeon's fee is divided with other physicians without the knowledge and consent of the patient. In its most

---

*A television documentary in 1977 described ghost surgery as surgery performed in a teaching hospital in which the actual work is done by the surgical resident and not the surgeon. The essential difference between this practice and what we have defined as ghost surgery is that in the teaching hospital instance the surgical resident is under the guided direction of a qualified surgeon who in all probability sees the patient preoperatively and postoperatively. The resident, moreover, is paid these days by the hospital on a salary basis. At issue in the television documentary was that the patient had not clearly been informed that the resident would be a key person on the case. There is an ethical issue here as well as a possible legal issue relating to civil liability under modern doctrines of informed consent.

pernicious form, it was a kickback from the surgeon to the referring physician as payment for the referral. One might describe it as a bounty system. But one might also describe it as a mechanism for discouraging surgery by GPs, saying to the GP, in effect: Don't do surgery because you are not really trained to do it, but to stabilize your income and to encourage you to refer patients, we'll give you a payment for every case referred. Fee splitting has long been a violation of the AMA's code of ethics, but it was believed to be widespread at least until the Second World War.

Fee splitting has also been carried out above board. In this instance, the family doctor refers the patient to a surgeon. The surgeon tells the patient that a medically qualified operative assistant would be desirable and that the surgeon would like the family doctor to be that assistant. In such a case, the division of the fee would be with the knowledge and, presumably, consent of the patient and would, therefore, not be a violation of the AMA's code of ethics. The surgeon's wish in this case might well be in the patient's interest. Then again, it could also be a splitting of the fee as payment for the referral. This practice is probably not significant today. Whether it was ever widely practiced, we doubt anyone can tell.

Unnecessary surgery is an issue that still troubles the nation. We shall deal with it later in the text. Suffice it to note here that specialists do what they are trained to do, and a surgeon is trained to treat medical problems surgically. There have undoubtedly been some unscrupulous surgeons who operated knowing that there were no medical indications for surgery, but probably more of the truly unnecessary surgery is due to inadequate diagnosis. We have used the phrase "truly unnecessary" because, as shall be noted in Chapter 6, much of the unnecessary surgery today is not factually based; rather, it is based on different judgments.

Some of the surgical leaders moved vigorously to address these evil practices through the American College of Surgeons (ACS). Besides opposing fee splitting and unnecessary surgery, the ACS also established standards for surgical training and developed a mechanism (fellowship) for recognizing those who were judged by the college to be acceptable surgeons. The AMA did not lag behind on the issue of fee splitting; it condemned it officially in 1913, stating that "any member of the American Medical Association found guilty of secret fee splitting or of giving or receiving commissions shall cease to be a member of the American Medical Association" (16, p. 953). But it had, in fact, acted even earlier, when in 1902 it supported the expulsion of fee splitters from local medical societies and in 1912 made fee splitting a violation of its ethical code. In working toward this position, the association's Judicial Council conducted a survey of prominent members of the profession. The results were reported by the Judicial Council: "It is interesting to note that in the replies given stating whether or not secret fee splitting was justifiable, there was 77.3 percent who answered in the negative, 13.4 percent who answered in the affirmative, and 9.3 percent who were doubtful" (15, p. 952).

The AMA's principles of ethics had always condemned unnecessary surgery, as had the profession from at least the times of Hippocrates. Although the AMA and the ACS condemned it, however, it was difficult to get a handle on the problem until the specialty of pathology was well developed and until the mandated recording of pathology reports on all hospital surgical cases in the 1950s by the hospital accrediting body (the Joint Commission on Accreditation of Hospitals [JCAH]).* The JCAH not only forced hospitals to monitor surgical practices but also sent inspection teams in as part of the accrediting process. Hospitals more or less had to go along if they wanted to be accredited, and this they wanted in order to get paid by Blue Cross and other health insurance companies. But even then the problem persisted, in large measure because of disagreements about the indications for surgical intervention.

---

*JCAH was renamed the Joint Commission on Accreditation of Healthcare Organizations (JCAHO) in 1987 to reflect its wider accrediting functions.

Contract and Group Practice

The desire for a reasonable and stable income prompted some physicians to enter contract and group practices. These arrangements were not like the unethical practices described above. They were open and above-board arrangements, and there was nothing about them that would suggest that the arrangements were in themselves injurious to patients, or that they were likely to be, or that they were in any way unethical. When they appeared as a threat to other practitioners, however, the cry of unethical practice was heard, and the organization that represented the aggrieved physicians—the state and local medical societies and the AMA—took up battle.

Although contract and group practices are commonplace today, are growing, and are accepted by organized medicine as appropriate and ethical ways to deliver medical care, many individual practitioners still resist what they perceive to be an unwise trend. These trends are represented today by salaried practice, Health Maintenance Organizations (HMOs), and Preferred Provider Organizations (PPOs). The controversies seem at first to be economic, that is, a threat to the incomes of the protesting physicians, but some very real issues lie behind the protests. We begin by defining contract practice and group practice, and then we look at the storms that surrounded their development.

Contract Practices

Certain industries (e.g., railroads, mining, lumbering, steel) employed company doctors to do preemployment health examinations, to treat occupational injuries, and in some instances to develop employee medical programs. These physicians were mostly salaried, that is, under contract. Medical societies opposed this type of practice (except when physicians were under contract to serve the military), which they regarded as exploitation because doctors bid against each other for the contracts, thus reducing the price of their services. The opposition of the medical profession over time discouraged employers from expanding medical services except in remote areas where physicians were generally unavailable.

Another type of contract practice emerged when mutual benefit societies, employee associations, unions, and fraternal orders flourished among immigrants in the early 1900s. These were often social organizations, and sometimes they made life insurance policies available to members. Some also contracted with physicians to provide medical care for their members (and sometimes their dependents) for a fixed yearly fee per member, thus, a capitation method of payment. These "benefit societies" thrived in the industrial areas of several states despite the opposition of most physicians. Although many of these contract physicians felt they were not paid enough for their services, some needed this type of contract, especially if they were younger and trying to establish their practices. Many local medical societies complained about poor-quality care by these contract practitioners, and there may have been some validity to their complaints.

These medical societies were also concerned about contract doctors undercutting them economically, doing work for less than they would normally charge on a fee-for-service basis. The AMA, which was as interested in upgrading the medical profession and preserving the independence of doctors as it was in improving medical education, also objected to contract practice. As Starr notes, the AMA in 1907 could see "no economic excuse or justification" for this type of practice, and it objected "to the unlimited service for limited pay and the 'ruinous competition' it 'invariably' introduced" (23, p. 208). This type of contract practice declined over time as the supply of physicians decreased and, as a result, there were enough patients for a physician to earn a living without resorting to it. However, it began to rise again with the development of HMOs and, more recently, of PPOs; these pose a threat to the traditional form of fee-for-service solo practice, which many physicians still feel serves the best interests of the patient as well as the physician's pocketbook.

Group Practice

Group practice, in which a number of physicians decide to practice medicine in a coordinated manner and typically in a single location, as distinct from the more traditional approach of solo (single physician) practice, has been a part of the American scene for a long time. The founding of the Mayo Clinic in Rochester, Minnesota at the end of the nineteenth century is generally cited as the beginning of organized group practice as we know it today, although there were some antecedents. Mayo was followed by other groups, among them the famous Ross-Loos Clinic in Los Angeles, which served the city water department employees and others under contract. Some operated on a loose fee-for-service basis as in solo practice, but as the groups became organized, many paid their member physicians a salary, sometimes also a percentage of the net business income or a bonus. MacColl notes that the quality of care in many of the early groups "was reasonably good, but there were others which did not reflect much credit on either the organizers or the physicians involved" (24, p. 12).

During the early period of group practice development, the AMA was somewhat ambivalent about it. Where groups existed, physicians outside the groups often expressed concern about the quality of care the groups provided, as well as concern about the competition from lower fees charged sometimes by the groups. Then, in 1932, a report was issued by a national committee, The Committee on the Costs of Medical Care, titled *Medical Care for the American People.*

The Committee was a prestigious group, chaired by a former AMA president, Dr. Ray Lyman Wilbur, who was at the time in President Hoover's cabinet as Secretary of the Interior. The Committee recommended, albeit with some medical and dental member dissent, that medical care should be provided by organized group practices and that "the costs of medical care [should] be placed on a group payment basis, through the use of insurance, through the use of taxation, or through the use of both these methods. This is not meant to preclude the continuation of medical services provided on an individual fee basis for those who prefer the present method" (25, p. 120). Later the report explained its reasoning regarding voluntary health insurance, noting that their plan is flexible, because "the same group of practitioners might render service to some patients on an insurance basis, to others on a fee-for-service basis, and to indigent persons in return for payments in full or in part from governmental or charitable bodies. Some of the professional men in such a group might continue to serve their former private patients, for a time at least, on a customary fee basis" (25, p. 124). As noted, the report was published in 1932. The report galvanized the opposition of the AMA to both group and salaried practice.

In 1933, the AMA declared that groups of physicians in salaried practice were considered unethical. It was unethical, as the dissenters had noted (25, pp. 156–157):

when there is solicitation of patients either directly or indirectly . . . when there is competition and under-bidding to secure the contract . . . when compensation is inadequate to secure good medical practice . . . when there is interference with reasonable competition in a community . . . when free choice of physicians is prevented . . . .

This change on the part of the AMA reflected widespread concern within the profession, which hit the boiling point in Washington, D.C., as well as in a number of other cities. The concern was professional as well as economic, although critics all too frequently focus on the economic component, ignoring the professional objections.

The AMA's involvement in state and local disputes generally stemmed from questions and issues raised by state and local medical societies. Typically, the latter had a problem for which they needed advice and they turned to the AMA; or the AMA's Judicial Council got involved whenever an aggrieved physician appealed an adverse decision rendered by the state medical society. A focal point here has been the AMA's *Principles of Medical Ethics,* which serves as a guide to state and local medical societies. The *Principles* was a document developed by physicians from the states and adopted by local state society representatives in the AMA House of Delegates. MacColl notes that "quackery, advertising, fee splitting, patient stealing, promoting fraudulent remedies and devices, and developing undue personal publicity have all been pretty well curbed through the application of these codes" (24, p. 136).

The AMA became directly involved in a local issue in the late 1930s, and was found guilty of restraint of trade in 1941. The case involved the AMA and the District of Columbia Medical Society in their actions relating to the Group Health Association of Washington (GHA). MacColl notes that opposition to the GHA by the D.C. Medical Society arose almost immediately after the GHA was organized in 1937. The society notified "all the physicians in the area that the plan was unethical. The GHA's salaried physicians were expelled from the Society, and a list of 'reputable physicians' was circulated to all the hospitals for their guidance" (24, p. 140). The D.C. Medical Society and the AMA were subsequently indicted, found guilty, and fined for having conspired to monopolize medical practice. MacColl goes on to note that the GHA physicians were later admitted to the Society and had no subsequent difficulty over hospital privileges. In other parts of the country, specifically Seattle and San Diego, the local medical societies and not the AMA were the defendants, and in each case the medical societies lost in their efforts to block development of group health plans.

Behind these medical society actions was the specter of the 1932 report of the Committee on the Costs of Medical Care (25). MacColl notes that after the AMA fine in the GHA case, the AMA disengaged from "further legal entanglement." He goes on to note that it fell to the local societies to interpret or misinterpret the code of ethics and that at times the interpretations were to serve the ends, and the fears and pressures, at the local level.

The objections to group practice at times took on rather nasty aspects. In metropolitan New York, for example, the Health Insurance Plan (HIP) was established in the mid-1940s as a demonstration project for national health insurance. HIP, the fiscal agent, contracted with medical groups, paying each group so much for each person on its list. How the group divided the money was up to the group. In return for the capitation payment, the group was responsible for providing comprehensive physician services, prevention, and treatment. For hospital care, most HIP subscribers were at that time covered by Blue Cross. Though the local medical societies might not have been able to keep HIP physicians from joining, they could ostracize them socially. For example, at a medical society meeting in the 1950s in Garden City, New York, at lunch the HIP physician sat alone while his "colleagues" enjoyed fraternal relations with one another. As late as the 1960s, HIP physicians were denied hospital privileges. The intensity of local medical feeling did not need AMA fuel, for HIP, at its inception, had proclaimed itself a demonstration project for a national system, and there were many physicians in New York who were accustomed to government systems before coming to the United States. In addition, the economic pressures on physicians in New York City were considerable, because many believed in the 1950s that New York City had an oversupply of medical practitioners. At every turn, HIP was challenged by non-HIP physicians. Blue Shield, which was sponsored by the medical profession, used paid salesmen and advertising, but when HIP did this, "the charge of unethical conduct was raised. Ben E. Landis, one of the HIP physicians, took the matter to the Judicial Council of the AMA, which ruled in his favor, finding that HIP was a legally organized plan and had as much right to advertise as did Blue Shield so long as the personal qualifications of the physicians were not promoted" (24, p. 139). By the late 1970s in New York, all wounds were healed, and HIP physicians were fully accepted by medical societies and hospitals. HIP no longer uses Blue Cross; it provides its own hospital coverage.

The AMA's Judicial Council, in addition to the Landis case, also reversed, on appeal, the earlier

expulsion from the Los Angeles County Medical Society of the developers of the Ross-Loos Medical Group.

In Baltimore, in contrast to New York, the state of Maryland, in consultation with the state and city medical societies, established a medical care program to pay physicians for care of the poor. Physician payments were on a capitation basis—so much a year for the complete care of each person on the physician's list. Outside Baltimore, a different program existed, paying physicians on a fee-for-service basis. Some years after the program became operational, some physicians, at what had evolved into a more conservatively oriented state society, raised objections to the system of capitation payments, but the city physicians were satisfied with the program at the time, and there was not much the state society could do about it.

To return to the *concept* of group practice medical service plans, in 1948, the Massachusetts Medical Society accepted free choice of medical group as the equivalent of free choice of physician; in 1959, the AMA ended its opposition by adopting the report of its Committee for the Study of Medical Care Plans, commonly referred to as the Larson Report. MacColl notes that the Larson Report advised medical societies "to exercise great caution in blanket condemnation and the use of the term 'unethical' " (24, p. 137).

Although many in the medical profession remain uneasy about contract and group practice and salaried practice, opposition has subsided. Organized medicine no longer opposes them, and each of these forms of practice is growing, as we shall see in Chapter 3. The change came about partly as a result of effective legal challenges against organized medicine, but perhaps more importantly as a direct result of a recognized physician shortage in the 1950s that would ensure fee-for-service, solo practice physicians an ample number of patients to maintain a good income, regardless of the presence of contract and group practice. By this time, group practice had also evolved and now was seen by its advocates as a way to regularize their hours, get easy consultation, and afford ownership of expensive technology that they could not justify economically by themselves, but could justify on a shared basis. All forms of medical practice could thus live together in harmony.

There is, however, a lingering legitimacy to the views advanced by those who oppose some of the modern-day manifestations of group and contract practice—the HMO and the PPO—because both put the provider at risk. This development occurred in the 1980s when we began to witness an oversupply of physicians competing with one another for patients. This competition came shortly after government and businesses had become greatly concerned over the rising cost of medical care. The worst fears of those still opposed to group and contract practice began to be realized: PPOs and HMOs became attractive to patients because they eliminated most of the charges they would have to pay, and they are attractive as well to employers and government, who pay for much of the health insurance, because they put a lid on the amount they would have to pay. The emergence of HMOs and PPOs is greatly altering the practice of medicine.

The AMA and Anticompetitive Behavior

The image of the AMA as a controlling group persists. It has been particularly evident in recent years in actions taken by the Federal Trade Commission (FTC) to restrict the activities of organized medicine. The FTC is concerned with restraint-of-trade practices, or forces and activities that interfere with the competitive forces of the marketplace. In 1976 it challenged the appropriateness of the Liaison Committee on Medical Education as the official accrediting body for medical schools, contending that AMA participation on the LCME might present a conflict of interest. The FTC conceded that it did not have any evidence of misconduct on the part of the AMA, but it argued nonetheless that the potential for misconduct existed. The FTC's challenge was not successful in getting the then U.S. Office of Education to get the AMA out of its participation in the accrediting process. The FTC,

in another case, found that the Michigan State Medical Society violated the federal antitrust laws when it urged its members to end their cooperation with Blue Shield and Medicaid because of irreconcilable disputes over their payment policies: with regard to Blue Shield, the plan proposed lower payments to participating physicians for vision and hearing care, and higher payments to nonparticipating physicians; with regard to Medicaid, the state ordered an 11 percent reduction in Medicaid payments. In still another case, the FTC went after the AMA and the Connecticut State Medical Society over the latter's ethical code statement on physician advertising. The FTC charged that the prohibition in the state society's code, and also in the New Haven County society's code, of false and misleading advertising constituted restraint of trade. Though the AMA *Principles of Medical Ethics* had already eliminated such prohibitions, the FTC apparently felt that, because the state society was affiliated with the AMA, the AMA was also rightfully a party to the complaint. The FTC view prevailed, and the AMA's 1982 to 1983 effort to get the Congress to prohibit FTC oversight of the profession failed.

Underlying these and similar controversies has been the search for some definition of what activities of organized medicine and of the other professions are appropriately subject to public scrutiny. The FTC, in its forays on accreditation and advertising, felt that the codes of medical ethics and the accrediting process might be professional cloaks for anticompetitive practices that were not in the public's interest. The profession, on the other hand, saw its activities and codes as important protections for the public. It seems to be agreed now that the business aspects of medical practice are to be more open to public scrutiny and control. The AMA, the state societies, and other medical groups now have to be more careful in what they say and do in order to walk the fine lines that have been drawn. One can expect that in the years ahead there will be more controversies as the rules are redrawn and professional practices adapt.

The AMA remains a potent, persuasive force on

the national scene, maintaining one of the most effective lobbying organizations in the nation's capital. On some issues, it represents the personal interest of its members, as do all other organized interest groups. On other issues, it represents the public as it advises elected and appointed officials on matters relating to the health of the people.

SUMMARY

In the early colonial period, most medical advice was given by lawyers, churchmen, and other learned people; having the ability to read, they could acquire some medical knowledge and use it for the benefit of those who had no alternative. The few physicians we had who were trained in medical school came from overseas. As the years passed, these physicians began to train others under an apprenticeship system. Not until 1756 did the first medical school, the College of Philadelphia, open in the colonies; it later became the University of Pennsylvania. At the time of the Revolutionary War it is estimated that there were only 3,500 medical practitioners in the colonies. Some, perhaps as many as 400, had some formal training, and only 200 held medical school degrees.

During the nineteenth century the number of medical schools proliferated, many at universities and colleges and many as independent financial ventures. The quality of the schools was mixed, as was the quality of the medical practice.

The better physicians, and particularly (but not exclusively) those who received training overseas, worked for reform, for an upgrading of the quality of both education and medical practice. One step taken was through the formation of various types of medical societies and associations at local and state levels, and, in 1847, at the national level with the formation of the American Medical Association. The AMA had as its primary goal the reform of medical education, and it worked continually toward the goal. Another step was the establishment of medical journals, vehicles for the dissemination of new knowledge and the continuing education of physicians. A third step toward reform came in

1876 with the formation of the Association of American Medical Colleges, which focused its efforts on the medical education process. Finally, toward the end of the nineteenth century, licensure of physicians and the testing of candidates for licensure became widespread. Each of these steps made progress, inching ahead in one area, yielding to stronger developments in another area, and renewing its progress at a later time.

By the end of the nineteenth century, the AMA was the instigator of the major reform efforts. The *Journal of the American Medical Association,* for example, began publishing in 1902 the failure rate of each school's graduates on state licensing exams. In 1904, the AMA created its Council on Medical Education, which picked up and carried the weapons of public exposure, embarrassment, inspection, and rating of the various medical schools. Its rating of schools exerted pressure to upgrade the curricula, the faculty, and the other resources allocated to the training of physicians. The AAMC also applied increasing pressure on its member schools.

But there was some feeling within this self-reform movement that what was needed was some confirmation of the work being done, confirmation by some outside body. The AMA's Council on Medical Education moved then in this direction, enlisting the support of the Carnegie Foundation for the Advancement of Teaching. The Carnegie Foundation was persuaded to undertake a study of medical education in the United States and Canada, commissioning one of its staff members, Abraham Flexner, to carry out this study, but to work closely with the AMA on it.

Flexner visited 155 schools and wrote a report, *Medical Education in the United States and Canada,* published in 1910. It was a searing critique of medical education at that time. Only three U.S. schools came through relatively unscathed: Johns Hopkins, Harvard, and Western Reserve. Flexner recommended that the number of schools be reduced from 155 to 31. Within 10 years of the report's release, the number was down to 85 and the quality of these was vastly improved. The report gave a boost to the efforts of the AAMC, which seized the advantage to strengthen its membership requirements. Foundation money began to pour into the better schools, and the reform of undergraduate medical education was largely complete.

Subsequent changes have been a rounding off of rough edges, such as the restructuring and formalization of the medical school accreditation process and the improvement in medical licensure testing and procedures.

Medical specialties evolved over time as physicians developed interests, and in turn special competence, in dealing with the medical problems associated with different parts of the body. The distinctions among physician, surgeon, and apothecary were, of course, of long standing. Major new emphases began during the nineteenth century, as physicians began to recognize the ineffectiveness of bleeding and purging and of most drugs then in use, as they identified specific pathology in different systems of the body, as anesthesia was discovered, and as new diagnostic instruments were developed. Physicians interested in some kind of specialty practice typically organized specialty societies and set standards for admission to their societies. One of these societies, the American College of Surgeons, played a particularly important role in establishing standards for surgical practice, and its role was especially important in raising hospital standards.

During the twentieth century the leading specialty societies joined forces with the AMA to sponsor national certifying boards in the various specialties. There are presently 20 *primary* specialty boards, each of which sets its own requirements for training and testing in order to become *board certified* or a *diplomate* in that specialty. In addition to these primary boards, there are three *conjoint* specialty boards, which are sponsored by two or more of the existing primary boards (rather than by the specialty societies and the AMA).

Licensure of physicians is not based on specialty training, but rather on the successful completion of a medical school program leading to an MD or DO degree *and* success in passing the state li-

censing examination. The NBME was established in 1916 and began giving examinations for medical licensure. Many states accepted the NBME test results; others used questions prepared by the NBME and determined their own passing grade. Because of this variation among states, the FSMB developed a licensure test called FLEX, using NMBE examination questions and the same passing grade, which was administered by each state. However, the great majority of applicants for medical licensure took the NBME examination until the early 1990s when a single, uniform examination for medical licensure called the United States Medical Licensing Examination (USMLE) was introduced and the NBME and FLEX examinations were phased out.

As the training and licensure systems became regularized, ensuring a reasonable level of professional competence, new problems arose in the practice of medicine. As physicians utilized and came to depend more and more on hospitals, the problems of fee splitting, ghost surgery, and unnecessary surgery arose. These were effectively dealt with by medical leaders who saw medicine as an honorable profession and not a business.

The need to earn a living prompted some physicians to enter into contracts with various organizations for the delivery of care, and also to form group practices, to secure or attract a sufficient flow of patients in order to stabilize their incomes. Forerunners of HMOs and PPOs, these moves were vigorously fought by the profession and by the AMA. Legal assaults on the AMA and on state and local medical societies, along with a shortage of physicians by the mid-1950s, combined to legitimize these forms of medical practice. But the resulting competitive environment raises a new set of problems as costs rise—the dangers of underservice and of overservice.

As one looks at the health system at any point in time, it seems riddled with weaknesses. However, when it is studied over a long period of time, enormous changes for the better can be seen, changes brought about by health professionals working through a variety of professional bodies.

Leadership within the medical profession, particularly within the AMA, has had an enormous positive impact. By and large, the changes that have been brought about were not sweeping; each change was merely an incremental, negotiated step that could be accepted and supported by most who might be affected. The role of government, except for the army and navy chiefs, is significant by its absence. The prevailing view of the times was that health matters were the domain of the physicians, that what they decided or wanted was appropriate. For this reason state licensing, like state boards of health, fell under the early control of the medical profession.

Shortcomings in our health system still exist, and change is occurring. As in the past, the change is usually a negotiated settlement, negotiated not because some do not want to act but because there are disagreements over how best to act.

DISCUSSION QUESTIONS

1. Why were the improvements in medical education, medical licensure, and medical practice not achieved more quickly?
2. Knowing what we do about the background of the Flexner study and how it was carried out, how would it be received if it were issued in 1994?
3. How desirable is it for physicians to have influence in the licensure of medical practitioners? What are the alternatives?
4. The American Board of Medical Specialties is a coordinated body representing the approved specialty boards. It has a number of cooperating or associate members: the AHA, AAMC, CMSS, FSMB, and NBME. What is the logic behind involving these associate member groups?
5. How did the AMA influence the practice of medicine?

REFERENCES

1. Packard, F.R.: *History of Medicine in the United States.* New York, Hafner Publishing Co., 1963.
2. Shryock, R.H.: *Medicine and Society in America, 1660–1860.* New York, New York University Press, 1960.
3. Corner, G.W.: *Two Centuries of Medicine. A History of the School of Medicine—University of Pennsylvania.* Philadelphia, J.B. Lippincott Co., 1965.
4. Stevens, R.: *American Medicine and the Public Interest.* New Haven, Yale University Press, 1971.
5. Shryock, R. H.: The Early American Public Health Movement. *Am J Public Health.* October 1937 (reprinted in Shryock, R. H.: *Medicine in America.* Baltimore, Johns Hopkins Press, 1966, p. 131).
6. Norwood, W. F.: *Medical Education in the United States Before the Civil War.* Philadelphia, University of Pennsylvania Press, 1944.
7. Burrow, J.G.: *American Medical Association—Voice of American Medicine.* Baltimore, Johns Hopkins Press, 1963.
8. Bonner, T.N.: *American Doctors and German Universities.* Lincoln, University of Nebraska Press, 1963.
9. Shryock, R.H.: *Medicine in America.* Baltimore, Johns Hopkins Press, 1966.
10. Johnson, V.: The Council On Medical Education and Hospitals, in Fishbein, M. (ed.): *A History of the American Medical Association, 1847–1947.* Philadelphia, W.B. Saunders Co., 1947.
11. Coggeshall, L.T.: *Planning for Medical Progress Through Education.* Evanston, IL, Association of American Medical Colleges, 1965.
12. Flexner, A.: *I Remember.* New York, Simon & Schuster, 1940.
13. Flexner, A.: *Medical Education in the United States and Canada,* bulletin 4. New York, The Carnegie Foundation for the Advancement of Teaching, 1910.
14. Ludmerer, K.M.: *Learning to Heal, the Development of American Medical Education,* New York, Basic Books, Inc., 1985.
15. Shryock, R.H.: The American Physician. *JAMA,* Vol. 134, May 31, 1947 (reprinted in Shryock, R.H.: *Medicine in America.* Baltimore, Johns Hopkins Press, 1966, p. 168).
16. Fishbein, M. (ed.): *A History of the American Medical Association, 1847–1947.* Philadelphia, W.B. Saunders Co., 1947.
17. Bond, A.K.: *When the Hopkins Came to Baltimore.* Baltimore, Pegasus Press, 1927.
18. Citizens Commission on Graduate Medical Education: *The Graduate Education of Physicians.* Chicago, American Medical Association, 1966.
19. American Board of Medical Specialties, *Annual Report & Reference Handbook—1982.* Evanston, IL.
20. *American Medical News,* December 12, 1977.

21. Quoted by Womack, N.A.: The Evolution of the National Board of Medical Examiners. *JAMA,* Vol. 192, June 7, 1965.

22. Derbyshire, R.C.: *Medical Licensure and Discipline in the United States.* Baltimore, Johns Hopkins Press, 1969.

23. Starr, P.: *The Social Transformation of American Medicine.* New York, Basic Books Inc., 1982.

24. MacColl, W.A.: *Group Practice and Prepayment of Medical Care.* Washington, D.C., Public Affairs Press, 1966.

25. *Medical Care for the American People: Final Report of the Committee on the Costs of Medical Care.* Chicago, University of Chicago Press, 1932; reprinted in 1970 by the U.S. Department of Health, Education and Welfare.

Chapter 2

Medical Education

The system of American medical education is faced with increasing criticism from within, as well as from outside, the medical profession. The criticism is not new, but is intensified both by the rapid growth in scientific knowledge that makes it more difficult than ever before for physicians to keep up to date, and by the economic pressures that are forcing physicians to change the ways in which they practice medicine—where they practice, how they practice, and how they are paid. This is causing a reappraisal by medical educators of the knowledge, skills, and personal qualities physicians need in order to practice medicine in today's world.

The goal has remained the same—to produce critical thinkers—but that is as difficult to accomplish in medical education as it is in other areas of education. Here we examine some of the efforts being made to improve medical education.

Physician training presently consists of four phases: premedical education, undergraduate medical education, graduate medical education, and postgraduate or continuing medical education.

Premedical Education

Premedical education typically consists of four years of study ending with a baccalaureate degree from a college or university. Most premedical students major in the sciences, although they can, in fact, major in almost any academic program as long as they take the specified science and other courses required by the medical school to which they apply for admission. About 8 percent of students entering medical school have advanced degrees.

Many students are attracted to medicine because it is a prestigious, well-paying profession, and the supply of physicians has, until recently, not exceeded the demand. Because of this, the competition for entrance to medical school is very intense. The American Medical Association's (AMA's) Council on Medical Education reports some interesting data (from which we have structured Table

2–1), on the competitive situation vis-à-vis medical school application and admissions (1).*

The number of medical schools and students continued to increase during the 1970s, but during the 1980s the number of students who applied and were enrolled in medical schools decreased. However, there has been a sharp increase in applicants in 1990 and in 1991 applications rose to over 33,000. The number of applications per person continues to hover above nine, reflecting a continuing recognition on the part of applicants of the difficulty of being admitted. Also, the premedical grade-point averages of those matriculating continue to fall in the A to B range.

Medical school admission is based, however, on a number of factors in addition to grade-point average. These include performance on the Medical College Admission Test (MCAT), which nearly all accepted applicants take, as well as recommendations and interviews. The MCAT is an objective

---

*Most of the data in this chapter are drawn from this report. The data were generated by AMA and AAMC staffs. This report is updated and printed annually in *JAMA*.

test that measures knowledge of science (biology, chemistry, and physics), ability to solve science problems, analysis and reading skills, and quantitative skills. In 1991 the MCAT was modified to strengthen the evaluation of skills such as critical thinking, verbal reasoning, and communicating, which have become more important as the vast expansion and change in medical knowledge requires physicians to rely less on rote memory. The new MCAT includes two nonscientific essays to help assess these skills.

Another weighted factor is the report to the medical school from the student's premedical advisers. In many schools, this confidential report is a committee report, which serves to minimize risks of bias. Interviews of applicants by the medical schools are also considered important by many as a means of asserting personality factors that tests and recommendations may not reveal. Not all schools or medical educators are satisfied with the interview because it is fraught with the risk of interviewer bias, and the search continues for other methods of assessing the personal qualities necessary for the best practice of medicine.

TABLE 2–1. Medical School Admissions

First-Year Class	Applicants	Applications per Individual	Number Accepted	Number Enrolled	Premed Grade-Point Average of Class* Percent			
					A	B	C	Unknown
1965–1966	18,703	4.7	9,012	8,769	12.7	76.7	10.6	—
1968–1969	21,118	5.3	10,092	9,863	16.8	75.9	7.3	—
1974–1975	42,624	8.5	15,066	14,963	39.3	50.8	3.0	6.8
1979–1980	36,141	9.3	16,886	17,014	47.5	48.2	1.8	2.1
1980–1981	36,100	9.2	17,146	17,204	45.8	50.2	1.8	2.2
1981–1982	36,727	9.3	17,286	17,320	46.4	50.9	1.6	1.1
1982–1983	35,730	9.4	17,294	17,230	44.7	52.9	1.9	0.6
1983–1984	35,200	9.1	17,209	17,175	42.4	55.1	1.6	1.0
1984–1985	35,944	9.2	17,194	16,992	41.7	55.1	1.6	1.6
1985–1986	32,893	9.3	17,228	16,929	45.8	48.4	1.9	3.9
1986–1987	31,323	9.4	17,092	16,779	41.8	48.4	1.9	3.9
1987–1988	28,123	9.5	17,027	16,686	46.6	49.4	1.9	2.1
1988–1989	26,721	9.7	17,108	16,781	44.6	49.0	2.1	4.3
1989–1990	26,915	9.5	16,975	16,749	43.7	52.7	2.3	1.3
1990–1991	29,243	9.1	17,206	16,803	45.0	52.4	2.2	0.4

SOURCE: Medical Education in the United States. *JAMA*, Vol. 266, No. 7, 1991.

*A—3.6–4.0 on a four-point scale; B—2.6–3.5; C—less than 2.6.

Nearly all leaders in medical education endorse the desirability of a broad liberal education in the arts, humanities, and social sciences, in addition to study in the biological and physical sciences during the premedical years. They recognize that such an education can enhance patient communication, improve understanding of the influence of social and economic problems on disease and convalescence, and enable physicians to acquire an understanding of the past that will help them contribute constructively to changes in society. However, because of the keen competition for admission to medical school, premedical students have tended to "play it safe" by emphasizing the biological and physical science courses at the expense of studies in other subject areas. Although medical schools are beginning to articulate more clearly and implement admission policies that give broadly educated applicants the same chance of admission as those with an intensive scientific education, this changing emphasis needs to be recognized more clearly by premedical counselors and by students preparing for medical school.

Illustrating the changes occurring in medical school admission practices, The Johns Hopkins University recently became the first medical school to make the MCAT an option rather than a requirement for admission. Hopkins' officials do not believe the MCAT is an accurate predictor of clinical performance or career outcomes, and they feel it forces students into a narrow, overly scientific education. The competition to achieve a high grade is intense. Premedical students may drop courses and curtail college or university activities during their junior year in order to study for the MCAT. Often it is the courses in the humanities that are dropped. Hopkins has set minimum science requirements so that students can obtain a broader undergraduate education, and since 1986 it has admitted students to its medical school solely on the basis of college transcripts, recommendations, and interviews.

Brown University has an innovative program that admits students to medical school directly from high school and merges the premedical and med-

ical programs into a seven-year program. Students in the program are encouraged to pursue courses in the humanities, arts, and social sciences. In an effort to broaden premedical education, the University of Pennsylvania has eliminated all course requirements for admission to its medical school. However, it still requires applicants to master the basic sciences and take the MCAT examination. Several other medical schools have eliminated course requirements, but they recommend courses, which causes many students to regard them as required. By making it easier for premedical students to take liberal arts courses, medical educators hope to produce more compassionate, humane physicians. Clearly there is a trend to prepare students for medical school with a more well-rounded education.

The *premedical student* is an undergraduate working toward graduation and a baccalaureate degree. Baccalaureate graduates who go on to graduate school in, say, nutrition or philosophy and who study for a master's degree or doctor of philosophy degree are, during this period of study, called graduate students. This is not the case for medical students. Although they typically hold a baccalaureate degree, in medical school they are considered undergraduates; hence, *undergraduate medical education* refers to medical schools and the training of physicians who will, on graduation, be awarded a Doctor of Medicine (MD) or Doctor of Osteopathy (DO) degree.

Graduate medical education refers to formalized training post-MD or post-DO in an approved internship or residency. *Postgraduate* or *continuing medical education* refers to formalized training on a short-course or short-term basis for physicians who have completed a period of graduate medical education; it generally includes refresher courses or intensive courses to develop new skills.

Undergraduate Medical Education

The typical medical school program lasts four years, covering 36 months of study. About 25 universities integrate their premedical and medical school programs and require less time to earn the MD degree.

Programs awarding the MD degree are accredited by the Liaison Committee on Medical Education (LCME), which is a joint committee established in 1942 by the AMA Council on Medical Education and the AAMC (Table 2–2). The legitimacy of accreditation by the LCME stems from its recognition for this purpose by its sponsoring bodies, and subsequently by the United States Secretary of Education and the Council on Postsecondary Education. Before 1942, the AMA was the only body to inspect medical schools. Not until 1969 did the U.S. Department of Education begin to recognize accrediting agencies.

Accreditation of the osteopathic medical schools is granted by the American Osteopathic Association (AOA), and its legitimacy in this role has also been acknowledged by the U.S. Secretary of Education and Council on Postsecondary Education.

Medical School Curriculum

Although the structure of medical education has not changed significantly for almost 50 years, new ways of teaching are being introduced to cope with the vast amount of information and the changing way medicine is practiced. The first two years of medical school have changed little. They are largely devoted to the basic medical sciences (anatomy, physiology, biochemistry, histology, pharmacology, microbiology, etc.), with lectures crammed full of facts given to a passive student body that hardly has time to memorize the information, much less to understand the relationship between facts and medical problems. The amount of scientific material to be learned has increased dramatically, and most schools have responded by adding the latest scientific findings in still more lectures. Many schools have incorporated electives and some patient contact during the first few years in response to student pressures. During the final two years students rotate through clinical clerkships in which they acquire clinical skills and give general medical care. Students are assigned patients on whom they

conduct histories, physical examinations, and some laboratory tests, and they are actively involved in the diagnosis and treatment of these patients under the supervision of the resident and faculty.

The clinical experience ranges from primary to tertiary care in a variety of inpatient and outpatient settings. Usually students do clerkships in internal medicine, obstetrics and gynecology, pediatrics, psychiatry, and surgery. Most schools allow students some elective courses or other clerkships during the final year. The number and duration of these vary from school to school. Society, government, and expanding knowledge continually pressure medical schools to add to the content of their curricula. However, the undergraduate years of medical education should emphasize a broad perspective of medicine. Medical school graduates are not expected to become experts in all subjects and are not prepared for immediate independent, unsupervised practice; they are prepared to enter a program of graduate medical education.

A 1984 report by the AAMC on the future of medical education, *Physicians for the Twenty-First Century* (2), recognized the need not only to modify admission criteria, but also to decrease the emphasis on memorization and passive learning in the curricula. It also made suggestions about improving the teaching of medical students, including one to reward good teaching as it rewards clinical research. Often professors at major teaching hospitals receive academic advancement and prestige from successful research rather than from teaching, as is true in other areas of higher education. In addition, most clinical faculty devote some time to private patient care, which has considerable financial rewards. Teaching sometimes suffers. As a consequence of research and private practice demands, much of the teaching in the clinical areas is thus relegated to residents (medical graduates in specialty training), who often lack the needed experience. Upgrading teaching is a difficult challenge in medicine, just as it is for higher education in general.

The AAMC report also stressed the need to address the humanistic aspect of medicine and

TABLE 2–2. Relationship Among Parent Organizations and CFMA, LCME, ACGME, ACCME

Parent Organizations Establish Policy

	ABMS, AMA, AHA, AAMC, CMSS (Council for Medical Affairs)	AMA, AAMC (Liaison Committee on Medical Education)	ABMS, AMA, AHA, AAMC, CMSS (Accreditation Council for Graduate Medical Education)	ABMS, AMA, AHA, AAMC, CMSS, AHME, FSMB (Accreditation Council for Continuing Medical Education)
Function	Review, develop, and recommend policy	Accrediting M.D. programs	Accrediting GME programs	Accrediting CME providers
Representatives	Two senior elected officers and the Chief Executive Officer of ABMS, AMA, AHA, AAMC, CMSS	AMA (6) AAMC (6) Public (2) Participants (nonvoting): Students (2) Federal (1)	ABMS (4) AMA (4) AHA (4) AAMC (4) CMSS (4) Resident Physicians Section AMA (2) Public (1) Fed. (nonvoting) (1)	ABMS (3) AMA (3) AHA (3) AAMC (3) CMSS (3) AHME (1) FSMB (1) Public (1) Fed. (nonvoting) (1)

SOURCE: *Annual Report & Reference Handbook—1987.* Evanston, IL, ABMS, 1987.

AMA, American Medical Association; AHA, American Hospital Association; AHME, Association for Hospital Medical Education; AAMC, Association of American Medical Colleges; CMSS, Council of Medical Specialty Societies; FSMB, Federation of State Medical Boards; ABMS, American Board of Medical Specialties.

the need for medical students to become competent in the computer area to manage the staggering amount of available information and to enhance independent learning. Most medical schools now require courses to facilitate a humanistic approach, courses designed to improve doctor-patient relationships, to enhance communication skills, and to grapple with social and ethical issues. Harvard Medical School, for example, has introduced an innovative curriculum to achieve a better balance between the scientific and humanistic aspects of medicine and the demands for better data management. About 20 percent of Harvard's medical students participated in this "New Pathway" program in 1986 (3). This program involves fewer lectures. Students are taught in small tutorials, they interact with patients during their first year, and they learn statistical and problem-solving skills while learning computer literacy in order to retrieve and assess information. Medical educators are watching the "New Pathway" program closely to see if it produces graduates with the proper mix of skills, knowledge, and attitudes to cope better with the challenges of modern medicine.

Although medical schools have considerable freedom to design and implement educational programs within the general criteria stated by the LCME, all schools provide an extensive knowledge of the basic biomedical sciences and exposure to the major clinical disciplines of internal medicine, obstetrics and gynecology, pediatrics, psychiatry, and surgery. The basic sciences provide the student with some comprehension of the complexity of human biology and a foundation for understanding new scientific advances. However, the studies calling for curricular reform appear to be having some effect as most medical schools are decreasing the number of didactic lectures while increasing problem-based and computer-assisted learning, and placing greater emphasis on social and ethical issues.

Whatever the curriculum, medical students usually were required to take parts I and II of the National Board of Medical Examiners (NBME) Examination (the "National Boards"). Part I was a two-day written, multiple-choice examination in the basic medical sciences. It tested not only knowledge but judgment and reasoning ability, and was often taken after the first two years of medical school. Part II was also a two-day written, multiple-choice examination, but it covered the clinical sciences and tested a broad spectrum of knowledge in each of the clinical areas. The NBME Examination satisfied the requirements in virtually all states for the licensure of U.S. medical school graduates. Many schools used the examinations to measure the effectiveness of their educational programs. An alternative licensing examination was the Federal Licensing Examination (FLEX), which was discussed in the previous chapter.

In 1992 the NBME Examination and FLEX were replaced by a single, uniform examination for medical licensure called the U.S. Medical Licensing Examination (USMLE), which was established by the NBME and the Federation of State Medical Boards of the United States (FSMB). As noted in Chapter 1, there are three steps to the examination. It uses multiple-choice questions to assess the knowledge and application of biomedical and clinical science necessary for supervised and unsupervised patient care. The third step, assessing unsupervised patient care, is taken after graduation and residency training.

In 1991 there were 126 U.S. and 16 Canadian medical schools fully accredited to award the MD degree. One additional school was fully accredited to offer the first two years of the medical curriculum. About 29,000 persons applied to medical schools in 1990. Of these, 59 percent were accepted. Once accepted, students are seldom dismissed for poor academic standing. Usually they are allowed to repeat all or part of the academic year if they are in academic difficulty. The decrease in the number of applicants during the 1980s is attributed to decreasing federal and state aid, a perceived oversupply of physicians, and a predicted decrease in physicians' incomes. The increase in enrollment in 1990 is difficult to explain, but may be caused by an economic climate that makes other careers such as business less attractive (1, p. 915).

Given the premise that any racial or ethnic group should have the same percentage of representation in medical school as the total population, Blacks, Native Americans, and Hispanics are underrepresented in U.S. medical schools. Blacks represent 11.7 percent of the total population, but only 6.5 percent of medical school enrollment; Native Americans represent 0.6 percent of the total population, but only 0.3 percent of the total enrollment in medical schools; and Hispanics represent 6.5 percent of the total population, but only 5.1 percent of medical school enrollment. These groups have been educationally disadvantaged in the past for a variety of reasons, including weak public high schools, few role models, and often little encouragement from the family to continue their education (1, p. 1016). High dropout rates among minority students in high schools and their underrepresentation in colleges and universities reduce the size of the applicant pool and make it virtually impossible for the percentage of minorities in medical schools to match that of the total population, despite intensive minority recruitment programs. Medical schools have academic support programs for those minorities admitted who need help. The increasing cost of medical school is a major factor in deterring potential minority applicants from considering medical school. Minorities often have debts from premedical education and have a higher than average debt for medical school. Contributing to this indebtedness is the shift in government financial aid for education from grants or scholarships to loans.

The percentage of women enrolled in medical schools remained between 9 and 13 percent until the enactment of federal legislation prohibiting sex discrimination in education in 1972. By 1990 the percentage of women medical students had climbed to 37 percent.

In addition to these 127 U.S. schools, there were 15 schools accredited to award the DO degree. There are no osteopathic colleges in Canada. Ac-

creditation of the DO colleges is granted by the AOA. There were 6,792 students enrolled in DO colleges in 1990, of which 32 percent were women and 6 percent were ethnic minorities. Admission to colleges of osteopathic medicine requires at least three years of preprofessional education at an accredited college or university, but almost all students admitted have baccalaureate or higher degrees.

Cost of Medical Education

The cost of training a physician is high, and tuition in most schools covers only a small portion. Nationally, tuition and fees constitute only 4 percent of medical school revenue for school and university activities (Table 2–3). On the assumption that medical revenue roughly reflects medical school costs, some argue that 96 percent of the costs of training physicians are thus subsidized. This is an important point to bear in mind, because it is in part the rationale for increased social control of medical practice—the income of physicians and how and where they will practice.

Because of the varied sources of funds and differing accounting practices, it is difficult to determine exactly what it costs to train a single physician. However, without subsidies, becoming a physician would be the privilege only of the wealthy. Because this is not a socially acceptable or desirable policy, and because the well-to-do probably cannot supply our physician needs in any event, subsidies of medical education have been commonplace. They are most apparent at public universities where tuitions are well below cost, with the legislatures appropriating tax monies to help keep the schools going and tuition costs down. Subsidies also exist in the form of scholarships and loans, enabling the tuition level to stay higher than it could otherwise be. Subsidies also come from patient income, from the monies received by the salaried faculty for patient care, and from federal appropriations. Further subsidies come from writing off education costs on the hospital charges for patient care. One of the largest subsidies comes

TABLE 2–3. Trends in US Medical School Revenues (Millions of Dollars)

Revenue Source	1970–1971		1980–1981		1989–1990	
	Amount	%	Amount	%	Amount	%
Federal research	438	25.6	1,446	22.5	3,869	20.6
Other federal	322	18.8	396	6.2	460	2.5
State and local government	323	18.9	1,452	22.6	3,750	20.0
Tuition and fees	63	3.7	346	5.4	816	4.3
Medical service	209	12.2	1,850	28.8	7,920	42.2
Other income	358	20.9	935	14.6	1,955	10.4
Total	1,713	100.1	6,425	100.1	18,771	100.0

SOURCE: *JAMA*, Vol. 266, No. 7, 1991.

from research grants and contracts from the National Institutes of Health (NIH) and other federal agencies. Although a comprehensive picture of the costs of medical education is not really possible, the Division of Operational Studies of the AAMC has provided some insightful data, which are shown in Table 2–3.

The figures in Table 2–3 relate to all medical school activities. How much of the medical school revenues is vital to the training of a competent physician cannot be ascertained. Any figure is bound to be largely judgmental. But it should be clear that when costs go up, and federal appropriations go down, a medical school heads for financial difficulty.

For a great many years after World War II, expansion in medical education was heavily fueled by federal monies coming in by way of research contracts and grants. These monies came from a variety of federal agencies, including the Defense Department, but the principal vehicle was the NIH. Freymann observes (4, pp. 86–87):

The seed of university-based medical research, originally imported from Germany, had been sown across the land by Flexner and the General Education Board between 1910 and 1940 and had been germinating all those years. NIH money only fertilized a field already sown. Furthermore, in any consideration of the deleterious effects federal research support had on education, one must never forget that NIH support almost single-handedly brought about the upgrading of the nation's medical schools which occurred between 1945 and 1965. Although research undoubtedly deflected the interest of many faculty members away from teaching, I agree with Chapman that "as a direct consequence of federal support of research and researchers, the medical student has, since the war, been actively exposed to and in direct contact with an infinitely broader galaxy of teachers than was the case before 1946."

The federal research monies paid the salaries of faculty (who were also permitted to teach) and secretaries; they bought equipment and even built buildings. Without these monies, expansion could not have taken place. These monies came not to the deans of the medical schools but to the individual researchers, which, of course, created a number of little kingdoms within each school. These centers of power carried enormous influence in shaping the course of medical education. The most adept could get the grants, and thereby hire more faculty, travel to meetings, and attract more residents, who were also paid out of grants. It certainly made the highly specialized areas attractive. Reinforcing this was the reward system. Medical schools reflected the universities of which they were a part; the rewards of promotion and salary increases went to those who pulled in the money and who published.

Freymann points out that before 1951 there were relatively few fulltime salaried faculty in American medical schools despite what Flexner recommended 40 years earlier. In 1954, out of 80 schools, 15 had no fulltime faculty; by 1968, 48 percent of the faculty had all or part of their salaries paid from federal funds (4, p. 87). "The proportion of each school's total salary budget derived from federal assistance ranged from 7 percent to 69 percent" (4, p. 91). Relatively small amounts of this federal money went directly for support of medical education; most of it was for research, which was indirectly used to subsidize the costs of medical education.

During the early 1960s change began to occur. There was a widely perceived doctor shortage, and Congress responded by passing the Health Professions Education Assistance Act of 1963, the primary purpose of which was to increase the supply of professional health personnel. The legislation provided direct federal assistance to medical schools in the form of construction grants, student loans, and financial distress grants. In 1965 the law was amended, partly because the medical schools were in financial difficulties, to provide direct institutional support for operating expenses on the condition that schools expand their enrollments to eliminate the doctor shortage. The Comprehensive Health Manpower Training Act of 1971 greatly increased support for operating costs plus a "capitation grant" of $2,500 per student for the first three years and $4,000 per student for the last year of medical school. However, schools that received capitation grants were required to increase their enrollment. As a result, the financial condition of medical schools greatly improved and their enrollments increased from 31,491 in 1962–1963 to 47,546 in 1972–1973 (50 percent). When the legislation expired in 1974 the doctor shortage was perceived to have disappeared, but when the legislation was finally renewed in 1976, the capitation grants were continued. This is a good example of the difficulty of terminating a government program when its objectives have been achieved.

The 1971 Comprehensive Health Manpower Act required for the first time that institutions carry out certain programmatic activities in addition to increasing student enrollment as a condition for receiving capitation grants. To qualify for the grants, institutions had to present a plan to implement projects in at least three of nine categories described in the legislation. Projects included activities such as promoting interdisciplinary training, establishing a team approach for providing health services, training new types of health personnel, including physicians' assistants, establishing programs in drug use and abuse and nutrition, and increasing the enrollment of disadvantaged students. This was the first time that the federal government had intervened in the internal program decisions of medical schools. The legislation also expanded student loan and scholarship opportunities and provided grants to initiate, expand, or improve professional training programs in family medicine.

The support of the federal government has decreased: the percent of medical school revenues from federal contracts and grants has decreased from 44 percent in 1970–1971 to 23 percent in 1989–1990 (Table 2–3). Included in the decrease was the elimination of capitation monies in the early 1980s, which caused difficult economic adjustments for medical schools. Revenues from state and local governments have increased, but their growth has slowed in recent years. In the past decade, medical schools and universities have assumed a larger role in providing their own financing, shifting from 16 percent of the revenues in 1970–1971 to 47 percent in 1989–1990.

The growing dependence on income derived from medical service activities—that is, on fee income earned by treating patients—draws faculty away from research, which has the adverse effect of slowing down activity designed to increase knowledge of better ways to treat patients.

Industry-sponsored programs, endowment income, and income from miscellaneous sources have decreased. Although tuition and fees account for only 4 percent of total medical school revenues, they are increasingly burdensome to students. There are a number of scholarship and loan funds available to medical students, but there has been a trend by the schools away from monetary awards based on financial need toward federally guaranteed loans from banks. By 1990 loans accounted for about 75 percent of all student aid. Almost 80 percent of medical school graduates have a mean amount of $46,200 in educational debts.

Osteopathic Medicine

About 5 percent of medical practitioners have become fully qualified to practice medicine by earning the Doctor of Osteopathy (DO) degree. Osteopathic medicine represents an approach to medical practice employing all the methods traditionally associated with physicians, for example, drugs, laboratory tests, X-ray studies, and surgery, but it advocates also the value of manipulative procedures in the diagnosis and management of disease and injury. The osteopath is a physician, licensed in all of the states to practice medicine and surgery. The osteopath is trained in essentially the same way as the allopathic physician (the osteopathic word for the physician trained in the MD schools) and in most of the same specialties.

As a school of medicine, osteopathy developed following the Civil War under the leadership of a former army physician, Andrew Taylor Still. Because his theories received little support from the established schools, Still branched off and opened the first osteopathic school in 1892. Others followed. The osteopathic schools took the same kind of drubbing from Flexner as did the allopathic schools, and osteopathic reform also began to take place.

Osteopathy was strong in the Midwest, where most of the schools were, and still are, located. Because it was a competing approach to medical practice, and because the AMA long sought a unified voice for medicine, there developed over the years considerable antagonism between the two groups. For many years osteopaths were unable to secure licenses in some states and were given limited licenses in other states. Today, however, the licensing barrier is down, and they are licensed in all states, with the same rights and responsibilities as the MDs. In eight states, they are licensed by an MD medical board, probably because there are not enough DOs in those states to justify a separate or a joint board. In 25 states there is a joint MD-DO board. In the remaining states, the osteopaths have their own licensing boards.

The fight between the MDs and DOs has subsided in recent years. Each group has now inspected each other's schools and satisfied themselves that each is worth associating with and that each could serve on the other's faculties and in the same hospitals. Before that, osteopaths had to develop their own hospital system. Occasionally, we hear of an allopathic hospital that will not give privileges to the osteopathic physician, but this is increasingly rare.

Although the AMA apparently wanted to absorb the osteopathic movement, the osteopaths felt it better to stay apart, believing that they could work for objectives they valued if they were outside the AMA framework. DOs were thus prohibited by the AOA from joining MD medical societies, but enforcement of this prohibition was apparently ignored in states where there were relatively few osteopaths, perhaps because it was believed that it is important for physicians to associate professionally with other physicians, and if there were not many DOs, then MDs would do! The AOA prohibition against DO membership in the AMA and other allopathic societies was dropped in the summer of 1979. In 1983 the AMA granted observer status in its House of Delegates to the AOA.

Is there any real difference between what an osteopath does and what an allopath does? Osteopathic philosophy speaks of understanding the whole person and treating the patient as a total unit. But the allopaths believe this also, so there is nothing unique on this score. Manipulative therapy is considered unique, but some of this seems to be part of physical medicine and rehabilitation (a speciality within allopathic medicine) and is used to some extent when the MD calls on the physiotherapist. It seems that the average MD is not trained to use manipulative therapy at this time, but some osteopaths assert that they really do not use it anyway.

What is clear, however, is that the osteopathic school, while encompassing all of the traditional medical specialties, does seem to stress family practice more than does the allopathic approach. Approximately 55 percent of the osteopaths are in primary care fields, whereas the percentage of allopaths in primary care fields is only about 45 percent. This difference, however, may be a passing one, because more and more osteopaths are selecting nonprimary care specialties, such as surgery, psychiatry, and obstetrics. In addition, there is growing pressure for and interest in the primary care specialties within allopathy.

Most of the data that appear here with regard to medical education relate to allopathy, because the published data by the AMA are more complete than the data available through the AOA.

It should be noted that the osteopath is very different from the chiropractor. The osteopath, like the M.D. is fully licensed to practice medicine and surgery; the chiropractor is not. The chiropractor uses manipulative procedures; some use physiotherapy, and some are permitted to take X-ray films for diagnostic purposes.

The osteopathic profession has more than doubled in the past 20 years. In 1967 there were 12,800 DOs; in 1991 there were 32,200 DOs, 15 percent of them women.

Development of New Schools

The decision of a university to start a new medical school cannot be made lightly. Apart from the cost of constructing the buildings, a medical school needs laboratories, classrooms, offices, and libraries. One important consideration in starting a medical school is, therefore, costs. Another consideration is whether or not the physicians graduated will be able to compete successfully for patients in developing an acceptable income level. The latter consideration has developed in recent years in many cities where physicians have had to compete for patients.

The AMA does not control the number of medical schools nor the number of students. Despite its role in the accreditation process, neither it nor the AAMC can prevent a school from developing. Neither may be happy about a new school, particularly if it means sharing available revenues, but both bodies are constrained by the accreditation criteria, which must be fairly applied. If they are not fairly applied, litigation can follow or complaints may be filed with the Office of Education, which could lead to the loss of LCME accrediting legitimacy.

The real control today on the development of new schools, as well as on the number of physicians new and old schools turn out, is money. One cannot enter the medical education game lightly.

Graduate Medical Education

Graduate medical education (GME) consists of a period of supervised training in a medical specialty in an approved clinical setting following graduation from medical school. Hospitals provide the large majority of GME opportunities, but state medical examiner offices, blood banks, ambulatory clinics, health departments, and mental health agencies are also involved. The laws on licensure vary from state to state and thus present a rather complicated picture. It should be noted, however, that although nearly all medical graduates complete some form of GME, it is required by 46 states for licensure of U.S. medical school graduates and by all states for graduates of foreign (international) medical schools.

The larger general hospitals, particularly those affiliated with medical schools or those that had approved residency training programs for specialty training, attracted the U.S. and Canadian medical graduates. Positions in smaller unaffiliated hospitals were filled mainly, if at all, by IMGs. In the former, there was usually a salaried full-time director of medical education who saw to it that the educational experiences of both interns and residents were appropriate. In the latter hospitals, the director of medical education typically filled that role on a voluntary or part-time basis. In both instances there was concern that the educational aspects of the program were being neglected while the services provided by the residents were being emphasized.

In 1991 there were over 6,000 accredited residency training programs in the United States. The largest number of programs was in internal medicine, followed by family practice, general surgery, and obstetrics and gynecology. Almost 40 percent of all residents were in training programs for internal medicine, family practice, or pediatrics (1, p. 934). Women accounted for almost 30 percent of residents, Blacks 4.7 percent, and Hispanics 5.6 percent. IMGs comprised 18 percent and graduates from osteopathic medical schools almost 4 percent. It is interesting to note that there were more women than men in first-year residencies in pediatrics, dermatology, and obstetrics and gynecology.

The number of hours residents should be on duty is controversial and was questioned again in 1987 when the state of New York investigated the number of hours residents worked following a mishandling of an emergency case after the residents involved had been on duty for an extended period of time. New York set rules to govern the working hours of residents in order to minimize the risk of future misadventures that might be attributable to residents being too tired to think clearly. The rules require an average 80-hour work week, shifts limited to 24 hours followed by 16 hours off. Surgeons objected because the rules could interfere with continuity of care, and they were granted a partial exemption. Implementation of the rules, which included increased supervision of residents, has increased hospital costs an estimated $226 million annually (5). Because of New York's action, some specialities have set less work hours for residents in their specialities, but no other state has taken action, perhaps because of the increased cost. The residency program is a learn-by-doing program and typically involves long hours. The average number of hours for first-year residents was highest in general surgery (84 hours per week). Internal medicine, pediatrics, and obstetrics and gynecology averaged 72 to 79 hours per week for first-year residents. In some specialities residents may be on continuous duty for 30 to 34 hours. Most specialties average 6 days a month with no duty.

Two recent studies of medical education have called for more resident training to take place outside of the hospital with ambulatory patients in a primary care setting because much of the preliminary work and treatment formerly done in hospitals is now done in ambulatory settings (6, 7). They also recommend that residency programs be the responsibility of medical schools. Easier said than done! Medical schools control undergraduate medical education, but hospital-based clinical faculty, national specialty boards, and residency review committees control residency training programs. It would be difficult to convince those responsible for graduate medical training to give up the responsibility.

Accreditation of Residency Programs

The process for reviewing, approving, and accrediting residency training programs requires, as with so many activities, coordination with a number of independent organizations and interest groups. Accreditation is granted by the Accreditation Council for Graduate Medical Education (ACGME). This council consists of four representatives from each of the most concerned or affected groups: the AMA, AAMC, ABMS, CMSS (Council of Medical Specialty Societies), and the AHA (American Hospital Association). In addition, there is a representative from the federal government, one from the "public," and two from the Resident Physicians Section of the AMA (Table 2–2).

The actual review and approval of each residency program is delegated by the ACGME to each specialty's residency review committee. On approval, accreditation is granted by the ACGME.

Securing a Residency and Becoming a Specialist

The National Residency Matching Plan (NRMP) is a computerized matching of resident applicants and approved hospital training programs. The aim is to meet the desires of the hospitals and the would-be residents to the greatest extent possible. The aims also are to eliminate, if possible, pressures and special inducements that tend to skew the distribution of interns and residents, leaving some hospitals with many unfilled slots and other hospitals oversubscribed.

The NRMP was introduced when there were twice as many positions available each year as there were graduating seniors. By the 1980s that ratio had changed because of the increased number of U.S. and foreign medical school graduates applying for residencies. The decrease in options in residency programs is beginning to concern some medical school graduates who are anxious to be accepted in top-quality programs, in a specific specialty, and in a desired geographic location. Acceptance into the "right" residency is considered as important as being accepted into the "right" medical school.

Traditionally, resident physicians have worked long hours for little pay while gaining the clinical experience necessary to practice medicine. In 1991 about 78 percent of hospital resident positions were filled by NRMP.

In 1991 first-year residents received an average annual stipend of $25,800. In part, the amount of resident pay and the decrease in "scut work" can be attributed to the development of house staff associations to improve working conditions. The decrease in the more menial tasks can also be due to increased pressure from the various residency review committees.

Table 2–4 is a list of approved examining boards in the various MD specialties and the subspecialties in which certification is currently possible. Table 2–5 lists the specialties and subspecialties in osteopathy. It should be noted that many osteopathic physicians complete their graduate training in allopathic residency programs. Most of the MD specialties examine DOs for certification upon meeting their respective requirements. Comparison of the two tables indicates remarkable similarities.

Preparation for certification by a specialty board is a major part of graduate medical education. As noted earlier, specialty boards are established voluntarily by the medical profession to assure the public that a board-certified physician has met the educational and assessment requirements to be identified as a specialist in a specific area of medicine. Certification is a voluntary process and is different from licensure, which is mandated by state legislatures. Even though certification is not a form of licensure, it is often required for certain appointments. Most residents aim toward certification by a specialty board.

The *Essentials of Accredited Resident Training Programs* spells out the general requirements for approval and accreditation of residency programs (8). The *Essentials* also describes the specific requirements that apply to the respective specialties. These special requirements are developed by the specialty's residency review committee and then adopted by the ACGME. Each accredited residency program is thus responsible for providing the training as specified in the *Essentials*. On successful completion of the residency program, the resident is eligible for specialty board certification. Certification thus comes not only from completing the residency program but also from being examined by the appropriate specialty board. On satisfying the speciality board, certification in the specialty is given. An increasing number of specialties periodically reexamine their members (Table 2–6). The training requirements for the MD specialties appear in Table 2–7.

Residency training is required for licensure in all states except Tennessee. Most states require one year of residency training, five require two years, and one state (Nevada) requires three years. In addition to completing a period of residency training, state licensing boards require applicants to have graduated from an acceptable school and to pass an acceptable licensing examination. Boards in all states except Texas and the Virgin Islands accept the certificate of the NBME, which the great majority of U.S. medical school graduates earn. For those that do not accept the NBME Exami-

TABLE 2–4. Specialty Boards (MD) and Certifiable Subspecialties, 1991

American Board Specialty	General Certifications	Certificates of Special Qualifications	Certificates of Added Qualifications	Dates Initial Subspecialty Offered
Allergy and Immunology	Allergy & Immunology		Diagnostic Laboratory Immunology	1986
Anesthesiology	Anesthesiology	Critical Care Medicine		1986
		Pain Management		
Colon & Rectal Surgery	Colon & Rectal Surgery			
Dermatology	Dermatology	Dermatopathology		1974
		Dermatological Immunology/ Diagnostic and Laboratory Immunology		1985
Emergency Medicine	Emergency Medicine	Pediatric Emergency Medicine		
Family Practice	Family Practice		Geriatric Medicine	
Internal Medicine	Internal Medicine	Cardiovascular Disease	Cardiac Electrophysiology	1992
		Critical Care Medicine		1941
		Diagnostic Laboratory Immunology		1987
		Endocrinology and Metabolism		1986
		Gastroenterology		1972
				1941
			Diagnostic Laboratory Immunology	1986
			Geriatric Medicine	1988
		Hematology		1972
		Infectious Disease		1972
		Medical Oncology		1973
		Nephrology		1972
		Pulmonary Disease		1941
		Rheumatology		1972
Neurological Surgery	Neurological Surgery		Critical Care Medicine	
Nuclear Medicine	Nuclear Medicine			
Obstetrics & Gynecology	Obstetrics & Gynecology		Critical Care	1985
		Gynecologic Oncology		1974
		Maternal & Fetal Medicine		1974
		Reproductive Endocrinology		1974
Ophthalmology	Ophthalmology			

TABLE 2–4. *(Continued)*

American Board Specialty	General Certifications	Certificates of Special Qualifications	Certificates of Added Qualifications	Dates Initial Subspecialty Offered
Orthopedic Surgery	Orthopedic Surgery		Hand Surgery	1989
Otolaryngology	Otolaryngology			
Pathology	Anatomic & Clinical Pathology	Blood Banking/Transfusion Medicine		1973
	Anatomic Pathology	Chemical Pathology		1950
			Cytopathology	1989
	Clinical Pathology	Dermatopathology		1974
		Forensic Pathology		1959
		Hematology		1952
		Immunopathology		1983
		Medical Microbiology		1949
		Neuropathology		1947
		Pediatric Pathology		1990
		Radioisotopic Pathology		1974
Pediatrics	Pediatrics	Adolescent Medicine		1994
		Infectious Disease		1994
		Diagnostic Laboratory Immunology		1986
		Pediatric Cardiology		1961
		Pediatric Critical Care Medicine		1987
		Pediatric Endocrinology		1978
		Pediatric Gastroenterology		1990
		Pediatric Hematology-Oncology		1974
		Pediatric Nephrology		1974
		Pediatric Pulmonology		1986
		Neonatal-Perinatal Medicine		1975
		Rheumatology		1992
		Emergency Medicine		1992
		Sports Medicine		1993

TABLE 2–4. (Continued)

Board	Certificate	Subspecialty Certificates	Added Qualifications	Year
Physical Medicine & Rehabilitation	Physical Medicine & Rehabilitation			
Plastic Surgery	Plastic Surgery		Hand Surgery	1990
Preventive Medicine	Aerospace Medicine			
	Occupational Medicine			
	Public Health and General Preventive Medicine			
Psychiatry & Neurology	Psychiatry	Child Psychiatry	Clinical Neurophysiology	1959
	Neurology		Geriatric Psychiatry	1992
	Neurology with Special Qualifications in Child Neurology			1991
Radiology	Radiology	Nuclear Radiology		1957
	Diagnostic Radiology			
	Radiation Oncology			
Surgery	Surgery	Pediatric Surgery	Hand Surgery	1975
			Surgical Critical Care	1986
		General Vascular Surgery		1982
			General Vascular Surgery	1988
Thoracic Surgery	Thoracic Surgery			
Urology	Urology			

SOURCE: *Annual Report and Reference Handbook—1991.* Evanston, IL, ABMS, 1991.

TABLE 2–5. Specialty Boards (DO) and Certifiable Subspecialties, 1991

American Osteopathic Board of	Subspecialty
Anesthesiology	
Dermatology	
Emergency Medicine	
Fellows of AAO	
General Practice	
Internal Medicine	Allergy & Immunology
	Cardiology
	Endocrinology
	Gastroenterology
	Hematology
	Hematology & Oncology
	Infectious Diseases
	Medical Diseases of the Chest
	Nephrology
	Oncology
	Rheumatology
Neurology & Psychiatry	Neurology
	Pediatric Neurology
	Psychiatry
	Pediatric Psychiatry
Nuclear Medicine	
Obstetrics & Gynecology	Obstetrical-Gynecological Surgery
Ophthalmology & Otorhinolaryngology	Ophthalmology
	Otolarynology
	Otorhinolaryngology
	Oro-facial Plastic Surgery
Orthopedic Surgery	
Pathology	Anatomic Pathology
	Cytopathology
	Forensic Pathology
	Laboratory Medicine
Pediatrics	Neonatology
Proctology	
Preventive Medicine/Public Health	Preventive Medicine & Aerospace Medicine
	Preventive Medicine & Occupational Medicine
	Preventive Medicine/Occupational-Environmental
Radiology	Diagnostic Radiology
	Diagnostic Roentgenology
	Radiation Oncology
	Radiation Therapy
	Roentgenology
Rehabilitation Medicine	
Surgery	General Surgery
	Neurological Surgery
	Plastic & Reconstructive Surgery
	Thoracic Surgery
	Thoracic Cardiovascular Surgery
	Urological Surgery

SOURCE: American Osteopathic Association.

TABLE 2–6. MD Specialty Board Recertification: Current Status and Requirements, 1991

Specialty Board: American Board Specialty	Date of Approval of Recertification	Written Exam for Recertification	License Required	CME Required	Recertification Interval (yr)	Total Number of Recertifications Issued to 1991	Time Limit Certificate‖
Allergy & Immunology	1977	Yes	Yes	Yes‡	6–10	449	1989—10 yr
Colon & Rectal Surgery	1988	Yes	Yes	Yes	8	—	1990—8 yr
Dermatology	1987	Yes	Yes	Yes	10	—	1991—10 yr
Emergency Medicine	1979	Yes	Yes	Yes	10	412	1990—10 yr
Family Practice	1969 by ABFP	Yes*	Yes	Yes	6–7	37,523	1969—7 yr
Internal Medicine	1973 by ABIM	Yes	Yes	No	2–10	8,621	1990—10 yr
Nuclear Medicine	1987	—	—	—	10	53	1992—10 yr
Obstetrics & Gynecology	1976	Yes	Yes	No	10	4,488	1986—10 yr
Ophthalmology	1986	—	—	—	10	—	1992—10 yr
Orthopedic Surgery	1980	Yes	Yes	Yes	6–10	329	1986—10 yr
Otolaryngology	1986	—	—	—	7	—	Indefinite
Pathology	1979	Yes†	Yes	Yes§	6–10	—	No
Pediatrics	1977	Yes	Yes	No	6	1,440	1988—7 yr
Physical Medicine & Rehabilitation	—	—	—	—	—	—	1993—10 yr
Plastic Surgery	1976	Yes	No	Yes	7–10	—	1985—10 yr
Psychiatry/Neurology	—	—	—	Yes	10	—	1994—10 yr
Geriatric Psychiatry	—	—	—	Yes	10	—	1991—10 yr
Clinical Neurophysiology	—	—	—	Yes	10	—	1992—10 yr
Surgery	1978	Yes	Yes	Yes‡	7–10	—	1976—10 yr
Pediatric Surgery	1981	Yes	Yes	Yes‡	7–10	—	1975—10 yr
Thoracic Surgery	1979	Yes	No	Yes	7–10	749	1976—10 yr
Urology	1980	Yes	Yes	Yes	10	35	1985—10 yr

SOURCE: *Annual Report and Reference Handbook—1991*. Evanston, IL, ABMS, 1991.

* Also requires satisfactory review of ambulatory (office) records as a prerequisite to the recertification examination.
† Required in one of three separate pathways.
‡ Type or number of hours unspecified.
§ Requirement for two of three separate pathways.
‖ Beginning in the years indicated, boards issued time-limited certificates.

TABLE 2–7. Requirements for MD Specialty Board Certification, 1991

American Board Specialty	GME Years Required to Certification			Full License Required	Creditable Federal or Military Experience	DO Acceptability	Fees and Charges for Certification Exam ($)	Written Exam	Oral Exam
	Preliminary Training Requirements	Specialty Residency Training Requirement	Total Years to Certification (Minimum)*						
Allergy & Immunology	3	2	5	No	—	Yes	1,000	Yes	No
Anesthesiology	1	3	4	Yes	—	Yes	850	Yes	Yes
Colon & Rectal Surgery	5	1	6	Yes	—	—	1,050	Yes	Yes
Dermatology	1	3	4	Yes	—	Yes	950	Yes	No
Emergency Medicine		3	3	Yes	—	Yes	1,355	Yes	Yes
Family Practice		3	3	Yes	—	Yes	500	Yes	No
Internal Medicine		3	3	No	Yes§	Yes	600	Yes	No
Neurologic Surgery	1	5	8	Yes	Yes	—	1,600	Yes	Yes
Nuclear Medicine	2	2	4	Yes	—	Yes	1,400	Yes	No
Obstetrics & Gynecology		4	6	Yes	Yes	Yes	1,025	Yes	Yes
Ophthalmology	1	3	4	Yes	—	Yes	1,265	Yes	Yes
Orthopedic Surgery		5	7	Yes	Yes	Yes	2,050	Yes	Yes
Otolaryngology	1	3	5	Yes	—	Yes	1,400	Yes	Yes
Pathology		4	4	Yes	—	Yes	1,000	Yes	No
Pediatrics		3	3	Yes	—	Yes	900	Yes	No
Physical Medicine & Rehabilitation	1	3	5	No	Yes	Yes	1,050	Yes	Yes
Plastic Surgery	3	2	7	Yes	—	—	2,550	Yes	Yes
Preventive Medicine	1	2	4	Yes	Yes	Yes	850/950	Yes	No
Psychiatry & Neurology		4	4	No	—	Yes	1,075	Yes	Yes
Radiology		4	4	Yes	—	Yes	1,050	Yes	Yes
Surgery		5	5	No	—	—	1,000	Yes	Yes
Thoracic Surgery	5	2	7	No	—	Yes	1,500	Yes	Yes
Urology	2	3	6½	Yes	Yes	Yes	1,350/1,600	Yes	Yes

SOURCE: *Annual Report and Reference Handbook—1991.* Evanston, IL, ABMS, 1991.

*Total may be greater than sum of Preliminary Training Requirements and Specialty Training Requirements due to practice experience requirements or other creditable experience.
†See published requirements under the specialty listed in the Directory of Residency Training Programs.
§Yes, if accredited residency training; no, if obligated service and practice-oriented.

nation, applicants for licensure must pass the FLEX, an alternative examination sponsored by the Federation of State Medical Boards.

Graduates of foreign medical schools face more complex rules. In general they must have graduated from a school listed in the World Directory of Medical Schools and have either an Educational Commission for Foreign Medical Graduates (ECFMG) or a Fifth Pathway certificate, as well as passing marks on the FLEX. Some states do not accept the Fifth Pathway certificate. Twenty-three boards require one year of graduate medical training, 12 require two years, and 19 require three years of graduate training for IMGs.

Graduate Medical Education Financing

The cost of GME involves resident salaries, the administration of the programs, and the increased cost of patient care (increased use of diagnostic services and length of stay) associated with the hospital's teaching function. As a result, the cost per case at teaching hospitals is estimated to be about 13 percent higher than at comparable non-teaching hospitals.

Until recently, financing GME was not a major problem. About 80 percent of residents' training costs was supported by patient care revenues, but now that costs are rising rapidly and are paid for largely by insurance and government programs, both government and insurance companies are looking for ways to reduce their costs. Private insurance companies are questioning the indirect support of GME that is built into patient charges. Federal and state governments, which were willing to subsidize GME when there was a shortage of physicians and when funds were more plentiful, are now searching for ways to reduce their support. Medicare (a federal government program that provides coverage toward the costs of medical care for the elderly) is now the major source of funds for GME. It subsidizes when the diagnosis-related group (DRG) payments reflect the cost of additional diagnostic tests and the longer patient stays that are necessary in teaching hospitals. The De-

partment of Health and Human Services is trying to cut those payments. Reimbursement to hospitals from Medicaid (a state-federal program to provide medical care for the poor) is hardly adequate to cover essential patient care, and yet government is also looking for ways to contain costs in that area.

Limited future funding is causing a careful reexamination of GME. Hospitals may reduce the number of programs they offer, and some hospitals may have to abandon resident training altogether. These programs are, however, essential to maintaining an appropriate supply for our society. How to finance these programs in a sound manner is one of the unresolved issues of this decade.

Continuing Medical Education

Lifelong learning is essential for members of the medical profession. For many physicians this occurs informally through reading journals, having conversations with colleagues, and attending presentations or discussions at medical staff or medical society meetings. In recent years there has been a move to encourage physicians to participate in approved continuing medical education (CME) courses or programs. In some instances physicians might participate voluntarily; in others, participation may be made a requirement for membership in state medical societies, for renewal of a license to practice medicine, or for retaining medical specialty certification. In 1947 the American Academy of General Practitioners (now, Family Physicians) became the first professional society to require members to participate in CME. The big push in CME came in the 1970s, when some state medical societies required it for membership maintenance and some states required it for relicensure. Requiring CME has been questioned by some, because there is no convincing correlation between CME and improved patient care.

It is generally agreed that the number of CME credits is no measure of a physician's ability. Nevertheless, CME participation in accredited programs is increasing. Some of the difficulties with

CME programs are identifying physician needs and integrating the material learned into the physician's practice. Institutions or organizations sponsoring continuing education can have their programs accredited and listed in *The Journal of the American Medical Association (JAMA)* and in other professional journals. Physicians are responsible for identifying their own CME needs and evaluating their own learning achievements. The trend is away from meetings in exotic locations and toward regional and local meetings and, more recently, toward videotape and individualized learning using computers.

As of 1991, 22 states and Puerto Rico required CME for relicensure. Ten state medical societies required it for maintenance of membership; in four of these states it was also a licensure requirement. Thus, in 28 states and Puerto Rico, CME was required for either retention of license to practice medicine or retention of medical society membership (1, p. 954). In addition, 15 medical specialties have a requirement for CME in order to retain certification in the specialty.

International Medical Graduates

The United States has always attracted graduates of foreign medical schools, who come for a variety of reasons: to escape wars, religious persecutions, and other repressions, as well as to seek new opportunities for adventure, economic well-being, and so on. In the eighteenth and nineteenth centuries, these physicians often provided a level of expertise very much needed in this land. Following the Second World War we began to experience a new wave of physician immigration, graduates of European schools who sought to establish a new life in the United States in large measure as a result of the dislocations resulting from the war or of the economic chaos that reigned in the postwar period. As Europe was reconstructed, the flow of physicians waned.

A new group of physicians began to come to the United States to establish new lives and to get advanced training; some came under the guise of advanced training, but hoped to stay. They came from Asia. During the 1950s and 1960s, the flow from Asia did not contribute much to the permanent physician supply in the United States, because our immigration laws were weighted heavily against Asians and Africans. Changes in 1968 and 1970, however, opened the gates to immigration from all countries. Physicians came in large numbers from a former American colony (the Philippines), from newfound military allies (South Korea, Thailand, Iran, Taiwan), and from India. We welcomed them, because they helped fill the physician shortage that we were beginning to experience as a result of a rapidly growing population, hospital expansions, and expansions due to research and technological advances that enabled physicians to help people in ways that were not previously feasible. The international medical graduates (IMGs), formerly called foreign medical graduates (FMGs), provided medical services in three important areas: residencies providing patient care in teaching hospitals that were unable to fill their residency positions with U.S. medical graduates; patient care for the medically underserved areas of the inner city; and specialties such as pathology and institutional psychiatry that have not attracted U.S. medical graduates. Many of these physicians came from medical schools that were relatively unknown to us, and many had language difficulties (though not the Indians, who, as a result of British imperialism, had received excellent English-language training). The unknown quality of the foreign schools raised legitimate questions about the adequacy of their student training and their graduates' competence. The language barriers caused communication problems between doctor and patient, as well as between the IMG and his or her American colleagues.

It should be emphasized again that Canadian physicians are not considered foreign trained. For a long time it was relatively easy for IMGs to come to the U.S. for graduate medical training and to remain in this country for an indefinite period of time. Although many foreign medical graduates had taken the medical knowledge and language reading ability test, which was developed in the 1950s by the ECFMG and is administered in many overseas locations, the test was advisory only and not legally binding. The failure rates were disturbingly high. It was also relatively easy for IMGs to enter the U.S. with or without ECFMG certification and take positions in places that did not attract enough U.S. medical graduates (e.g., state mental hospitals and inner-city indigent hospitals). Then, in 1974, the Coordinating Council on Medical Education reported an increasing concern that the U.S. had become overly dependent on IMGs to provide medical services, especially in hospitals. The report also stated that the IMGs coming from so many different countries, cultures, and educational institutions were not screened vigorously enough and might jeopardize the health and safety of the patients they treated. Testimony before a Congressional committee in 1974 described the variety of practices that were occurring and the serious questions about the quality of care being provided by many of the IMGs (8, pp. 126–129). Some states, because of the physician shortage in certain areas, issued temporary licenses. In Illinois in 1977, for example, all 127 temporarily licensed physicians working in the state mental hospitals who took the licensure examination failed it; another 63 did not even take it. Most of these Illinois "physicians" were foreign born and all were foreign trained (9).

The data and the official reports that focused on the IMGs problem, along with the emerging realization by others that there could be an excess supply of physicians by the 1980s, resulted in amendments to the Health Professions Educational Assistance Act of 1976 (PL94-484), which placed restrictions on the number of IMGs entering and remaining in the U.S. In addition, the legislation mandated that IMGs who wished to enter the United States as immigrants on the basis of their medical skills and qualifications would have to pass parts I and II of the NBME Examination, or their equivalent, and be competent in written and oral English. The Visa Qualifying Exam (VQE) was subsequently developed and certified as equivalent. Failure rates were high—80 percent for 1977 and 1980. IMGs performed better on the clinical portion than on the part testing basic medical science knowledge.

In 1984 a new test, the Foreign Graduate Examination in Medical Sciences (FMGEMS) replaced the VQE for ECFMG certification. ECFMG certification is necessary for graduates of foreign medical schools who want to be licensed and practice in the United States. At the present time, IMGs who are not U.S. citizens are required to pass either the FMGEMS or the new United States Medical Licensing Examination (USMLE) to become certified. Both tests have basic science and clinical science components. They are also required to pass an English-language proficiency test for certification.

To be eligible to take the basic science portion, applicants must have completed at least two years at a medical school listed in the *World Directory of Medical Schools*. To take the clinical portion, the applicant must have graduated from such a school.

In 1989 only 16 percent of those taking the medical science part and only 30 percent of those taking the clinical science part of the FMGEMS passed. In both parts foreign citizens did better than U.S. citizens who trained at foreign schools.

In 1986, there were about 6,000 alien IMGs in residencies in the U.S., or about 8 percent of the total number of residents.

U.S. Foreign Medical Graduates

About half of the IMGs today are U.S. citizens who were unable to gain admission to a U.S. or Canadian medical school and so took their training in foreign countries. Virtually all plan to practice in the U.S. The exact number of those studying abroad is not known, but fewer are now accepted in residency programs. In 1984 there were 1,831 U.S. citizen IMGs (USIMGs) accepted in residency programs in the United States, but in 1990 only 929 were accepted—a 61 percent decrease. This is due in large part to the efforts of U.S. medical organizations and the government to limit the numbers of both USIMGs and IMGs, because there is still uncertainty about the adequacy of their training.

Most of the U.S. nationals studying in foreign medical schools are concentrated in schools located in Mexico and the Caribbean. The accrediting bodies in those countries do not assess schools by the same criteria as are used for U.S. and Canadian medical schools, and all but a few of these schools are proprietary. It is generally believed that they lack the resources and teaching facilities, particularly the clinical teaching facilities, to provide an adequate undergraduate medical education. Because of the weak clinical teaching facilities, some students transfer to U.S. schools to complete their undergraduate training. Other countries attract U.S. students, especially Italy, Hungary, and Spain. Students there also frequently seek to transfer to a U.S. school to complete their training. In 1990–1991 there were 117 students who transferred to U.S. medical schools from foreign medical schools, a decrease of 60 percent in the last four years. To help the U.S. schools evaluate the transfer applicants, the AAMC conducts the Medical Sciences Knowledge Profile (MSKP), a two-day examination designed to assess knowledge of medical sciences of students seeking advanced placement. The use of test results and the criteria for advanced placement vary among the U.S. medical schools. However, transfer to a U.S. school is not easy, and as the above figure suggests, few are accepted.

U.S. as well as alien students who complete their undergraduate medical education in a foreign country must pass, as noted earlier, the FMGEMs or steps one and two of the USMLE before entering an accredited residency program in the U.S. Of the USIMGs who took the ECFMG examination in 1989, only 30 percent passed.

Many U.S. citizens in foreign medical schools opted for the Fifth Pathway program but the program has been declining steadily and is only offered by seven medical schools in the United States. The Fifth Pathway program provides a one-year clinical clerkship to U.S. citizens who completed their premedical training in the United States and who graduated subsequently from foreign medical schools. These people must pass a screening examination designated by the U.S. school offering the program, have an acceptable MCAT score, and earn an acceptable premedical grade-point average. A personal interview is also required. In 1991 there were 290 applications for the Fifth Pathway program, from which 67 students were accepted. The number of Fifth Pathway applicants in 1986–1987 dropped to less than half the number of applicants two years before.

All of the measures seek to discourage U.S. citizens from seeking medical undergraduate education abroad, to restrict the number of alien IMGs, and to increase the quality of IMGs who train and practice in the U.S. The preexisting deficiencies of policies and practices regarding IMGs are apparent, but the solutions depend on the formulation of a clear national policy and the cooperation of many interrelated organizations. The role of the IMGs in the U.S. medical system is likely to continue to decrease.

SUMMARY

The training of physicians is a continuing process and can be viewed as consisting of four parts: premedical education, undergraduate medical education, graduate medical education, and postgraduate (continuing) medical education.

The premedical phase is that period of study in a college or university during which the student prepares himself or herself for medical school. Though most premedical students study or major in biology, almost any major will suffice so long as the student fits the necessary science courses into his or her course of study. There is more flexibility in premedical studies than most premedical students recognize.

Competition for admission to medical school is intense and requires a high level of achievement in course grades, high scores on the Medical College Admission Test (MCAT) that most premedical students take, as well as good recommendations and, in most cases, a successful interview at the medical school.

Once in medical school, the student pursues a four-year course of study. In some instances this can be completed in three years by going through the summer period. The four-year course of study has a preclinical or basic medical science component in which the student studies such subjects as anatomy, physiology, pharmacology, medical microbiology; and a clinical science component that includes studies in such patient-oriented matters as medicine, surgery, pediatrics, family practice, psychiatry, obstetrics, and so on. Historically, the preclinical component was studied during the first two years and the clinical subjects in the third and fourth years. However, in the past two decades there has been a tendency on the part of most schools to be more flexible so that the students can secure patient contacts early in their studies.

The term "medical" schools is used here to refer to schools that train physicians and award the student the degree of MD (Doctor of Medicine) or DO (Doctor of Osteopathy) on completion of the course of study. For all practical purposes, these two approaches to the training of physicians are identical.

On graduation from medical school, the degree is awarded by the school, but this does not give the physician the right to practice. To practice medicine and surgery, a physician must take and pass the licensing examination that is administered by the appropriate examining board of the particular state government in which he or she wishes to practice.

Graduation from medical school and being licensed, however, are still not deemed sufficient for modern, independent medical practice. In addition to the degree and a license, it is generally believed that all physicians need an additional period of supervised clinical experience, and this is now secured by nearly all physicians, either before or after being licensed, through some form of graduate medical education. Most states will not grant a license until additional training is taken. This phase of the medical education process is the graduate education component and is known as the *residency* period. It leads to certification as a specialist. Most new physicians today pursue the residency to completion and to certification in a specialty. Some physicians interrupt their residency after one year and go into practice, but most of these generally return after a while to complete their specialty training. The period of residency training lasts at least three years and may require much longer periods of time depending on the specialty.

The final phase of the medical education continuum (postgraduate or continuing medical education) is that period in which the physician pursues a variety of educational experiences in order to keep up to date. Increasingly, specialty boards and societies and state medical associations are requiring physicians to take a certain number of approved continuing medical education courses in order to retain membership. Some specialty boards have begun to retest their members periodically.

DISCUSSION QUESTIONS

1. Should admission to medical school require such high performance in premedical courses and on the MCAT? What are the alternatives?
2. Does the accreditation of medical schools by the LCME give too much power to the AMA and to the AAMC? Would accreditation by some other body be more appropriate?
3. Should the allopathic and osteopathic schools of medicine have a common accrediting body, and should only one type of degree be awarded?
4. Since physicians pay only a small percentage of the cost of their training, do they have any responsibility for providing medical care to those who cannot afford it? If so, how much and what kind of responsibility do they have?
5. To what extent should medical research be used to subsidize medical education?
6. Which of the reforms in the medical school curricula are most important for the training of physicians?

REFERENCES

1. Educational Programs in U.S. Medical Schools. *JAMA*, Vol. 266, No. 7, 1991.

2. Physicians for the Twenty-First Century. Washington, D.C., AAMC, 1984.

3. Goodman, L.J., Brueschke, E.E., Bone, R.C., Rose, W.H., Williams, E.J., Paul, H.A.: An Experiment in Medical Education. *JAMA,* Vol. 265, No. 18, 1991, pp. 2373–2376.

4. Freyman, J.G.: *The American Health Care System: Its Genesis and Trajectory.* Baltimore, Williams & Wilkins, 1974.

5. *American Medical News,* April 22/29, 1991.

6. Ebert, R., Ginsberg, E.: The Reform of Medical Education. *Health Affairs,* Vol. 7, No. 2, Supplement, 1988.

7. *Clinical Education and the Doctor of Tomorrow.* New York Academy of Medicine, 1988.

8. AMA: *Essentials of Accredited Resident Training Programs,* Chicago, American Medical Association, annual.

9. *American Medical News,* March 7, 1977.

Chapter 3

Medical Practice

Extraordinary changes are taking place in the practice of medicine in the United States. After decades of "business as usual" physicians are now faced with a decline of professional autonomy, increased competition among themselves, and changes in the methods of payment for their services. Although much of this change can be attributed to cost containment efforts that seek to provide more efficient, effective medical care, and to the alternative delivery systems that have developed, the growing supply of physicians is also a major factor.

There were 615,421 physicians in the United States in 1990, or 244 physicians for 100,000 people—more physicians than ever before (Table 3–1). The number of practicing physicians is expected to continue to increase throughout the 1990s.

A high physician/population ratio does not necessarily mean better medical care, as can be seen in such countries as the former Soviet Union and Hungary, where the physician/population ratios are among the highest in the world (1,2).

The effect of the increasing U.S. physician/population ratio is fewer potential patients for each physician, which intensifies competition among physicians and is causing some physicians to form group practices and others to accept salaried positions with hospitals and managed care organi-

TABLE 3–1. Physician Supply
for Selected Years

Year	Total Number of Physicians	Physicians/ 100,000 People	Total Population/ Physician
1960	260,484	142	703
1970	334,028	161	623
1980	467,679	202	494
1985	552,716	228	440
1987	585,597	237	423
1989	600,789	240	416
1990	615,421	244	404

SOURCE: American Medical Association: *Physician Characteristics and Distribution in the U.S.* Chicago, 1991.

zations. One needs a supply of physicians that is adequate for a population so that it has easy access to care and so that the full state of medical science can be applied. The number of physicians needed will be affected by the level of our knowledge and technology: new knowledge and new technology permit physicians to do what was previously not possible, and the need for more physicians becomes necessary. But determination of need is complex and, one might say, elusive. It is affected not only by the limits of our knowledge and our technology but also by the age characteristics of the population (the elderly having greater needs), by the existing health problems that are recognized by the population as problems, and by public decisions about which health services should be covered by insurance or government programs and what level of investment should be made in research and facilities. It is also affected by the extent to which physicians are willing to use other health workers, by the population's willingness to accept other kinds of practitioners, and by the expectations of the population. Thus, there is no correct number of physicians any more than there is a correct amount of money to spend on health care.

About 40 percent of physicians are in the primary care areas of internal medicine, family and general practice, pediatrics, and obstetrics and gynecology. The majority of U.S. physicians are younger than 45 years of age, with most of these being in the 35- to 44-year age group. More than 16 percent of practicing physicians are women, and about 20 percent are international (foreign) medical graduates. The average physician, according to a survey by the American Medical Association (AMA), spends 48 hours a week in direct patient care and sees an average of 121 patients a week. In response to the competitive environment, many more physicians are holding evening and weekend office hours. The average earnings for physicians in 1991, after expenses and before taxes, were $170,600. More and more physicians are being employed by others, with almost half of

younger doctors and women being in that category.

Solo Practice

Historically, most physicians were in the *solo practice of medicine,* that is, they practiced alone. However, that is changing, as most young physicians prefer working in group practices or health maintenance organizations (HMOs).

The chief criticism of solo practice is that the physician practices in an unchallenged setting wherein he or she is not accountable to peers for either comprehensiveness or quality of care. The physician, instead, has only to satisfy the patient; as a lay person, the patient is not in a position to judge either completeness or quality. In such settings, critics note, sloppy and inappropriate care can develop too easily. This is a widely held belief by those who are not in solo practice. Critics of solo practice typically go on to say that the quality of care in group and hospital-based practices is superior to that provided in solo practice. This, too, is a widely held belief by those not in solo practice, but data to support this conclusion are hard to obtain.

Most physicians are paid a *fee for service,* but that is changing. Critics assert that fee for service encourages a physician to overservice because the physician is paid for each service. This may mean added units of service during each visit, or it may mean unnecessary followup visits, and there are no controls except the conscientiousness of the physician and the limits of patient tolerance. Abuses of Medicare and Medicaid and of some health insurance policies lend support to these criticisms.* But how widespread the abuses are, no one really knows. These abuses, however, can exist

---

*Medicare, the federal government's largest health program, provides health insurance to those age 65 and older who receive social security benefits, and also to the permanently disabled and to those with end-stage renal disease. Medicaid is a joint federal-state program that finances health care for the poor.

in group practice settings just as easily, particularly in the ordering of extra services for which charges can be made. But whether extra visits or services are ordered because they are judged to be clinically necessary, to safeguard against possible malpractice suits (the physician practicing in this instance what is known as *defensive medicine*), or to earn the extra payments is not easily determined except in the most glaring cases of abuse. Increasingly, such patterns of medical practice are being computer monitored by the organizations that pay Medicare and Medicaid claims, as well as by those handling other health insurance payments. Such surveillance, it is hoped, will control abuses.

It is fairly agreed within professional circles that physicians have not been as sensitive to cost implications as they might be. Their training never focused on what services cost; they just ordered tests and services to explore all avenues as part of the learning process. Recognition of this weakness in physician education has prompted some to argue for introduction of this issue into the educational process.

Fee for service can be viewed positively as a symbolic contract, binding the physician to the patient in terms of attention, care, and confidentiality. If the patient does not like the physician's attention or the way the care is delivered, the patient can go elsewhere. Though patient choice is built into most large group practice arrangements, there are bureaucratic constraints that may govern regardless of who the physician is.

Fee for service is also a vehicle for strengthening the confidentiality of patient records: if the patient contracts with a physician for certain services, the contract being consummated by payment of the fee, the patient has a right to confidentiality. No one has a right to that information without the patient's consent. Typically, patients authorize release of information in order to have the fee covered by insurance, but if the patient asks no one to pay the fee, then the patient is assured by contract that no one will have access to that information. This is not a matter of theoretical concern.

Many patients do not submit claims to the insurance company because of the possibility that their employers might gain access to that information. Many workers do not consult company physicians for some ailments for the same reason. Can one be absolutely certain that the boss would not be able to pressure the company physician into releasing the medical information on an employee?

Finally, on fee for service, we might note that historically physicians charged on a *sliding fee scale,* the poor paying (if at all) less than the more affluent. With the widespread growth of health insurance, and now Medicare and Medicaid, sliding fee scales are much less common.

Group Practice

Although most physicians are in solo practice, a rapidly growing number are in group practice—either in a group made up of physicians of the same specialty or in a multispecialty group. Group practice is normally defined as constituting three or more physicians who have organized to practice together, typically sharing offices, personnel, equipment, and other expenses. How they are paid varies from fee for service, to salary, to share of the group's income. The income of group practice physicians tends to be a little higher than that of solo practitioners because of economies achieved by the group from the sharing of support personnel and other resources. The appeal of group practice comes not only from these economic advantages; other major factors are ease of consultation with colleagues, intellectual stimulation, coverage on nights and days off, and the opportunity to retain control of their practices at a time when professional autonomy is under attack from government, business, insurance companies, and managed care plans (see below). This is perhaps best illustrated by the fact that more than 90 percent of the groups are owned by physicians.

Although most of the groups contain a single specialty and consist of only three or four physicians, some are quite large, with more than 50 or even more than 100 physicians. The larger groups tend to be multispecialty.

Group practices are expanding in size and increasingly they compete for patients with one another, with solo practitioners, and with hospital-based physicians. Over half of the groups have now contracted with prepaid health plans. Despite the fact that they compete with the hospital's own ambulatory clinic, these groups can have considerable influence on hospitals, because they control the admission of a significant number of patients to a particular hospital.

Managed Care

Managed care is a recent term, used for programs that seek to control or "manage" the use by patients of physicians and other health care services. It is a type of prepaid health plan or insurance program in which the enrollees receive medical service in a coordinated manner to eliminate unnecessary services. Typically, enrollees must have a primary care physician's or a utilization review person's approval before receiving care from a specialist and before being hospitalized on a nonemergency basis. There are a variety of managed care programs, ranging from HMOs and preferred provider organizations (PPOs) to preadmission reviews required by some traditional health insurance companies. All have a common goal— to reduce health care expenditures while maintaining the quality of care. At least half of all practicing physicians are involved in at least one managed care program.

Managed care is revolutionizing medical practice. Traditionally, physicians, with their patient's approval, decided the tests, treatment, and amount of hospitalization the patient was to receive. With managed care, the health care purchasers (employers, government, insurance companies) are increasingly involved in the treatment decision-making process.

Eighty percent of enrollees in managed care plans rated them as high as traditional insurance

plans (3). The two major types of managed care are HMOs and PPOs, which together provide health care benefits to 38 percent of the nation's employees. They are described below.

Health Maintenance Organizations

HMOs are organized systems that provide comprehensive health services to a voluntarily enrolled population for a fixed, prepaid, usually capitated fee, that is, so much paid for each person enrolled, hence a *per capita* or *capitation* payment. A specific set of health care benefits is provided, using the services of physicians, other health care professionals, hospitals, and outpatient facilities for the periodic (usually monthly) payment, regardless of the number and complexity of services provided to the enrollee.

Although the phrase "health maintenance organization" is relatively new, the idea of paying for services on a fixed fee or capitated basis appears throughout U.S. medical history. It became most prominent, however, during the 1940s with the development on the east coast of the Health Insurance Plan (HIP) of Greater New York, and on the west coast of Kaiser-Permanente. Expansion of the HMO approach was modest—some would say slow—until the 1970s, when the costs of health care began to soar and when these costs became a concern both to government and to the business community. The federal government took the initiative in 1973 with passage of the Health Maintenance Organization Act, which provided financial incentives for the development of what then became known as HMOs. The government saw in the HMO approach a way to control rising costs of health care, a sizable portion of which it paid for through Medicare and Medicaid. The HMO approach thus shifted the risk arising from increased costs caused by heavy utilization from the government to the provider of services.

Despite subsidies, HMO growth was slow, but by the 1980s HMO enrollment increased in part because of the continued rising cost of health care (Table 3–2). Despite the ending of federal subsi-

TABLE 3–2. Growth of HMOs, 1981–1990

Year	Number of HMOs	Persons Enrolled/ Million
1991	550	38.6
1990	569	36.5
1989	591	34.5
1987	700	29.0
1985	393	18.9
1983	280	12.5
1981	243	10.3

SOURCE: National HMO Census 1986, Interstudy. *American Medical News,* Jan 1, 1988, May 27, 1991, and July 6/13, 1992.

dies, HMOs began to develop all over the country, spurred on by the prevailing idea that through competition costs could be controlled. Businesses found them appealing because, like the government earlier, the HMO seemed like a good way to put a lid on rising costs; no longer would the employer or the insurance company pay without limit. Now there could be a limit, and if the costs rose above that limit, the HMO would have to absorb them. Declining hospital bed occupancy—i.e., lots of empty beds, and a large supply of physicians (some said, an oversupply)—gave the HMOs the necessary leverage to compete for business, offering employers lower costs, and offering hospitals and doctors an assured flow of patients for maintenance of their incomes.

Quality of care was, of course, not supposed to suffer, but as the HMOs competed with one another for their share of the market, some critics feared HMOs would begin to curtail services in order to keep their costs low: making patients wait for appointments, ordering fewer laboratory and X-ray tests, reducing the amount of nonemergency surgery, signing up only those employee groups that appeared to be better than average—in other words, begin to ration medical care. One is reminded of the early opposition to contract practice, described in Chapter 1.

More than 15 percent of the population belonged to HMOs in 1990. The highest concentrations of enrollees are in California, Minnesota, Massachusetts, Oregon, and in the large metropolitan

areas. The number of HMOs grew so rapidly during the 1980s that many did not have the management skills or the number of enrollees that were necessary to survive. Many of the HMOs merged or disappeared during the late 1980s, resulting in fewer HMOs with a steady, but slower growth in the number of persons enrolled (Table 3–2). Only 15 percent of HMOs have more than 100,000 enrollees. HMOs are causing a restructuring of the way health care is marketed, delivered, and financed in almost every metropolitan area of the country.

There are many varieties of HMOs, but they can be categorized into five types:

- *Staff model* HMOs employ physicians directly, provide care through central offices, and pay physicians by salary.
- *Group model* HMOs contract with one independent, multispecialty group practice to provide physician services. The HMO pays the group practice a negotiated per capita rate and the group practice determines what each physician will be paid—typically a salary plus incentive payments.
- *Network model* HMOs resemble the group model. The only difference is that the HMO contracts with more than one independent multispecialty group practice.
- *Individual practice association (IPA)* HMOs contract with an association of individual physicians in solo practice or with group practices to ensure the provision of services to HMO members. Payment schemes vary from capitation to fee for service, as well as variations on these types of payment. Unlike the above HMO models, IPA physicians usually provide services in their own offices and see other patients in addition to their HMO patients. About 60 percent of the HMOs are IPAs.
- *Point-of-service* HMOs, sometimes called open-ended HMOs, are the most recent model. This model provides enrollees the option of choosing doctors and hospitals outside of the HMO if they pay a portion of the costs.

No study has shown one model to be superior to the others, but the group model seems, to date, to yield a larger profit than the others; although the cost of the care they provide is greater, their administrative costs are less. The staff model, which makes up about 10 percent of all HMOs, has higher costs per enrollee; many serve older patients. The physician-controlled IPAs have drawn heavy criticism for being poorly managed, permitting overutilization, and not having enough cash reserves. Critics say IPAs are run to protect private physicians and not according to sound business procedures.

The structure of HMOs is changing and becoming more diversified. Some are beginning to offer plans with copayments and deductibles and, increasingly, the point-of-service option (4). Although the majority of HMOs are nonprofit, there is a growing number of for-profit HMOs.

The reduction in health care expenditures for HMO members is mainly due to a reduction in hospital admissions, not physician services. HMOs reported a yearly average of 372 inpatient days per 1,000 members under age 65, compared to the national average of 692 days for other health plans. Despite lower costs, employers are not saving as much money as they had hoped, and they continue to press to keep costs down without sacrificing quality. Even though HMO premiums continue to increase more than employers expected, they are still turning to them rather than traditional insurance plans in an effort to contain costs. In 1991 HMO premiums increased 10 percent while traditional indemnity plans increased 25 percent (5).

HMOs use a number of utilization management activities to control unnecessary use and costs of health care that include:

• Primary care physicians as "gatekeepers," which means that patients must have the approval of their primary care physician before seeing a specialist, having diagnostic tests, or being admitted to the hospital.
• Concurrent utilization review of services that patients receive while they are still in the hospital or being tested.
• Retrospective utilization reviews of services patients received in the hospital after they are discharged.
• Prior authorization for inpatient care.
• Primary care physician profiles. In almost 50 percent of HMOs, the number and types of services physicians

performed for specific conditions are compared to other physicians (6).

Traditional insurance companies and PPOs also use some of the same utilization management activities.

Membership in HMOs typically offers some advantages for enrollees, such as a predictable cost for health care, broader coverage for more routine care (e.g., physical examinations), and no claim forms to fill out and submit. Disadvantages often cited are having to choose a physician affiliated with the HMO, the need to get approval before hospitalization or specialty care, and the possibility that their chosen primary physician may not be available.

Physicians may find HMOs advantageous because they offer a guaranteed income if in a staff, group, or network model; those in an IPA model may appreciate the possibility of expanding their patient base. Disadvantages for physicians that are often cited include some loss of autonomy, minimal input into quality assurance and utilization review criteria (except in the IPA model), possible alteration of referral patterns, increased outside influence on treatment decisions, and possible reduced earnings (3). Although HMOs are expected to grow and increase their enrollments, they are facing increasing competition from another type of managed care—preferred provider organizations (PPOs).

Preferred Provider Organizations

PPOs are primarily a phenomenon of the 1980s and have grown dramatically.

A PPO is an arrangement in which a limited number of health providers—physicians, hospitals, and others—agree to provide services to a defined group of people at a negotiated fee-for-service rate, which is usually less than their normal rate. There are incentives for enrolled people to use the preferred providers, because the cost of provider services are fixed and, except for routine office visits, they are typically paid for in full. If the enrolled person goes to a nonpreferred provider, a lesser payment is paid (typically only 80 or 90 percent), and the patient must pay the balance.

PPOs have attracted enormous interest as a way to contain costs while retaining the patient's choice of physician and retaining the fee-for-service type of payment. PPOs may be sponsored by insurance companies, employers, Blue Cross and Blue Shield, hospitals, or physicians. Most hospital and physician-sponsored PPOs are formed in response to economic competition, as a mechanism for capturing and securing a share of the market lest they lose patients to other physicians, hospitals, HMOs, or other PPOs. Hospital-sponsored PPOs are generally larger than those that are physician-sponsored PPOs.

The success of PPOs depends on the recruitment of cost-effective physicians and hospitals. The competition must be strong enough for these providers to be willing to negotiate discounted rates for PPO members. PPOs, like HMOs, also depend upon management activities to keep costs down. They may include prior authorization for hospital admission, concurrent and retrospective utilization reviews, mandatory second opinions for surgery, planning for discharge from the hospital, and physician practice profiles (4). Another factor for success is the provision of a set of incentives that channel patients to PPO providers rather than outside ones. An attractive feature of PPOs is their flexibility, which makes them able to respond rapidly to market conditions.

Physicians like the PPO's feature of maintaining fee-for-service, office-based medical practice. Many physicians see PPOs as a way to compete with HMOs. As suggested earlier, they see an opportunity to enlarge their patient base or to preserve their current one. Like the IPA model HMO, PPOs typically allow member physicians to treat patients not enrolled in the PPO. Some physicians, moreover, have participation agreements with more than one PPO. However, some PPOs in California now have "exclusive service contracts" that prohibit physicians from signing contracts with other health delivery groups.

Physicians lose some of their autonomy and must accept some controls in PPOs, just as in HMOs. The responsibility for utilization review may lie with hospitals, insurance companies, administrators, or outside physician groups, leaving PPO physicians less opportunity to influence the design and operation of reviews. Another disadvantage for physicians is that fee schedules are usually discounted, so more patients must be seen or fees to non-PPO patients must be increased if their level of income is to remain the same.

PPOs appeal to patients because they allow selection of any doctor and hospital for care. If they prefer to use a nonpreferred provider, they have to bear some share of the costs. Admittedly, the additional amount they pay may effectively deter them from exercising that option.

Employers and other purchasers of health care hope to realize cost savings from the discounted fees and the reduced use of inappropriate services through utilization reviews. Also, they can have greater influence in deciding which benefits to offer.

Both PPOs and HMOs are expected to continue to grow at the expense of traditional forms of medical practice. Their costs are significantly less and they have been increasingly accepted by consumers and physicians, despite the instability due to recently announced premium increases and the likely closing of some HMOs. PPOs and HMOs are in intense competition, and they are both altering the plans they offer to respond to the demands of health care purchasers. Often the differences between them become blurred. The future for managed health care delivery systems will probably be a combination of the positive features of both PPOs and HMOs. Physician payments are coming under closer scrutiny as health care purchasers look for additional ways to reduce costs; this could have a dramatic impact on the traditional, unrestricted, fee-for-service system of payment.

The future undoubtedly holds contention and frequent litigation, because vital professional and public interests are at stake, and antitrust issues will be raised with increased frequency as hospital staff privileges are denied physicians, as physicians are excluded from participation in some HMOs and PPOs, and as complaints arise over what are claimed to be anticompetitive practices and price fixing. For example, an IPA model HMO filed an antitrust suit against Blue Cross and Blue Shield (commonly referred to as "the Blues") in Rhode Island, where the Blues controlled more than 80 percent of the private health insurance market. The physician-controlled IPA charged that the Blues engaged in anticompetitive activity when they announced that they would not pay physicians more for a service and would not offer a payment mechanism more favorable than any other health care purchaser. This was in response to the IPA's withholding 20 percent of its payments as a reserve against heavy utilization and consequent costs. The Blues proposed to do the same. The IPA claimed that the Blues were monopolizing health care services and were able to set prices that would eliminate competition. The Blues denied a monopoly and defended their action as a legitimate cost-containment measure—to be a prudent buyer, and thereby to get the best deal for their subscribers (7).

Competition resulting in lower costs has been the main concern of managed care plans, but recently quality of care and how to measure it have become major concerns.

Quality Assessment

Quality of care has become a significant issue in health care, for both purchasers and providers who worry that competition and cost-containment efforts may reduce the quality of medical care. Managed care programs, in particular, are thus coming under close scrutiny, and leaders in the HMO and PPO movements are working with others to develop appropriate measures for monitoring quality as well as efficiency.

Methods of measuring quality include more rigorous peer reviews, ambulatory care treatment standards, and clinically based measures that constitute appropriate care. For example, standard diagnostic and treatment protocols for some common conditions have been developed by the American Board of Internal Medicine and Blue Cross

and Blue Shield. These kinds of standards should help ensure an acceptable quality of care and should serve to reduce the number of unneeded procedures. These developing standards should have benefit for all practicing physicians, not only those associated with managed care programs. Any physician not adhering to standardized procedures would have to be ready to explain why—either to colleagues in the managed care program or to an insurance company that is asked to pay for the physician's services. On the other hand, physicians following standardized protocols would be more able to refute charges of medical negligence if their patient's outcome was poor.

Clinical outcomes are becoming the chief measure of quality of care. One of the chief components of systems that measure quality of care is classification of hospitalized patients according to the severity of their illness. Measuring the severity of illness accurately is a very difficult task, but a number of insurers, employers, and reviewers are using illness severity systems to generate data for improving peer reviews and for comparing clinical outcomes.

Many physicians have resisted attempts to evaluate their clinical treatment and are not convinced that the quality of medical treatment can be quantified. They have tended to sit on the sidelines while the systems are being developed. Rather than condemn the systems, however, they are being urged to play a major role in evaluating them. As the president of the National Academy of Sciences' Institute of Medicine, an MD wrote: "We should be more professional in how we examine and evaluate what we do. That is, how do we measure the quality of care that is delivered, both by the physician and by the system, and how do we deal with those circumstances in which the performance is not up to standard? There is no perfect quality assessment mechanism. If we argue that we will not introduce quality assessment unless it is perfect, then, simply, somebody else will impose assessment on the medical profession, and we again will have given up our professional responsibility" (8).

Costs of Medical Practice and Physicians' Earnings

It costs a considerable amount of money to maintain a medical practice. In addition to personal income on which taxes must be paid, the self-employed physician also has to meet expenses for maintaining an office. In 1990 an average of about 45 percent of the total (gross) income of self-employed physicians was used for professional expenses. The average expenses included nonphysician wages (36%), office (22%), malpractice insurance premiums (10%), medical supplies (11%), medical equipment (5%), other expenses (16%). Equipping the most simple doctor's office can cost $30,000 to $60,000 and some specialty offices can cost over $100,000. Self-employed physicians must charge a fee that will not only cover their office expenses, but provide them with a personal income.

Medicine is the highest-paid profession in the United States. The average physician's net income (after expenses, before taxes) reached $170,600 in 1991, a 4 percent increase over 1990. Specialists with the highest average earnings were surgeons, radiologists, and anesthesiologists. One fourth of all surgeons in 1990 earned $300,000 or more, with orthopedic and cardiac surgeons sometimes earning over $500,000. Those with the lowest average income were general or family practitioners, pediatricians, and those specializing in internal medicine (Table 3–3). The average net income growth exceeded inflation during the 1981–1990 period.

Physicians' fees vary according to specialty, geographical location, type of visit (first visit or followup visit), and the procedures performed. About 24 percent of all physicians are employed by groups such as HMOs, hospitals, and group practices.

The AMA in its analysis of physician incomes suggests that when adjusted for inflation, the net income in 1989 exceeded the inflation rate by 2.5 percent. However, incomes of very few people actually keep pace with inflation in recent years.

There is growing concern about the rise in physician fees and a general unwillingness to accept the validity of the AMA analysis, certainly an unwillingness at the very least to accept it as justification for further fee inflation. The concern over physicians' fees has increased as the gap widens between practitioner charges and the amounts allowed by third-party payers (health insurance firms and government programs). A number of U.S. and Canadian economists advance what is called the *target income hypothesis.* This hypothesis contends that physicians set their sights on a given income level, and that they adjust their fees to reach it. When the demand for services is down and threatens attainment of the desired income, fees are raised; alternatively, they provide more services, which could be for the purpose of augmenting income rather than for more comprehensive and appropriate medical care. Supporters of this hypothesis point to the rise in physician incomes despite increased competition for patients as the number of physicians increases. Surgery is often cited in this regard, where fees have apparently increased to compensate for low demand. Others argue that the more critical factors in rising physician incomes may be increased demand and productivity resulting from the provision of additional, appropriate diagnostic and therapeutic services as a result of new knowledge and new technology; fear of possible malpractice suits (the practice of *defensive medicine*); the ability of more people to seek medical care because increasingly more of the cost is covered by direct payments, insurance, or government programs; and a rapidly aging population with correspondingly increased morbidity. With some specialties, particularly radiology and pathology, not only is there increased utilization of these services (because of new knowledge and technology as well as for protection against possible malpractice suits) but also, when specialties are hospital based, incomes of physicians in these specialties are typically derived from a percentage of the business generated; negotiating skills and monopolistic factors may be operating here.

Physician incomes are a subject of some debate

TABLE 3–3. Physicians' Average Net Income 1983–1990 (in Thousands of Dollars)

	Average Net Income					
	1983	*1985*	*1987*	*1989*	*1990*	*1991*
All physicians	104.1	112.2	132.3	155.8	164.3	170.6
Specialty						
General Practice	66.9	77.9	80.3	95.9	102.7	111.5
Internal Medicine	94.6	102.0	121.8	146.5	152.5	149.6
Surgery	144.3	155.0	187.9	220.5	236.4	233.8
Pediatrics	70.8	76.2	85.3	104.7	106.5	119.3
Obstetrics/Gynecology	118.1	124.3	163.2	194.3	207.3	221.8
Radiology	144.3	144.3	180.7	210.5	219.4	229.8
Psychiatry	79.2	87.2	102.7	111.7	116.5	127.6
Anesthesiology	141.6	142.7	163.1	185.8	207.4	221.1
Pathology	114.4	124.8	124.6	154.5	172.5	197.7

SOURCE: American Medical Association: *Socioeconomic Characteristics of Medical Practice.* Chicago, 1993 and earlier editions.

even within the medical profession. Internists have long argued that their cognitive skills and resulting services are undervalued as compared to the payments made for surgical skills and procedures and for technological procedures performed by radiologists and pathologists. To correct the wide variation in physicians' fees and to encourage more medical students to enter the lower-income primary care specialities, Congress legislated a new way to pay physicians for services to Medicare patients. It authorized that payments to physicians be made based on a relative value scale that is based on three main factors:

• Total work performed by the physician for each service.
• Practice costs, including the cost of malpractice insurance.
• Cost of specialty training to perform the service.

The relative value scale is based on a model developed by a Harvard research group. Medicare's payment schedule is determined by the relative value scale, which relates the value of each medical procedure to others, a dollar conversion factor, and a geographical factor. It is known as the Resource Based Relative Value Scale (RBRVS) and it redistributes money among physicians by increas-

ing the amount paid for cognitive services (listening, diagnosing, explaining, and advising patients) and decreases the amount paid for invasive procedures (e.g., surgery) and diagnostic tests. Thus, family doctors can expect their income from Medicare patients to increase about 13 percent while surgeons' fees would decrease. For example, the average payment for coronary bypass surgery for Medicare patients in 1991 was $3,181; in 1992 it was $2,892; and in 1996 it is expected to be $1,925. This decrease is not because coronary bypass surgery is less important, but because the procedure has been overvalued in relation to other medical procedures. Payment according to RBRVS began in 1992 and will be phased in over a five-year period. Some insurance companies are also using the RBRVS to revise their payments to physicians.

Few object to physicians being well paid for their services, but there is a growing feeling that some physician incomes are excessive, be they from inflated fees or increased productivity, and that, given that their education is heavily subsidized and their practices are dependent on subsidies as represented by the community hospitals in which they generate most of their income, there should be a stronger social control on their earnings unless the profession can find some effective mechanism to discipline itself.

Malpractice and Professional Liability

Medical professional liability (medical malpractice liability) continues to be an important issue. About 38 percent of all physicians have incurred at least one claim during their careers. Over one half of all obstetrician-gynecologists and surgeons have had at least one claim filed against them (9). However, the rate of medical malpractice claims (lawsuits) has begun to decline in recent years (Table 3–4). The rate has declined in all geographical areas and in all specialties except psychiatry.

Several reasons have been given for the decreased number of malpractice claims. Physicians have become more careful. They are keeping better records so that they can defend themselves in court. They are improving their communication skills to enhance the physician-patient relationship and to help patients to understand better the risks involved in procedures. It is well known that there are fewer lawsuits when the physician-patient relationship is good. Also, physicians are trying to reduce the risk of lawsuits by practicing "defensive medicine," which involves ordering more diagnostic tests than may be necessary for a diagnosis but

which also contributes to the rapidly increasing cost of medical care. Another development that promises to decrease the number of lawsuits and the amount of malpractice premiums is the adoption of standards of care by some specialty groups. For example, the American Society of Anesthesiologists adopted a standard in 1990 that requires its members to use certain devices to measure the level of oxygen in the blood, which it estimates could have prevented serious injury or death in almost one third of the cases in which anesthesiologists were accused of malpractice. In Maryland, as another example, obstetrician-gynecologists' premiums were reduced about 35 percent when they agreed to follow certain standards of care such as specific procedures for handling breech deliveries and hypertension during pregnancy. In addition, some states have passed laws to penalize patients who make frivolous claims. Both hospitals and the government are increasing efforts to identify doctors with a history of malpractice. In 1990 the federal government established a national computer file to keep track of doctors who were successfully sued for malpractice and those who have been disciplined for incompetence.

The high cost of medical malpractice insurance is a significant factor contributing to the increase in physicians' fees. After rising sharply for more than a decade, insurance premiums are leveling off and in some states are declining. This decline is attributed to a reduction in the number of claims and to laws passed in about half of the states limiting the amount or type of damages that can be recovered in malpractice suits. Still, the average annual malpractice premium for physicians in 1989 was over $15,000. Specialties such as anesthesiology, surgery, and obstetrics and gynecology are more than double that. Since 1989 premiums have continued to drop and in some states have dropped more than 30 percent. More than half of all doctors in private practice are insured by physician-owned companies, usually state medical societies, which try to keep premiums at a minimum. Medical liability rates vary greatly for different geographical areas (Table 3–5).

TABLE 3–4. Percentage of Physicians Incurring Malpractice Claims by Specialty, 1985, 1989

	1985	1989	Average Annual Rate of Change in %
All Physicians*	8.5	6.6	−8.1
Specialty			
General/Family Practice	5.5	4.9	−3.1
Internal Medicine	5.4	5.5	0.6
Surgery	13.6	9.9	−10.0
Pediatrics	6.6	5.4	−6.5
Obstetrics and Gynecology	20.0	13.2	−12.9
Radiology	11.2	5.0	−23.6
Psychiatry	2.9	4.4	14.9
Anesthesiology	7.5	5.9	−7.7

SOURCE: American Medical Association: *Socioeconomic Characteristics of Medical Practice, 1986.* Chicago, 1990/1991.

*Includes physicians in specialties not listed separately.

TABLE 3–5. Medical Liability Premiums by Geographical Area, 1991

Specialty	Los Angeles Area California	Miami Area Florida	Long Island New York
Family Practice Minor Surgery	$ 8,400	$ 32,600	13,200
Neurosurgery	51,400	183,300	118,100
Obstetrics and Gynecology	38,000	149,000	101,200
Orthopedic Surgery	32,300	110,900	37,900

SOURCE: AMA Dept. of Professional Liability and Insurance.

Medical Discipline

There are several groups that attempt to protect the public from incompetent physicians. They include medical societies, state licensing boards, specialty boards, peer review organizations (PROs), and hospital boards. None has worked very well. To drop a physician—a surgeon or other specialist—from the hospital is in effect forcing that physician out of the community, because he or she would be deprived of a livelihood, which, like going to jail, is not decided lightly but only after the most rigorous trial. There is always the risk that the physician will sue the hospital either for terminating privileges or for failing to give a good recommendation to the next hospital. More often than not, what happens is that the hospital curtails privileges or restricts the physician to practice areas in which the physician is less likely to be negligent.

In the past if physicians faced disciplinary action or had their hospital privileges revoked, they simply went to another hospital or state and continued to practice without the new hospital knowing of their past record, but this is becoming increasingly difficult to do. The federal Health Care Quality Improvement Act of 1986 makes it difficult for incompetent physicians to move from state to state without their previous professional records being known. The law requires that hospitals and other institutional providers report certain actions against physicians to the appropriate state licensing board. It also established a National Practitioners' Data Bank, which began operation in 1990 and stores information on disciplinary actions taken by the state medical boards, hospitals, or professional groups against individual physicians. Hospitals are required to check with the Data Bank before hiring or granting hospital privileges. Access to the data is restricted so that it is not used by lawyers for malpractice claims. Importantly, the law offers protection to persons participating in professional review activities from being sued, except in cases in which they knowingly provided false information.

Medical society efforts to discipline physicians have not been very effective, and we often hear lay people complain how physicians cover up for one another, and how the medical society serves to defuse situations and to protect the physician. To some extent this is true, but to what extent we cannot reliably determine. Discipline by the medical society is largely meaningless if the physician can continue to practice. It is believed that some of the most negligent physicians are not even members of the medical society.

As a nation, we seem somewhat ambivalent about medical societies. On the one hand, we want them to discipline their members, but to be effective at that they have to have meaningful sanctions, and we seem reluctant to grant societies those powers. Moreover, as noted above, they have no power over physicians who are not members.

The real potential power in discipline rests in being able to suspend or revoke medical licenses, but the state laws in this area have historically been weak.

As pressure grows to weed out incompetent physicians, state legislatures are beginning to give medical licensing boards more power and money to do their job. Nationally, medical licensing boards reported 2,957 license revocations, probations, suspensions, or other disciplinary actions in 1989. Of these, only 500 were revocation of licenses to practice medicine. Even so, only a small percentage of the nation's incompetent physicians (estimated to be 5 to 15 percent of all physicians) will be disciplined by the boards. An unknown number of these physician problem cases will be handled in some of the less formal ways, as noted above.

At the federal level, government-funded Peer Review Organizations (PROs) are located in the states and are required, among other responsibilities, to review Medicare complaints of inadequate care. These organizations are composed of physicians who review the complaints and, if appropriate, recommend sanctions to federal officials. More than 97 percent of the complaints taken to PROs are resolved without a recommendation of sanction. Between 1984 and 1987, only 79 sanctions were imposed nationally, and no sanctions were imposed in 25 states. No one—the government, the AMA, or consumer groups—is satisfied with the PROs. However, the medical profession is attempting to improve the performance of both the state medical licensing boards and the PROs, realizing that if physicians do not effectively identify, evaluate, and discipline incompetent physicians within the profession, outside groups will take over the job. There are serious concerns, however, that the medical profession is unable to discipline itself. This is illustrated by two recent, widely publicized cases. In one case for 22 years a physician in Ohio performed surgery to restructure the genitals of hundreds of women without their consent while they were under general anesthesia for other procedures. The surgery was not recognized as a valid procedure and often caused sexual dysfunction, scarring, and chronic infections, and sometimes corrective surgery was needed. The hospital where the doctor operated, the surgical team, and some gynecologists were aware of the malpractice, but

took no steps to stop it. Ten lawsuits by women had to be dropped because physicians refused to testify against him. Several physicians reported the physician's actions to the state medical board, which took no action until the Governor, pressured by some women, wrote a letter to the Board. Only then was his license revoked.

In another case a Virginia gynecologist deceived women into thinking they were pregnant, and lied to them about having a donor insemination program and used his own sperm to inseminate them without informing his patients. He was able to maintain his practice for 12 years before a physician filed a complaint with the state medical board although it was clear to many area physicians that he was practicing fraudulent medicine. After 18 months the physician signed an agreement with the state medical board that barred him from practicing medicine for five years. Virginia law requires physicians to report unprofessional conduct to the state medical board, but for years none did. Why? Some physicians took no action because they feared the reported physician would sue them and they would have to go to court to defend themselves. Most states provide some legal protection for reporting doctors, but they might still have to go to court to protect themselves. Other physicians said they didn't feel comfortable filing a complaint because they didn't have enough information. Whatever the reasons, there are many physicians practicing whose colleagues know are incompetent, impaired, or unethical. If the profession will not monitor itself, others will have to do it.

Until recently, hospitals and their medical staffs were not as diligent as they might have been, in part because they were immune to liability. But now that hospitals may be legally liable under the doctrine of corporate negligence for the malpractice of physicians providing care in their hospitals, the pressure is on to scrutinize matters more intensely. We might note that the shortcomings were not due to desire to cover up or to condone but to the difficulty of challenging a colleague in any field of endeavor, particularly if one has to stick to facts. Often the facts are not all there, and the case of malpractice is not that clear-cut; much of what is left is judgment, and judgments differ; these differences are the fuel for litigation. Under the doctrine of corporate negligence, one must have a mechanism for providing consultation to attending physicians when necessary and for assuming that only competent physicians are allowed to practice in the hospital.

Strengthened peer review mechanisms all contribute to the development of data bases that will enable hospitals and their staffs to monitor and discipline physicians with assured fairness and that will reduce the likelihood of damage suits by the physician who is called to task. There is always the risk, of course, that the disciplined physician might enlist the talents of the Federal Trade Commission (FTC), accusing the hospital and medical staff of restraint of trade.

Another control is developing in the relicensure and recertification procedures being developed by the states and by the specialty boards.

Another form of control also exists—the fall-off of referrals—but to what extent it operates is not known. If a family physician judges that a particular specialist's care is not up to standard, then the family physician routes his or her patients to a specialist in whom confidence is held.

The extent to which there is malpractice is not known. We hear of those cases in which the patient or survivors sue or complain. We do not hear of the cases in which the patient is never aware of the possibility, because of the confidence the patient has in the malpracticing physician whose bedside manner is a model for patient assurance. One has to be careful in judging malpractice, for like unnecessary surgery, which might be viewed as a form of malpractice, physicians of good faith differ about what is and what is not malpractice.

Primary Care Physicians

A *primary care physician* was defined in 1975 by the Coordinating Council on Medical Education (CCME) as one who provides an individual or family with continuing health surveillance along with the needed acute and chronic care he or she is qualified to provide and referral service to specialists as appropriate. General and family practitioners fall within this category, as do pediatricians, internists, and obstetrician-gynecologists, although not everyone would agree about this last group.

In many countries, specialists rarely provide primary care. In those countries, pediatricians and internists serve primarily as consultants, devoting their time almost exclusively to the practice of their specialty. In the United States and a few other countries, however, most of these two specialties have evolved into primary care practice; most pediatricians and most internists provide primary care. Relatively few devote their time solely to practice of the specialty. However, the pediatrician typically limits his or her clientele to a certain age group; the internist typically does not handle some things that a family practitioner might handle, such as obstetrics and pediatric problems. So, too, with obstetrics and gynecology, which has evolved largely as a primary care specialty, in this instance not for general care but for categorical care for obstetrics and/or gynecological problems, with female patients going directly to the specialist without referral.

The definition developed by the CCME still leaves much to be desired. Other specialties handle a considerable amount of routine primary care that in other settings might be handled by a family practitioner or other health professionals. In this regard, we need to note the tendency of many people to self-diagnose and self-refer to a specialist—psychiatrist, surgeon, dermatologist, orthopedist—when, in fact, the family practitioner or other primary care medical specialist might well be able to handle many of the problems. We might note the frequent use of ophthalmologists and orthopedic surgeons when optometrists and podiatrists might well suffice. We might also note that the specialities of public health and general preventive medicine do a considerable amount of primary prevention that to some extent reduces the need for primary care.

Rural and Inner-City Medical Practice

However one chooses to define primary care physicians, rural areas and inner cities have had considerable difficulty in recruiting and retaining them.

The lack of appeal for rural practice stems from fear of professional isolation: lack of professional interactions, inaccessibility of hospitals, absence of consultation and continuing medical education opportunities, lack of opportunity for spouse, and cultural deprivation (no theater, no concerts, no lectures, limited adult education activities, etc.). The physician today and his or her spouse are urbanites by virtue of their long periods of education and training in urban professional settings, and the adjustment to rural living, though sometimes inviting in moments of idyllic dreaming, has not been successful in most cases. There seems to be greater chance of retention if the physician is originally from a rural area, but no one yet has devised a generally valid formula for the successful establishment of rural practices. Professional as well as personal isolation are factors that are very real, and the former is reinforced to some extent by medical school faculty and preceptors in residency programs who caution about going to the very rural areas lest a physician promptly get out of touch with medical developments. Some also feel that insurance payments, which pay rural physicians less, may also be operative, but the data on this view are sparse.

There is some ambiguity in the word "rural." One federal agency set the definition at a population of 35,000 or 50,000. Other agencies have used other, usually lower, figures. It might be noted that rural communities at the 35,000 and 50,000 level, and many even smaller, seem now to be successfully recruiting physicians. The reasons for their successes are several: There are more physicians available, and the supply/demand factor operates to secure a more even distribution; the large urban settings are congested and are plagued by high costs and high crime rates; the assets of urban life are not as remote as our road networks improve; the small communities have sought to make their areas attractive to primary-care and other physicians by developing for their communities the best hospital facilities their communities can support, and sometimes more than they can support. It is worth noting that when the U.S. Department of Health and Human Services (HHS) proposed planning guidelines for hospitals, the guidelines would have hit these more rural hospitals, because of their tendency for low occupancy; the resulting outcry from rural America forced HHS to backtrack a bit, for these hospitals are not only all that these communities have, but they are also often the needed ingredient to make those areas attractive for professional practice.

Inner-city problems are somewhat different. In large cities, the poor have not always used private doctors. Their needs, historically, were largely handled by the indigent and voluntary hospital outpatient departments and emergency rooms. As people moved to the suburbs, the physicians went where their paying patients were. Other factors encouraging the out-migration of physicians and discouraging the in-migration of new physicians are the high cost of office and parking spaces, transportation hassles, and crime. In addition, the cities are far more litigiously inclined, and malpractice insurance rates are generally higher. The movement of physicians out of the cities has become a matter of concern, because the poor under Medicaid are now entitled to private physician care, but the changed consumer expectations often find the cities short of medical manpower. Solving this shortage problem is not easy.

The Emphasis on Primary Care

Part of the recent emphasis on primary care physicians is economic. The rising costs of health care make the principal payers, that is, industry through health insurance premiums and government, want some mechanism to control costs. They believe that one way to control costs is to decrease the use of specialists by encouraging primary care physicians to treat mild illnesses rather than refer to expensive specialists. When specialists and primary care physicians treat patients with comparable illnesses, specialists hospitalize patients more often, write more prescriptions, and order more diagnostic tests (10). Of course, when an illness is complicated or severe, treatment by specialists is appropriate. Primary care is also the area of medicine that provides the majority of preventive services such as counseling about healthful life-style changes, immunizations, and detection of illnesses before they become serious, all of which are becoming more important in maintaining good health.

As mentioned earlier, managed care organizations often use primary care physicians as "gatekeepers" to prevent the unnecessary use of specialists. Medical students are being encouraged to enter primary care fields by the increased payment for their services by Medicare and some insurance companies using the RBRVS.

Family Practice and Surgery

One of the most spirited and continuing professional debates concerns surgery and the family practitioner. Before the time of the American College of Surgeons (ACS), and for many years after, the general practitioner did about everything, including general surgery. In many communities in the United States, particularly in the more remote areas, family practitioners still do a great amount of general surgery, such as appendectomies, herniorrhaphies, cholecystectomies, hysterectomies, vein ligations, and hemorrhoidectomies. They have done these procedures for years and they see no reason to give up such surgery. Besides, in many communities, there is no board certified surgeon to do the work. The surgeons, on the other hand, strongly believe that, except in emergencies or in remote locations where a surgical specialist is not available, surgery should be performed by one trained in surgery.

The American Academy of General Practice (AAGP), the predecessor of the American Academy of Family Physicians (AAFP), found in a 1969 survey that 39 percent of its members did major surgery. Estimates in 1973 were that the percent-

age, including major surgery in their practices, was down to 20 to 25 percent (11). Though physicians in general or family practice may be doing less major surgery overall, 88 percent of them were reported in 1982 to be performing some ambulatory surgery, which generally consists of the less complicated surgical procedures (12).

As the number of surgeons grows, and as they spread throughout the country, many have moved into areas in which surgeons had not been before; understandably problems arise. In Kalispell, Montana, a surgeon states, "I've been here five lovely years, three of which were struggling years. In Kalispell, there's a very good relationship with the family physicians. I'm willing to give them some gallbladders just to get them to be here and provide coordination in family practice" (11, p. 71).

The varying viewpoints in this Montana town were expressed by others as well. One surgeon said:

A GP should do some surgery. But I don't think he has any business in the belly. A woman who had her gallbladder taken out by a GP developed pain, jaundice, and diarrhea 20 years later. I found a cystic duct remnant with two stones in it. That wouldn't have happened with many surgeons. I'm willing to help a GP with a GP operation, but not a big operation. A GP who feels he's competing with me for hernias will not send me his stomachs, he'll send them to Spokane instead.

Another surgeon observed that "four board-certified surgeons in town are too many."

A general practitioner of long standing in the community said that he gave up surgery "the day a board man arrived." Another GP, who had had some surgical training, observed (11, p. 71):

As more surgical specialists have arrived, the GPs have drawn the line on what they do themselves. In my view, we now have to stay out of the stomach and bowel, complicated bile duct surgery, and the more complex orthopedic surgery. But I still do about 85 percent of my own surgery. It isn't just us, but our patients' wishes that have to be considered.

Finally, a family practitioner stated, "In my mind our group is doing some general surgery because it's part of the continuing care we give. Our patients feel confidence in us."

The ACS has, of course, long sought to curb surgery by those not trained to do it except as noted above. The ACS is also concerned about itinerant surgery.

Itinerant surgery occurs when a surgeon performs surgery at a distance from the usual place of practice and relies for diagnosis, preoperative preparation, and postoperative care on another physician who is not as well qualified, even though the other physician may have been trained by the surgeon. The ACS feels that this is not in the best interests of the patient and that it may lead to ghost surgery (13). Others argue that in the more rural parts of the country, this practice is a necessity. As one Nebraska official put it, "The ACS doesn't understand that about half our ninety-three counties are medically underserved by federal standards. . . . If itinerant surgeons weren't allowed to compensate for this shortage, either rural hospitals would fold, or rural FPs would start doing the surgery" (14). Fellowship in the ACS is, of course, separate from certification by a specialty board. The content of family practice residencies requires, however, some training in a variety of other specialty areas, including surgery (15). Specifically:

The resident must receive training in pre- and postoperative care, basic surgical principles, asepsis, handling of tissue, and technical skills to assist the surgeon in the operating room. The program should provide the opportunity for residents to develop the technical proficiency to perform specific surgical procedures which family physicians may be called upon to perform. If the residents expect to include surgery as a major aspect of their practice, additional training must be obtained.

The ACS attitude toward this was clearly stated some years earlier by its director, C. Rollins Hanlon, MD, FACS (16):

The College receives a number of letters from Fellows initiated by pressure on them to provide surgical training

or surgical privileges for family practitioners or family practice residents in hospitals. The Fellows have properly resisted such pressure for inappropriate surgical privileges.

One can see this pressure as part of a larger movement to downgrade the quality of surgical care, often under the guise of federal cost containment, by abolishing educational standards at various levels in the field of medical care, substituting in their place the vague and dangerous criterion of "tests of competence."

But, it is an even more dangerous delusion to assume that professional expertise, especially in surgery, can be provided by a once-over-lightly type of on-the-job training, or by exposure comparable to an extended rotating internship.

Dr. Hanlon went on to attack the aggrandizing efforts of the family practitioners and even rejected the necessity to train them for preoperative and postoperative care. On this he said:

The College has long maintained that leaving the patient in the care of a general practitioner not adequately prepared to recognize and handle post-operative complications is a critical component in the deplorable practice of itinerant surgery. This is the type of care I would be delighted to lose sight of by stamping it out.

One can view this controversy as a professional debate in which the surgeons, following in the tradition of the ACS, continue to stress the importance of strict qualifications for those engaged in surgery, and in which the family practitioners, on the other hand, assert that surgery is not the preserve of the surgeons, that the family practitioners, to be a true generalist, must be able to function supportively in this area and in some cases even do the surgery. One can also view this as an attempt on the part of the surgeons to protect their domain both economically and professionally at the very time that residencies are under attack, that the number of surgeons is called excessive, and that public concern increases over the amount and cost of surgery.

An interesting series of questions arises from this controversy: To what extent should family practitioners do surgery? If they should not do surgery, and at least 88 percent are estimated to have surgery as part of their practices, what does this say in terms of the number of surgeons who should be trained? How can one say whether we are "oversurgeoned" or not, unless the first question is answered?

The Appeal of Specialization

There are many reasons why physicians specialize: Specialists, to begin with, have always been held in high regard by the population. The specialist was something special, a person who could do things that lesser mortals and general physicians could not do, a person whose special skills also warranted a higher fee. The very best of these specialists were professors on the faculties of medical schools.

There has always been, of course, a certain aura that surrounded the physician, a mystique that was more pronounced for the specialist who had special knowledge and skills that saved lives, eased pain, and improved functioning.

The medical student has to choose in which area of medicine she or he will practice. Many factors may enter this decision process, but because most of the faculty are specialists, the pressure to respond to one of those specialty role models is ever present. We should not forget that specialization has a certain intellectual appeal. It enables the curious to know more and more about the problems that afflict the human being. Because the problems are complex, the curious have to specialize in order to understand them.

Other factors may enter. A person's own medical history or that of the family frequently channels a physician's interest. For some specialties, very high incomes are ensured or orderly personal lives are more possible because of fewer emergencies and irregular hours.

Most of the factors that affect the location of primary care physicians also influence practice location choice of specialists. Hospital access, however, may be even more critical for the spe-

cialist, in terms of the supportive services that may be necessary for the effective practice of her or his specialty. Studies have also shown that specialists tend to locate in areas close to the place where the residency is taken. There are some good reasons for this. The new specialist is familiar with the clinicians in the area and tends to know and be comfortable with other specialists for referrals. Conversely, because the new specialist is known by many of the physicians, the new specialist can anticipate some helpful referrals. Notwithstanding the pull to practice in urban settings, during the past decade the overall increase in the supply of specialists, the spread of technology, and the disadvantages of urban life have influenced the movement of new specialists to outlying areas.

Medical Society Memberships

Most physicians find it valuable to belong to the county or city medical society in the area in which they practice and to their state medical society. Only slightly more than half elect to join the AMA. A variety of factors influence the latter choice. Many disagree with the AMA's policies (although the association probably truly represents the views of its members), others are more interested in their specialty society, and still others are concerned about the rising costs of membership, particularly in view of the many other memberships a physician feels he or she must maintain. The AMA dues in 1992 were $375. Pennsylvania Medical Society dues were $375. Add to these the local society dues and specialty society dues, and the total can easily reach over $1,000 per year.

Approximately 78 percent of all osteopaths belong to the American Osteopathic Association (AOA). AOA is, of course, a much smaller body with a smaller constituency; it is less active in the political arena, and it does not engage in the breadth of activities that the AMA does.

Membership in the local and state societies is more vital for the practicing physician. These organizations serve a number of purposes. First, and perhaps most important, these organizations enable the physician to meet his or her colleagues, to learn about the skills and abilities of other physicians, and vice versa. This is a vital element in building the practice of a specialist, enabling other physicians to evaluate the specialist for the purpose of referring patients to him or her. Second, society membership facilitates an intellectual interchange among physicians, which has always been a key element in the continued learning process of physicians. Indeed, this has been formalized in most societies, whereby the society sponsors regular continuing medical education programs, an increasingly important and necessary activity for professional practice. Many local medical societies and all state societies also issue medical journals for dissemination of knowledge and other matters of concern to the profession. Third, medical societies provide an organizational focus for representation of medical viewpoints about matters affecting the health of the population and about other matters of interest or concern to them. Related to this is that if any government, industry, or other body wishes to communicate something to the medical community, the medical society is perhaps the most effective vehicle. Fourth, membership often enables the physician to receive such financial benefits as group life, health, and malpractice insurance. A fifth function of the medical society is social.

Laws and society rules governing memberships vary from state to state. Some states allow membership in the local society only. Other states have a unified local/state membership.Some have a unified local/state/AMA membership. Generally, membership in the state society or AMA requires membership in the lower units. One AMA exception is direct AMA membership for federally employed physicians. Only five states require state medical society members to belong to the AMA.

Physicians often belong to other medical societies, depending on their interests and on their specialties. Among the many other societies is the National Medical Association (NMA), an association representing the special interests of black physicians.

It was suggested above that the policies of the AMA probably reflect the views of its members, thus making it a very democratic organization. We can begin to understand this if we look at the lowest level of medical society organization, the county or city medical society.

When the physician first enters practice, he or she tends to join the local and state medical societies for reasons that have been cited. The local society carries out a variety of society activities; these vary from one society to another. They might include working with the local health department to assist it in carrying out its functions; for example, assisting the health officer with an immunization program, or helping with athletic physicals. Other activities could include making representations to the local government on behalf of some voluntary agency that is seeking government help; assigning representatives to serve on the boards of directors of various community agencies; investigating complaints against physicians involving medical ethics or malpractice; organizing continuing education programs for members to help them keep up to date; participating in public and school health education programs; or editing the local medical journal or newsletter. The local society has its officers and is entitled to send a certain number of delegates to the state medical society's legislative body, often called the House of Delegates. Each of these activities—some to serve the public's interest, some the medical profession's interest—requires time on the part of the local members. If the physician participates, accepting her or his share of the society's workload, the physician can be influential and help shape the policies that are formulated by the local body and the positions taken by the local delegates to the state society. If the physician ducks local assignments, the physician's influence is reduced accordingly. The story is told about one group of physicians who could never activate their local society around a particular set of issues that concerned them; one society member observed about that group of physicians: "They never assumed a role in society affairs, they never came to meetings except when they wanted the society to do something for them, so it should have been no surprise to them that the membership was lackluster in its responses."

As in most voluntary groups, leadership falls to those who take the time, who make the effort to help the organization. All too often, the critics of medical societies remove themselves from meaningful participation and are, therefore, unable to exercise influence.

State medical associations or societies are similarly structured, except that their legislative bodies are not the total membership present and voting, as at the local levels, but are instead the House of Delegates from the constituent local medical societies. State society delegates meet usually once or twice a year to conduct the legislative business of the association and at other times when it becomes necessary. The state associations tend to have a broader range of activities and larger paid staffs. (Large local medical societies have well-paid executives, usually nonmedical; state societies have larger nonmedical staffs to execute the directives of the House of Delegates and officers. Some state societies may employ physician executives.) The state associations concern themselves mainly with state issues: advising and negotiating with state agencies, testifying and lobbying at the state legislative sessions, proposing new policies and new legislation, negotiating as appropriate with the state hospital association, helping to devise solutions to problems that have an impact on society members, organizing the annual meeting of the association for the conduct of association business, and encouraging continuing medical education activities. State medical journals also represent an important medium of communication to association members, with scientific articles, book reviews, editorials, communications from the state health agencies (which may consist of reporting on new health problems, new state services, as well as rules and regulations regarding diseases that must be reported to the state, etc.). Some of these journals are of exceptional quality, the *New England Journal of Medicine* (the journal of the

Massachusetts Medical Society) being one of the world's leading medical journals.

Much of the work of the state medical societies is carried out by committees drawn from the general membership. The committees are assisted by the paid staff, and the committees serve generally in an advisory capacity to the House of Delegates or to carry out the mandates of the House. Here again, the ability to influence the state society or association depends on the willingness of the membership to get involved.

Each state society elects a certain number of delegates to serve as its representatives in the AMA's House of Delegates. The AMA functions as do the state societies except that, as a national body, it deals mostly with national issues, and it has a larger staff with many more functions to perform.

The activities of the AMA are far ranging. It is one of the largest publishers in the world. Its journal, *JAMA,* comes out weekly, and has subscribers in 132 countries. *JAMA* is also published monthly in five languages—German, French, Flemish, Italian, and Japanese—and bimonthly in Chinese. These editions have, as one might expect, different contents. *JAMA* is also one of the world's leading medical journals. In addition to *JAMA,* the AMA also publishes nine specialty journals; a weekly newspaper *(American Medical News),* which deals largely with socioeconomic issues that are of interest to and may affect physicians; directories; and research and policy advising reports on a wide variety of socioeconomic and scientific issues that affect the practice of medicine. Its publishing activities are also directed toward the consumer in the form of books and health education pamphlets.

In cooperation with the GTE Corporation, it has developed and is now expanding its Medical Information Network, which is a computerized system that gives physicians immediate access to data from *AMA Drug Evaluations, Current Procedural Terminology* (CPT), *Current Medical Information and Terminology* (CMIT), as well as other types of information. Nearly 40 percent of the AMA's budget is devoted to medical education and scientific policy development and dissemination activities.

As a national organization it participates with a number of other national organizations on committees and councils to reach agreement on issues that affect each and on which agreements need to be reached if the health system is to work well and to improve. Some of these groups (LCME, ACGME, ACCME) were mentioned in an earlier chapter. The AMA is also active in negotiations with various federal agencies, as well as on more mundane matters that affect the practice of medicine. It plays a key role in helping to shape federal legislation through testimony before congressional committees and direct lobbying with individual members of Congress. The AMA is widely recognized as being one of the most effective lobbying groups in Washington. It might be noted here that physicians are significant contributors to political campaigns individually and through their political action committees.

The work of the AMA is carried out from its headquarters in Chicago and from an AMA office building in Washington.

As noted in Chapter 1, the AMA frequently has been involved in state and local disputes stemming from questions and issues raised by state and local medical societies. Because of its involvement, the organization has frequently been charged by the FTC and others of seeking to restrain trade and to maintain its monopolistic position. The FTC has also attacked the AMA, but not in court, over what the FTC perceived to be undue medical influence in the medical school accreditation process, and it has attacked the one-time AMA prohibition of advertising by physicians.

Critics of the AMA also attack it as a control center, pulling strings at all corners of the nation and dictating policies to the state and local levels. The criticisms are particularly severe regarding stances taken by the AMA that appear, to the critics at least, as an excessive concern for protecting the economic interests of physicians and preserving the right of physicians to practice medicine with minimal social control.

One has to respond that the AMA has no control. It has considerable influence, but in the final analysis it does not control the right of a physician to practice medicine, nor can it direct a state or local medical society to do what the AMA wants. What gives the AMA power—and it is persuasive power or influence—is the fact that it generally represents the wishes of its members around the country as expressed through actions of the House of Delegates, which governs the work of its officers and staff.

The power of the AMA is somewhat diminished by the fact that only about half of all physicians are members. It can no longer speak with as unified a voice in medicine, because many specialty societies have set up lobbying groups to concentrate on their own interests, which are not necessarily those of the AMA. Some disunity among physicians, according to the chairperson of the AMA Board, stems from controversy about the fees that should be paid to different types of physicians (17). This fragmentation among physicians comes at a time when other health lobbies (for example, the American Hospital Association) are becoming stronger and have views that may differ from those of the AMA. Thus the AMA, though still influential, has become less able to resist the many changes that are being made in medical practice.

Medical Ethics

It is customary for physicians to recite the Hippocratic Oath upon graduation from medical school. This oath is the doctor's' traditional pledge regarding treatment of patients. It says, in part, "I will use the treatment to help the sick according to my ability and judgment, but I will never use it to injure or wrong them." This served as sufficient guidance in the past when there were few options in treatment and physicians were relatively helpless in the face of many diseases. However, in the past few decades "advances in medicine have produced new treatment options for many illnesses and injuries which, even when they cannot produce recovery, may greatly affect the circumstances of life and death" (18, p. xi). Making medical decisions in the light of recent technology can be very difficult, and the help of philosophers, the clergy, lawmakers, and ordinary citizens is often sought by the medical profession, because the decisions go beyond medical judgment and involve moral issues about which "serious and responsible people hold a diversity of views, even contradictory ones, and they can present valid moral defenses of the positions they hold" (18, p. xii).

Amid these changing circumstances, the modern physician must struggle with a wide range of moral and ethical issues ranging from high technology medicine and the care of dying adults and disabled newborns to use of cost-containing measures. Questions that were once settled among the physician, patient, and family have now become controversial issues, debated by society and increasingly ending in the courts. New questions arise as high technology medical treatment results in the ability to prolong life and dying almost indefinitely and makes extensive organ transplantation possible. Medicine can no longer afford to do all that it is capable of doing, and outside groups, including the courts, are trying to influence medical treatment. Often pressure groups and legal opinions conflict with the physician's judgment about the proper course of action for a patient, and the physician is forced to think not only of the ethical choices, but also of the legal consequences of his or her actions. Philosophers, clergy, physicians, lawyers, social scientists, and society often disagree among themselves on medical ethical issues. The physician is in the uncomfortable position of having few clear-cut guidelines to apply to many of the new medical situations. Some examples of the more prominent issues follow.

- When, if ever, is it permissible to withhold or withdraw artificial nutrition (in the form of tube feedings) from dying or irreversibly comatose patients? Some physicians and lay people believe that artificial feeding can be considered a medical procedure and may be stopped in rare instances when the burdens for the patient outweigh the benefits. Others believe that feeding, even tube feedings, should never be discontinued and fear the cost involved could influence the decision. The courts give conflicting messages. In the case of a 48-year-old firefighter who told his wife he did not want to live with artificial life supports, the court prohibited the removing of feeding tubes saying that feeding tubes differ from other life-support treatments such as mechanical ventilators. In another state, the court came to the opposite conclusion. The court ruled in the case of an 84-year-old nursing home patient that artificial feeding, like mechanical ventilators, could be discontinued provided certain explicit procedures were followed. In 1986, the AMA issued guidelines that state that it is not unethical to discontinue "medication and artificially or technologically supplied respiration, nutrition or hydration" for patients in an irreversible coma, even if death is not imminent, if certain safeguards are met.

- When, if ever, is it permissible to withhold treatment from a deformed newborn? This issue came to national attention when a child known as Baby Doe who had Down's syndrome and an esophageal malformation was not treated. The baby died of starvation when the parents, upon the advice of their doctor and with court approval, refused to give permission for surgery that might have enabled the child to eat. The federal government moved to restrict the decision-making powers of physicians and parents, first by issuing government regulations (which were struck down in court) and then by passing the Child Abuse Prevention Amendments of 1984. The regulations that implement the law were revised several times in response to criticism by the medical profession and others. In 1986 the AMA successfully sued to set aside federal regulations that mandated the nature of care for severely impaired infants in favor of physician-patient, locally developed standards of care. Although the final regulation is more flexible than the original, many believe that doctors have been made more fearful of the legal consequences of their treatment of infants and are likely to overtreat and cause newborn intensive care units to become so overcrowded with newborns who may never recover that infants who might benefit from treatment may not be able to gain access.

• When, if ever, is it permissible to withhold or alter medical treatment based on the ability to receive reimbursement for the treatment? Less dramatic but no less cogent is the issue of access to medical care on the basis of the ability to pay. Millions of Americans are not covered by private health insurance or government programs. As the numbers of uninsured, underinsured, and cost-containment measures increase, the ability to shift the costs of uncompensated care to paying patients decreases, and medical care providers must determine how they are going to deal with nonpaying patients. A frequent example cited is of the pregnant woman whose delivery is imminent but who is not accepted at hospitals or by physicians because she is unable to pay for her services. Some groups believe that medical care is a "right," but this idea has never been converted into law or practice in the U.S. Others regard medical care as a commodity to be purchased.

Other areas of concern that are under study include the ethical issues relating to AIDS and the potential for altering genes to treat disease. These and other complex dilemmas that confront the practice of medicine in today's world are being studied at places like the Hastings Center in New York. They are being debated on television, in newspapers, and by society at large. At the federal level, a Biomedical Ethics Board and Biomedical Ethics Advisory Board were established in 1985 to report to Congress on ethical issues relating to health. While all of this study and discussion continues, physicians must make decisions on these issues now.

SUMMARY

Most physicians are self-employed either in solo or group practice. Most are paid a fee for service. These are the time-honored methods of practice and payment.

An increasing number of physicians are working in group practice, which is generally defined as three or more physicians—of the same specialty or of different specialties—who choose to practice together. They do this for a variety of reasons, including ease of consultation with colleagues, coverage on nights and days off, sharing of equipment and support personnel, and intellectual stimulation. Physicians in group practice typically charge a fee for service, but how they divide the income varies. In addition to the growth of group practice, an increasing number of physicians are also entering hospital-based practice. Here again, the patient typically pays a fee for service, but how the physician is paid varies from fee for service to straight salary, to salary plus a percentage of the income generated. In a growing number of group practices, the group contracts with a population to provide complete medical services in return for regular payments whether the enrolled person uses the service or not. These kinds of groups are often known as *health maintenance organizations,* and they place great emphasis on prevention. Physicians working in such settings as these typically are salaried. There are, in addition, newer forms of managed care such as open-ended HMOs, IPAs, and PPOs.

Most physicians find it valuable to belong to the county or city medical society in the area where they practice, and most also belong to their state medical society. Only slightly more than half elect to join the AMA, for a variety of reasons: many disagree with the AMA's policies (although the association probably represents the views of those who are its members); others are more interested in their specialty society; some are concerned over the rising costs of membership, particularly in view of the many other memberships they feel they must maintain.

Membership in the local and state societies is another matter. These organizations serve a number of purposes for the practicing physician. First, and perhaps most important, these organizations enable the physician to meet his or her colleagues and to learn about the skills and abilities of other physicians and vice versa. This is a vital element in the building of a specialist's practice and in the referral of one's own patients. A second element in society membership is that it facilitates intellectual interchange among physicians, which has always been a key element in their continued learning process. This has been formalized in most societies with the society's sponsoring of regular continuing medical education programs. Third, these medical societies provide an organizational focus for representation of medical viewpoints on matters affecting the health of the population, as well as on matters of interest or concern to physicians. Related to this is the fact that if anybody—government, industry, or others—wishes to communicate something to the medical community, the state or local medical society is perhaps the most effective vehicle.

Physicians often belong to other medical societies depending on their interests and on their specialties.

Until recently physicians tended to set up practice close to the institutions at which they did their graduate medical training. In recent years there has been a perceptible movement away from these centers of learning to areas beyond the suburbs. An increasing number are moving to the smaller communities because of the quality of life and other opportunities they afford. But the very small, rural communities are still having difficulty attracting physicians and retaining them. Professional and spouse isolation are the key elements that make physician practice in the more rural areas uninviting.

The AMA's activities range far and wide. Most people perhaps know it best as a prominent and very effective Washington lobbying group that represents the interests of American physicians. Some of its lobbying is in support of legislation and policies that are important to the health of the American people, and some is for things that benefit its membership. Its activities go well beyond this, however; it is one of the world's largest publishers, publishing professional journals, directories, research reports, and newspapers. It also publishes books and pamphlets directed toward the public. Its research activities provide scientific and clinical guidance to physicians, and it is the main source for information on how and where physicians practice, on what their incomes and expenses are, and on other socioeconomic factors. It continues its long-standing tradition of seeking to improve the quality of both medical education and medical practice.

There are issues that figure prominently in the medical practice arena, and one can only touch upon a few of the most pertinent. One of these issues is the changing manner in which physicians practice, and in particular some of the more experimental forces as represented by IPAs and PPOs. Another issue is the rising income level in some of the specialties. A third issue is the role of family physicians, and in particular the extent to which surgery should be a part of their training and practice. Another issue is the cost of malpractice insurance.

DISCUSSION QUESTIONS

1. To what extent should the subsidized costs of training a physician allow social control of where and how a physician will practice, and the type and amount of remuneration for that physician's services? What about the subsidization of other professional education?

2. Are the payments for physician cognitive skills and services, as found in and provided by the medical specialties, undervalued when compared with the payments for surgical specialties and for technological skills offered by radiologists, anesthesiologists, and pathologists? If so, what should be done about it?

3. If you were selecting a family physician:
   a. Would you prefer your physician to be trained as an MD or DO, in what specialty if any, and what reasons do you have for your preferences?
   b. In what kind of practice or practice setting (solo, single or multispecialty group, hospital-based) would you prefer your physician to be, and why?
   c. How would you prefer your physician to be paid for his or her services (fee for service, salary, salary with a productivity or bonus component, or some other method), and why?

4. Does your area have enough, too many, or too few physicians?

a. If too many physicians, what have been the implications for people in your area? What if anything needs to be done about this situation?

b. If too few physicians, in what specialties are there shortages? What are the reasons for this? What can be done about it?

5. Are physician fees and incomes too low, just about right, or too high? If too low or too high, what should and can be done about them?

6. To what extent is the AMA a positive force on the national scene? A negative force? How would you like to see the AMA change?

7. If you were a physician, would you join the AMA? Why?

8. Should the AMA be held accountable for actions by a state medical society?

9. What can and should be done about the high cost of malpractice insurance?

10. Are the informal checks on physician competence (continuing medical education, recertification, threat of malpractice suits, control over hospital privileges, family physician referrals) adequate to deal with the issue? If not, how should the informal mechanisms be strengthened? Should the formal mechanisms be strengthened?

11. Should people have a "right" to medical care in the United States?

12. Is withholding medical treatment ever justified?

REFERENCES

1. Raffel, N.K.: Health Services in the Union of Soviet Socialist Republics, in Raffel, M.W., ed.: Comparative Health Systems. University Park, Penn State Press, 1984.
2. Raffel, M.W., Raffel, N.K.: The Medical Care System of Hungary. J Med Pract Manag, Vol.4, No.2, 1989.
3. American Medical News, March 13, 1991.
4. Morrison, E.M., Luft, H.S.: Health Maintenance Organization Environments in the 1980s and Beyond. Health Care Financ Rev, Vol.12, No.1, Fall 1990.
5. Darling, H.: Employers and Managed Care: What Are the Early Returns? Health Affairs, Vol.10, No.4, Winter 1991, p. 149.
6. Langwell, K.M.: Structure and Performance of Health Maintenance Organizations: A Review. Health Care Financ Rev, Vol.12, No.1, Fall 1990, p. 75.
7. Kirchner, M.: Can This IPA Beat the Blues. Med Econ, June 8, 1987.
8. Their, S.O.: Reexamining the Principles of Medicine. Health Affairs, Vol.6, No.4, Winter 1987.
9. Slora, E.J., Gonzalez, M.L.: Medical Professional Liability Claims and Premiums, 1985–89. Socioeconomic Characteristics of Medical Practice 1990/1991, Chicago, AMA.
10. Greenfield, S., Nelson, E., Zubkoff, M., Manning, W., Rogers, W., Kravitz, R., Keller, A., Tarlov, A., Ware, J.: Variations in Resource Utilization Among Medical Specialties and Systems of Care. JAMA, Vol.269, No.12, March 25, 1992, pp. 1624–1630.
11. Medical World News, September 21, 1973.
12. SMS Report, Socioeconomic Monitoring System. Chicago, AMA, 1982.
13. Statement on Principles. Chicago, ACS, 1981.
14. Medical World News, March 17, 1980.
15. Special Requirements for Residency Training in Family Practice, Directory of Residency Training Programs for 1983/1984. Chicago, AMA.
16. Hanlon, C.R.: Bulletin, American College of Surgeons, February 1978.
17. American Medical News, January 22/29, 1988.
18. Harron, F., Burnside, J., Beauchamp, T.: Health and Human Values, A Guide to Making Your Own Decisions. New Haven, Yale University Press, 1983.

Chapter 4

Nurses and Other Health Professionals

Nurses

Nurses are "the hearts and hands of health care" (1). Nursing is a unique profession in that it is the only one that is 97 percent female and is controlled by women. Almost 70 percent of nurses work in hospitals. They also work in community clinics, doctors' offices, long-term care facilities, schools, patients' homes, and the armed forces. Experienced nurses are recruited by insurance companies, peer review organizations, and pharmaceutical companies. Some have their own independent practices. The nursing profession is undergoing rapid change in the educational and training programs for nurses and in the tasks that nurses perform.

Nursing began as a helping profession in the United States with training programs associated with general hospitals. The pattern that developed dominated the nursing field until after the Second World War: Nurses were trained for three years in special schools associated with hospitals. On successful completion of the course of study, the graduating student was awarded a diploma, and on passing the state licensing examination, the nurse became a registered nurse, or RN. Only about 40 percent of RNs today are graduates of *hospital diploma schools of nursing*. This percentage, however, is decreasing as diploma programs close because of their cost to the hospitals, because of professional pressures, and because the number of graduates from college nurse education programs is rising. This changing scene will be discussed after we briefly examine the various types of nursing programs.

Hospital diploma school programs typically had a large nursing service component, that is to say, the training was heavily weighted in favor of on-the-job training rather than academic training. From the beginning, these programs served as a form of labor exploitation, because much of the student's time was spent on the wards nursing patients, for which they received no compensation, save perhaps room and board. As these programs evolved, more and more adopted stronger academic components; in some states, the students took some of their courses at local colleges and universities.

During World War I, a number of university nursing programs were developed that granted, instead of a diploma, a baccalaureate degree. On passing the same state licensing examination taken by the diploma school graduates, the baccalaureate graduate also became an RN. Baccalaureate programs have experienced a rapid rise, and these graduates now constitute nearly 30 percent of the total registered nurse population and is rising. The total RN population holding associate degrees is rising (Table 4–1).

A third type of nurse training program began to develop during the 1950s in community colleges. These programs last two to two-and-a-half years. Upon completion, the student is granted an associate degree; on passing the same state licensing examination taken by the diploma school and college or university graduate, the student becomes a registered nurse. Over half of the graduates from RN programs today are from associate degree programs. About 25 percent of the total number of practicing RNs hold associate degrees.

There are, therefore, three basic pathways to becoming an RN. Each has an academic component; each uses hospital facilities for clinical training; and each graduate becomes registered by taking a common state examination administered by the state board of nurse examiners. It is generally acknowledged that the clinical (on-the-ward) training in the diploma programs is of longer duration than in the other types of programs, that the baccalaureate and the associate degree grad-

uates frequently do not have sufficient clinical training, and that this must be augmented by in-service training when hired by a hospital. There are, of course, great variations among programs, with strong and weak programs in each pathway. The baccalaureate approach is distinctive in that it alone has a public health nursing component. In addition, a baccalaureate degree (in nursing or some other field) is necessary if an RN wishes to pursue graduate training. There is considerable debate over the comparative operational competencies of the graduates from the different types of programs, and there have been attempts to categorize the programs. The data to support the various categorization attempts are far from conclusive because of the great variability among programs within each pathway and the variability of admission requirements by the programs. Nurses, whether trained at the diploma, associate degree, or baccalaureate level, have similar roles and functions in hospitals and generally receive the same salary (2).

The nursing profession has been embroiled in a long and unproductive controversy among themselves over what is adequate educational preparation for nursing. Since 1964, the American Nurses' Association (ANA) has advocated that only nurses with baccalaureate degrees should be called professional nurses. However, because most nurses enter the profession with either an associate degree or a diploma, the ANA, in 1985, called for the establishment of two levels of nursing practice—a level called *professional nurse* for those nurses holding a baccalaureate degree and a level called *technical nurse* for those holding an associate

TABLE 4–1. Graduations from Registered Nurse Programs

Type of Program	1970		1980		1990	
	Number	Percent	Number	Percent	Number	Percent
Diploma	22,551	52.3	14,495	19.1	5,199	8
Associate	11,483	26.6	36,034	47.7	42,318	64
B.S. nursing	9,069	21.1	24,994	33.1	18,571	28

SOURCE: National League of Nursing.

degree. Efforts to change state licensing laws to reflect this difference have not been very successful.

There is clearly a movement on the part of nurse leaders to get the diploma schools to close because, they believe, nurse training should be part of an educational system and not under the control of a hospital or of any other profession. Diploma schools are closing, and although professional pressures are operative, the cause is primarily costs. The costs of diploma education can no longer be buried in general hospital costs and covered by Blue Cross and other insurance payments. The views of nurse leaders vis-à-vis diploma education have to some extent spilled over into the classroom, and baccalaureate students frequently are persuaded to view their roles in nursing as more professional, that is, to view themselves as leaders in nursing and as people having a deeper theoretical understanding of nursing practice than the others. When baccalaureate graduates have not been able to gain perspective on this in work situations, it has sometimes led to conflicts with the diploma nurses as well as with hospital administrators. An experienced diploma nurse is not likely to feel kindly toward a recent graduate from a baccalaureate program who expresses such views, nor is a hospital administrator, who is concerned more with nursing performance. This lack of consensus over issues concerning the educational preparation of nurses has caused disarray within the nursing profession and has affected its image and its relationship with other organizations.

There is perhaps a deeper issue here, and that is that nursing seems to be a profession in search of identity. Part of this is manifest in the conflict nursing has with the medical profession. Long dependent on medical practitioners, long under their control—and still so in hospitals and doctors' offices—nurses have begun to seek more independence. They want to define a role that puts them on a par with physicians and not subservient to them.

Part of the search for professional identity has led nursing to decrease its participation in certain functions that were historically a part of nursing, such as diet therapy, medical social work, medical records, recreation therapy, ward administration, and bedside nursing. A great deal of this change was, of course, necessary because of the growing complexity of the health field. No longer could a nurse have all the knowledge and skills necessary to cover these functional areas. Specially trained people emerged to cover those functions. But spinning off those functions raised the question: What is nursing? Bedside nursing was historically a key nursing function. In a very real sense, it was more fundamental to nursing than all of the other functions. Now, however, a great portion of bedside nursing is being taken over by the licensed practical nurse (LPN) and the nurse's aide. If bedside care and other things are given up, what is there left to legitimize nursing as a profession?

This question has led nurse leaders to identify different roles. Accepting the proposition that the diploma nurse is a disappearing breed, nurse leaders have begun to see the associate degree nurse as a technical nurse capable of handling whatever functions remain to patient care in hospital and doctor's office, and the baccalaureate nurse as the leader and teacher. Some nurse leaders are even beginning to talk about the professional nurse as being one who earns a master's degree as a specialist in a clinical area of nursing (e.g., pediatrics, public health, medical-surgical nursing, intensive care) or as one who holds only a doctorate, not in sociology or higher education but in one of the developing doctoral programs in nursing. Some argue that professional nursing should not only be concerned with "sick care" but also with "wellness," that is, with the steps needed to keep from getting sick. Others argue that there is a unique role for nursing that relates to helping people cope with conditions that medicine is unable to cure or help.

However, much of what goes on today in terms of the search for professional identity is also a reaction to domination by physicians. That domination was very real, and it reflected the dominant attitudes of society, attitudes that were accepted by a large segment of the female population, including the nurses. Although some of the medical rhetoric of the past sounded sexist, to accept that language uncritically would cause one to misinterpret reality. The physician wanted to dominate, to be captain of the therapeutic team, because the physician always had been. This domination was not sexually motivated, for even today male lawyers and male health administrators frequently complain of physician domination. Many physicians appear to know it all and to dominate even beyond their areas of competence. But this is, in part, a result of the status of the physician in society and a result of the training process, which creates a positive, decisive person who must often make life-and-death decisions and live with the results of those decisions. The physician, by selection and training, is bright, aggressive, and decisive, and this sometimes may be hard to deal with, but the imperial-type physicians of the past have long since passed away. Their successors have some of the same traits, but they no longer demand as much subservience; they know they have limits; they know that other health professionals exist and have knowledge they must heed. Most do listen; most compromise and accommodate. It is a changed, and still changing, world.

Change is very prominent in the large teaching hospitals where nurses today are doing things that neither they nor physicians ever thought would be nursing functions. They are performing tasks that are new as well as those that were once done by physicians. Though the *theory* of nursing may not have taken such events fully into account, nursing is being *operationally* redefined. There is, of course, no iron-clad definition of what a nurse or a physician is. The terms and the things they describe are human devices applied to a world that is forever changing.

Another attempt to address nursing issues was the formation of the National Commission on Nursing in 1980. This was an independent commission composed of leaders in the fields of nursing, hospital administration, medicine, government, academia, business, and hospital trustees.

They concluded that nurses should be given more responsibility for patient care and be involved along with physicians in decisions affecting patient care. The commission recommended that nurses be included in policy-making in hospitals and be responsible for resources to assure high-quality care (2). They found the nursing profession to be fragmented and urged nurses to agree on common policies in nursing education, credentials, and standards for practice. The commission recommended that the nursing profession develop a curriculum to include a common body of knowledge and skills and a related credentials procedure. They endorsed the trend toward baccalaureate degrees and advanced degrees for clinical specialization, administration, teaching, and research.

A commission to implement these recommendations has met with little success. Meanwhile, better educated, more assertive nurses try to expand their role in the changing, more technological atmosphere of health care. They have established independent practices and are seeking direct reimbursement for services from third-party payers. They have pushed for legislation that would authorize nurse-sponsored organizations to be reimbursed under Medicare Part B for home health visits and a number of other outpatient services. Organized medicine [the American Medical Association (AMA) and other medical professional groups] have to date successfully opposed such legislation. Another area of conflict is the struggle over new regulations to increase restrictions on certified nurse anesthetists; nurse anesthetists believe this is an attempt to eliminate them from the field, leaving medical anesthesiologists in full control of the practice of anesthesia.

Strains between physicians and nurses continue to exist as the nursing role expands and the relationship with physicians becomes more of a collaborative partnership, with nurses being a part of the clinical decision-making process. In 1983, the AMA House of Delegates adopted a statement, designed to ease some of the friction, stating that nurses should not be expected to follow blindly all medical orders and that a nurse may take action contrary to standing orders to protect a patient in an emergency if a physician is not available. The resolution was sending a message to physicians that the nurse has a responsibility to use judgment, too.

Factors Affecting the Supply of Nurses

There are over two million registered nurses in the United States, of which 80 percent are working either full- or part-time. Nevertheless, there is serious concern about a national nursing shortage. The severity of the shortage depends upon the geographical location and types of nurses needed. Although the national shortage is around 11 percent, the shortage in some parts of the country reaches 15 percent. The shortage is most noticeable in hospitals. Some large urban hospitals employ nurses from other countries to help alleviate the shortage.

Several factors contribute to the nursing shortage in hospitals. First, there is an increased ratio of nurses to patients because of increased technology and sicker patients. The ratio has increased from 50 nurses per 100 patients in 1972 to 91 nurses per 100 patients in 1986—an 82 percent increase (3, p. 642). Also, wages and working conditions contribute to the shortage. The wages of hospital nurses compare poorly to female professional and technical workers in other fields. Although the starting salaries of nurses are now comparable to those of college graduates, the maximum average salary is much lower. Women who plan to work a number of years do not find the pay raises and career ladders in nursing that exist in many other professions women now enter. In other words, women today have many more career options in which the economic rewards are greater, their contributions are better recognized, and the hours are more regular. In addition to the low pay and difficult hours, there are other dissatisfactions: short staffing, which prevents nurses from giving optimal care; superiors (especially physicians) who do not listen to or respect their professional abilities; and a lack of authority to make decisions they feel qualified to make. It is interesting to note that according to the National Commission on Nursing, the chief complaint among hospital nurses is a lack of recognition of the services they provide rather than poor wages.

Although nursing school enrollments increased in 1991, there had been a significant decline during the 1980s which contributed to the shortage. Part of the enrollment decline can be attributed to a 50 percent decline in government subsidies to nursing students and nursing schools since 1973. However, a strong publicity campaign, increased salaries, the creation of some career ladders, and an economic recession that makes other professions less attractive has reversed the decline.

Hospitals have taken several measures to improve the recruitment and retention of RNs. Along with substantial salary increases, they are offering flexible staffing, extra pay for nights and weekends, and child care. Hospitals are also restructuring nursing duties to relieve some of the drudgery by decreasing the time spent on non-nursing activities such as housekeeping, bookkeeping, and secretarial chores. Some hospitals have introduced a case management approach to nursing, where a nurse is assigned to a patient and follows the care of the patient for the entire hospital stay. However, more and innovative changes still must be made if the supply of nurses is to meet the demand.

Before these problems can be solved, the dilemmas that have plagued it for more than 110 years—what nursing is, who should practice it, with what preparation, and in what setting (1)—must be addressed. When the nursing profession agrees upon these questions, it can speak with a unified voice to address the larger issues facing it.

Young people are not likely to be attracted to nursing until its image is improved, and until nurses are given appropriate recognition for the vital role they play in health care. Central to any strategy that seeks to improve the situation of nurses and thus alleviate the shortage is the need to recognize the interdependence of nurses, physicians, hospital administrators, third-party payers, and patients. Unless all of these groups are involved in helping to chart nursing's future, it is unlikely that nursing's problems, including the physician-nurse conflicts, will be solved, and until they are solved the care of patients will be adversely affected (4, p. 651).

Clinical Specialists in Nursing

The complexity of the health field results in large measure from the rapid growth of knowledge. We know more and more today, and health practitioners are able to do more. But coping with this new knowledge has forced specialization in nursing as in medicine. Nurses with a baccalaureate degree may undertake graduate study, usually toward a master's degree, in a variety of clinical areas to develop the needed special competence for teaching, for supervision, and for advanced practice. Most of these graduate programs include a formalization, in an educational setting, of developments that occur in practice, just as diploma and, later, baccalaureate educational programs constituted a formalization, in an educational environment, of what was being learned on the job, on the hospital wards.

In addition to training in such clinical specialties as pediatric, obstetric, medical-surgical, psychiatric, anesthesia, and midwifery nursing, there have developed a number of specialized programs, such as public health nursing and nurse practitioner nursing programs. Some nurse practitioner programs train nurses to work on their own in private practice or as equals on a health care team; other programs train nurses to provide primary care in rural and other settings.

Public Health and Community Nursing

Public health nursing, with its focus on preventing disease and promoting health in the community, offers an alternative to hospital care of the sick. It also provides nurses with an opportunity to work more independently than in the hospital. For the most part, public health training is generalized to enable a single well-trained nurse working in the community to recognize and cope with multiple problems that may arise in a family. Generalized training is based on the premise that people and families, rather than diseases or physical situations, should be served. There is some specialized training in such areas as industrial or full-time clinic nursing.

Most state health departments have separate bureaus or divisions of public health nursing, in which public health nurses are employed as advisors to local health departments, boards of education, voluntary health agencies, and other state agencies. They also may conduct in-service training and promote services that are available through the local public health nursing programs.

At the local level, public health nurses are employed by local health departments, where their primary tasks relate to disease prevention and health promotion; and by agencies such as visiting nursing associations, which are primarily concerned with rendering home nursing care to the sick. When employed outside of public health departments, the public health nurse is frequently called a community nurse. The nomenclature, however, is not precise. Some public health departments also call their public health nurses, community nurses.

As the health care system becomes increasingly complex with a proliferation of public, private, and proprietary health service agencies that target specific population groups, there is some concern that the health of the entire community is not being addressed. Health departments and others, for example, are often affected by reimbursement mechanisms and the growth of federal- and state-mandated categorical programs that promote a narrow focus of services. Many nurses without public health preparation work in community settings, and this has resulted in some confusion about what public health nursing is. The Public Health Nursing Section of the American Public Health Association is concerned that public health nursing be defined as more than community nursing and offers the following definition with its emphasis on the health of the entire community (5):

Public health nursing synthesizes the body of knowledge from the public health sciences and professional nursing theories for the purpose of improving the health of the entire community. This goal lies at the heart of primary prevention and health promotion and is the foundation for public health nursing practice. To accomplish this goal, public health nurses work with groups, families, and individuals as well as in multidisciplinary teams and programs. Identifying subgroups (aggregates) within the population which are at high risk of illness, disability, or premature death, and directing resources toward these groups, is the most effective approach for accomplishing the goal of [public health nursing]. Success in reducing the risks and in improving the health of the community depends on the involvement of consumers, especially groups experiencing health risks, and others in the community, in health planning, and in self-help activities.

Nurse Practitioner

Another expanded role for nurses is that of the nurse practitioner who is trained to provide *extended* nursing services in primary care such as history taking, physical examination, ordering laboratory tests, and assuming responsibility for medical management of selected cases with emphasis on primary care. Typically, nurse practitioners graduate from a two-year master's program, but some graduate from shorter certificate programs. Nurse practitioners generally specialize in one of three types of care: infant and child health care, maternity care/family planning, and adult health care. The majority are employed in ambulatory clinical practices, largely community-based clinics. Almost 20 percent are employed in physicians' private practices with few in hospitals and long-term care facilities. The most important reasons nurses give for becoming nurse practitioners are the chance to have a greater influence on patient care and the opportunity for additional learning.

According to the ANA (6):

The median age of nurses graduating from nurse practitioner programs is 30 years; therefore, many of these individuals have a good practice base behind them. Most nurse practitioner graduates choose settings where maldistribution of health care services exists. Experience to date shows that they tend to reside longer in their respective communities and hopefully will become life-long residents.

The nurse practitioner delivers health care which includes not only physical assessment, but also assessment of the emotional and developmental status of an individual and the family as well as an analysis of health behavior.

Nurse practitioners deliver care in a variety of settings including but not limited to homes, ambulatory care centers, [health maintenance organizations], schools, industries, and physicians' offices. Statistics indicate that a large number of nurse practitioners are in rural states and the majority practice in clinics providing direct primary care.

Nurse practitioners practice independently and have a collaborative arrangement with a physician. A collaborative arrangement indicates a cooperation in the management of a patient's health care problem, when necessary. It is assumed that a nurse practitioner functioning "interdependently" has a physician available for ready consultation and that she/he can refer patients easily. Such physician services, whether on site or by telephone or other means, must, of course, be reimbursable under all third-party payment plans. In this way, the client benefits from both the nursing perspective and the medical perspective. The nurse role and the physician role are not merely greater and lesser degrees of a single role, but are coordinate and complementary in providing high-quality primary health care. Each role constitutes a different emphasis of practice. The nurses' emphasis is on the psychosocial needs of patients rather than just the pathological; its emphasis is on preserving wellness, not just curing illness; its emphasis is on the whole patient and on coordinating total health care rather than giving just isolated bits of care.

Almost one third select positions in which they have autonomy. The role of the nurse practitioner has been well accepted by the community, but less by physicians and other health providers. This is because of the changing nature of the physician-nurse relationship, which in the case of the nurse practitioner fluctuates between physicians having supervisory roles and a collaborative role. Along this line it is interesting to note a 1980 study that, when nurse practitioners performed physical examinations, they consulted physicians in one fourth of the cases, and when they were deciding whether to manage a patient or refer the patient to a physician, they consulted a physician in one third of the decisions. Some of the frequency of consultation depended on the availability of the physician, either physically on the premises or by telephone. Nevertheless, as the nurse practitioner continues to make independent judgments, there is some apprehension among other health care providers, particularly as nurse practitioners move from areas in which physicians have been in short supply (inner cities and rural areas) to more affluent locations.

Organizations representing the nation's 22,000 nurse practitioners have been pressuring for an expanded role in health care with greater independence, including third-party reimbursement and prescription-writing privileges. Many physicians, in the current climate of physician oversupply and increased physician competition, view these as intrusions on their turf and oppose them. In fact, nurse practitioners provide some services that can be viewed as substitutes for physician services, so they appear to be another source of the competition facing physicians.

One new place where the nurse practitioner may find a role is in the nation's nursing homes, where, preliminary reports show, they can offer high-quality care under physician supervision. The nursing home environment is a growing area of need and is not threatening to the few physicians working in that area.

Nurse-Midwives

The number of nurse-midwives is increasing in the United States. Although only about 2 percent of the babies born each year are delivered by nurse-midwives, the increase is having an impact on maternal care and the evolving relationship between physicians and nurses. Midwives delivered most newborn Americans until World War I, when medical advances and the acceptance of hospital deliveries resulted in a dramatic decline in the practice of midwifery. In the mid-1960s there were fewer than 300 midwives, but in 1992 there were more than 3,000 certified nurse-midwives. They are trained in programs approved and certified by the American College of Nurse-Midwives. Most work in hospitals where they provide maternity and gynecologic care to women who do not have private physicians. However, a growing number are entering private practice with other nurse-midwives or physicians, or are working for maternity services that are run by nurse-midwives They have traditionally practiced in poor city neighborhoods and in rural areas. Recently, they have increasingly attracted well-educated, middle class women who want to participate in decisions about their care; nurse-midwives in private practice tend to offer personalized, family-centered, low-intervention maternity care. In private practice, nurse-midwives work in collaboration with physicians to whom they refer high-risk patients and those with complications.

Even though they have physician backup, there is considerable opposition from physicians to nurse-midwives opening their own practices. In many instances they and their collaborative physicians have been refused hospital privileges, the authority to admit and care for private patients. This has led in some instances to an increase in out-of-hospital childbirth centers. Another obstacle has been the reluctance of insurance companies to cover patients who use independent midwifery services. However, legislatures in approximately 10 states have recently required companies to reimburse nurse-midwives. Also, in January 1983, nurse-midwives became eligible for Medicaid reimbursement. A midwife-attended birth in a birthing center costs about 50 percent less than a hospital birth.

Doctoral Programs in Nursing

A growing number of nurses are pursuing doctoral education. Most of these doctorates are in fields other than nursing, for example, sociology, psychology, and higher education, principally because until very recently there were only a few doctoral programs in nursing. For some time it was questionable whether there was sufficient knowledge in nursing to justify nursing doctorates, but nurse leaders seem to have answered this in the affirmative and programs are developing.

Nursing Education Approval, Accreditation, and the National League for Nursing

Nursing programs—LPN, diploma, associate degree, and baccalaureate degree—must be approved by an agency of state government if graduates are to be permitted to take the licensing examination. The *state board of nurse examiners* is typically the name of the agency in a state that handles this. This National League for Nursing (NLN) provides a mechanism for academic accreditation over and above the state approval process. The NLN focuses principally on educational programs from LPN, diploma, associate degree, baccalaureate, and advanced degrees. Some disagreement exists with ANA about accreditation of continuing education programs. RNs who are graduates from NLN-accredited programs normally can have their licenses endorsed by other states.

Graduate programs in nursing can be professionally accredited by the NLN. Approval of graduate programs is usually beyond the scope of state government authority. In addition to NLN accreditation, specialty subcomponents of a master's program are sometimes also accredited by a nurse specialty body.

The American Nurses' Association

The American Nurses' Association is a professional association for RNs that establishes and imple-

ments nursing's political and legislative programs, promotes a professional and equitable work environment for nurses, and develops standards that ensure high-quality patient care. It also approves organizations for providing continuing nursing education. The ANA works to increase nurses' pay and negotiates with hospitals and other health care institutions wages and conditions of employment for nurses. It actively lobbies lawmakers and regulators whose decisions impact on nursing concerns. The ANA is a professional organization with a primary focus on nursing practice. It is broadly based and accredits nursing continuing education programs.

Licensed Practical Nurse

The licensed practical nurse (LPN), or the California and Texas licensed vocational nurse (LVN) developed from the nursing shortage that followed World War II when hospitals began to hire them in place of more expensive RNs whenever possible. However, this trend subsided as technological procedures increased and patients who were admitted to hospitals were sicker. LPNs are trained to provide a variety of nursing services to non-acutely ill patients and to assist RNs with the more seriously ill. The LPN training takes, on the average, 12 months to complete and is usually part of public vocational school programs, although some LPN programs are run by hospitals, community colleges, and community agencies. Except in a few community college programs there is no upward mobility for LPNs in nursing, unless they start in one of the other nursing programs from the beginning with no transfer credits. Since the early 1980s the number of LPNs employed by hospitals has dropped, and they are being replaced by RNs (Table 4–2).

Physician Assistants

Physician assistants (PAs) practice medicine with supervision by licensed physicians. As members of the health care team, PAs provide a broad range

TABLE 4–2. Number of Nurses Employed in U.S. Hospitals

Year	Total	RNs		LPNs	
		Number	Percent	Number	Percent
1990	1,077,695	875,714	81	201,981	19
1987	1,042,589	841,351	81	201,238	19
1985	1,007,107	789,670	78	217,437	22
1983	1,029,975	770,863	75	259,112	25

SOURCE: American Hospital Association.

of medical services that would otherwise be provided by physicians (7).

There are more than 20,000 PAs, whose work includes performing physical examinations, ordering and interpreting laboratory tests, diagnosing problems, determining treatments, and other medical procedures. Most PAs work in primary care areas such as family practice, internal medicine, emergency medicine, pediatrics, and obstetrics and gynecology. About 25 percent work in surgery, often acting as first or second assistants in major surgery.

The PA profession was started in the mid-1960s in response to a perceived doctor shortage in order to increase access to medical care and reduce the cost of the services. The first PA training program was started at Duke University in 1966. Originally, most PA programs were designed to capture hospital corpsmen or medics who were leaving the armed forces. Because many of these people had some formal training and usually a considerable amount of experience, it was felt that their talents could be effectively employed in civilian health care. Within 10 years less than half of PAs had a military background and today the vast majority are men and women with no military experience.

There are over 50 accredited educational programs for PAs that are accredited by the Committee on Allied Health Education and Accreditation on behalf of the AMA. Programs are usually affiliated with colleges, university schools of allied health, or medical schools. Almost all programs require one or two years of college with courses in biology and chemistry, but most have a baccalaureate degree. Applicants also should have some previous

health care experience and many are RNs or other allied health professionals.

PA training programs are usually two years in length and are taught mostly by physicians. The first year is devoted to an understanding of medical sciences and the second year involves clinical experiences in the areas of family medicine, internal medicine, surgery, pediatrics, psychiatry, obstetrics and gynecology, and emergency medicine. Three quarters of PA programs offer a baccalaureate degree and eight have master's degree programs.

Most states require PAs to pass a national certifying examination given each year by the National Commission on Certification of Physician Assistants. To maintain certification PAs must take continuing medical education and a recertifying examination every six years. There are more than 20,000 practicing PAs in the United States, more than double the number of just 10 years ago.

Over three quarters of PAs practice in outpatient settings such as doctors' offices, clinics, and HMOs. They often work in rural areas that might not have access to health care otherwise. PAs are qualified to perform between 75 and 80 percent of the most common duties done by physicians and are allowed to prescribe medications in more than 30 states (7). About one quarter practice in inpatient settings, mostly in surgical specialties.

PAs have become attractive to hospitals seeking to reduce costs. There is less money for resident training, and in some crowded specialties in which the number of residents should be reduced, PAs could take on some of their duties. Many hospitals endorse the use of PAs as house staff, because they can be trained for a very specific role and, unlike residents, they stay in that role. A number of studies have shown they can work safely and cost-effectively in hospitals, and their role is expected to increase greatly in that area. Just as with nurse practitioners, physicians are concerned that the PAs' expanding role may reduce the need for physician services and increase the competition among physicians. Nevertheless, with the socio-economic forces changing health care delivery, PAs (as well as nurse practitioners) are likely to play a larger role in the health care system. The differences between nurse practitioners and PAs should be noted. Their training and orientation are different. PAs are more medically oriented, whereas nurse practitioners place more emphasis on patient education and wellness. Both groups seek to extend Medicare coverage for reimbursement of their services.

Pharmacists

Pharmacy is an ancient profession. Certainly it was prominent in seventeenth century England; the practitioners were apothecaries who ran shops and compounded various drugs and medications. The pharmacist today, however, is rarely called on to compound a drug or medication, which now comes packaged from the manufacturer.

There are about 160,000 pharmacists in the United States. They are the third largest group of health care professionals, exceeded only by physicians and nurses. About 75 percent of pharmacists practice in community pharmacies, two thirds as salaried employees and one third as proprietors. In this setting, their main function is to dispense prescription orders written by physicians, dentists, and other prescribers. In addition to the management and administration of the pharmacy, they also make available to the public thousands of items used in health care, ranging from drugs and chemicals to compound prescriptions to sickroom supplies. Increasingly, community pharmacists are spending more time on patient care functions, such as clarifying the patients' understanding of

dosage, advising patients of potential drug-related conditions, and referring patients to other health care resources.

Pharmacists are basically specialists in the science of drugs. They understand the composition as well as the physical and chemical properties of drugs and their impact on both well and sick persons. Therefore, they are able to make recommendations regarding drug therapy to physicians and patients.

Hospital pharmacy is an expanding area. Pharmacists and hospitals are responsible for systems of total control of drug distribution, designed to ensure that each patient receives the appropriate medication in the correct form and dosage at the correct time. They are also an authoritative source of drug information for physicians, nurses, and patients. There are a number of specialized areas within hospital pharmacy such as nuclear pharmacy, drug and poison information, and intravenous therapy. Hospital pharmacists are seeking to change the pharmacy from a *supply* department, which is a product-oriented technical function, to a patient-oriented clinical service in which the pharmacy would be a department of drug experts who would be more involved in monitoring and counseling on matters relating to drugs.

In 1990 there were about 30,000 students enrolled in the 75 schools of pharmacy that are accredited by the American Council of Pharmaceutical Education. Of these, over 11 percent were minority students. Women made up more than 60 percent of the pharmacy students. There was a steady decline in enrollments from 1975 to 1983, as capitation grants from the federal government decreased. Since then enrollments have increased each year. Pharmacy schools, like schools of nursing and medicine and other health training programs, had received capitation grants from the federal government on the condition that they increase enrollments. Enrollments have decreased as capitation funds decreased.

Students are accepted in the pharmacy schools after graduation from high school. There are two first professional degree programs that usually qualify graduates for the licensure examination. The large majority of students enroll in a baccalaureate degree program, which is customarily a five-year program that awards the Bachelor of Science in Pharmacy (BS Pharmacy). There is also a doctor of pharmacy program that usually requires six years to complete; these graduates are awarded the Doctor of Pharmacy (PharmD). Both of these qualify the student to take the National Association of Boards of Pharmacy Licensing Examination (NABPLEX), which must be passed before practicing pharmacy in all states. Each state also requires applicants to take a special examination on the legal aspects of pharmacy practice in that state. A small number of students pursue the Pharm.D. degree after completing the BS Pharmacy program.

Recently, there have been comprehensive curricular changes in pharmacy schools with less emphasis on drug product information and more on the application of that information to the care of the patient. The concept of clinical pharmacy was promoted by the federal government, which required it for capitation grants. The concept requires that the student learn not only how a pharmaceutical product is prepared and how it acts in the body, but also how to counsel patients on the correct use of pharmaceuticals and to become more involved in drug selection process and patient-oriented services.

After graduating from pharmacy school, some students take residency training in institutional pharmacy practice, which is sometimes required for employment both in hospital pharmacy practice and for clinical faculty positions at pharmacy schools. The accrediting body for those programs is the American Society of Hospital Pharmacists.

Dentists

There are currently about 141,000 practicing dentists in the United States, or approximately 56 dentists per 10,000 population. Most of the nation's dentists are in private practice and about 82 percent are general practitioners. Sixty-nine percent of the private practitioners are in solo practice and the rest work with one or more other dentists. The average net income derived from private practice was about $91,000 for solo practitioners and about $97,000 for all independent dentists. Undergraduate predental education and the first two years of their four-year dental school training are very similar to that for medical doctors. Graduates from dental schools are awarded either a DDS (Doctor of Dental Surgery) or DMD (Doctor of Dental Medicine), depending on the school. There are 55 U.S. dental schools, for which the American Dental Association is the accrediting agency. To be licensed, candidates must pass a national written examination *and* pass a clinical examination conducted by licensed dentists from the individual states or from a regional grouping of states. Delaware has a slightly different licensing procedure, which includes an internship.

The widespread use of fluorides has dramatically reduced the incidence of tooth decay in children and has changed the nature of dental practice. Since the 1970s, tooth decay in American children declined 37 percent, according to the National Institute of Dental Research. More time and effort is now spent on other dental problems such as the management of periodontal (gum) disease, which causes about 70 percent of all adult tooth loss, and cosmetic dental procedures.

Approximately 17 percent of dentists are specialists, the most common ones being orthodontics (teeth straightening), oral and maxillofacial surgery, and periodontics (treatment of tissues or gums supporting teeth and underlying bone). To be a certified specialist in the above areas a dentist must have two years of advanced education (three for oral and maxillofacial surgery), in addition to the D.D.S. or D.M.D. degree, and an additional three or four years' experience in the chosen specialty before taking an objective examination and, on passing, securing approval of the chosen specialty board.

Optometrists

An optometrist is a doctor of optometry (OD). The OD degree should not be confused with the DO, the latter being the degree conferred to a doctor of osteopathy, nor should the optometrist be confused with the ophthalmologist, who is a medically qualified physician (MD) with a specialty qualification for diagnosis and treatment of eye conditions. The optometrist is trained and licensed by the state to examine, diagnose, and treat eye and vision conditions; to prescribe and fit eyeglasses, contact lens, and low-vision aids; and to provide vision therapy services.

Optometrists serve as a major point of entry into the vision care system and may refer patients to ophthalmologists or other physicians for treatment of ocular and systemic diseases. Optometry differs from ophthalmology. Optometrists provide the vast majority of primary care services for eye care. Seventy percent of optometrists are self-employed, mostly in solo practice. However, the trend is toward associate or partnership arrangements, which is at least partly due to the high cost of equipment needed to set up a solo practice. There were about 27,000 active optometrists in the United States in 1992. They are trained today at 16 schools of optometry, which are accredited by the Council of Optometric Education. The length of optometric training is four years. Though most schools require at least two years of preoptometric study in a college or university, most optometric students (more than 70 percent) begin professional studies after completion of a baccalaureate degree. Over the past decade, there have been changes in the curricula to emphasize a more comprehensive, holistic approach to patient care. Students are taught how to take a complete medical history and to understand the effects of systemic diseases on the ocular system. Most state licensing boards now accept for licensure the results of a national board examination and also require continuing education as a condition for license renewal, but there is increasing concern in optometry, as in other professions, that participation in continuing edu-

cation courses is no guarantee of competency in practice and of incorporating the latest developments into daily practice. One way an optometrist demonstrates clinical proficiency is by becoming a Fellow of the American Academy of Optometry, which requires careful examination of clinical skills. Fellows of the Academy can be awarded *diplomate* status in specialty areas (e.g., contact lenses, binocular vision, and perception) following further tests.

Allied Health Personnel

The term allied health includes a large number of health-related areas of work that assist, facilitate, and complement the work of physicians and other health professionals. There are 28 allied health training occupations for which there is AMA program accreditation. Accreditation is granted by the AMA's Committee on Allied Health Education and Accreditation (CAHEA), which works collaboratively with the various specialty societies, allied health organizations and societies, educational associations, the American Hospital Association (AHA), and various federal agencies. As with other accrediting bodies, legitimization comes from recognition by the Council on Postsecondary Accreditation (COPA) and the U.S. Department of Education. Table 4–3 lists the AMA-accredited program areas and the number of programs accredited in each category.

There are many other allied health programs accredited by bodies other than CAHEA, such as programs in physiotherapy, occupational therapy, health education, medical dietetics, dental hygiene, and graduate programs in health administration. In addition, there are a large number of other allied health occupations for which there is, at this time, no formal program accrediting process except that some of them are parts of regionally accredited academic institutions. There is a continuing shortage of most allied health personnel, especially in hospitals. Although many new graduates choose the hospital as their first place of employment, many later go into outpatient or other nonhospital

TABLE 4—3. Number of CAHEA-Accredited Programs by Occupational Type and Institutional Sponsorship, 1992

Occupation	Number of Institutions
Anesthesiologists' assistant	2
Cardiovascular technologist	4
Cytotechnologist	48
Diagnostic medical sonographer	47
Electroneurodiagnostic technologist	14
Emergency medical technician-paramedic	77
Histologic technician/technologist	39
Medical assistant	197
Medical illustrator	6
Medical laboratory technician (Associate Degree)	214
Medical laboratory technician (Certificate)	42
Medical record administrator	55
Medical record technician	115
Medical technologist	410
Nuclear medicine technologist	109
Occupational therapist	74
Ophthalmic medical technician	11
Perfusionist	31
Physician assistant	51
Radiation therapy technologist	111
Radiographer	680
Respiratory therapist	263
Respiratory therapy technician	165
Specialist in blood bank technology	28
Surgeon's assistant	3
Surgical technologist	118
Total	2,980

SOURCE: American Medical Association: *Allied Health Education Fact Sheet,* Chicago, 1992.

TABLE 4—4. Allied Health Personnel: Percentage of Full-time Hospital Vacancies, 1991

Occupation	%
Physiotherapists	17%
Occupational therapists	14%
Radiation therapy technicians	13%
Cytotechnologists	12%
Speech pathologists	11%
Nuclear medicine technicians	8%

SOURCE: *American Medical News,* May 18, 1992

settings where the pay is better and the work conditions more appealing. Hospitals have raised salaries and offered overtime pay, incentive bonuses, and innovative scheduling to recruit and retain allied health personnel. Contributing to the shortage is an inadequate number of graduates from many programs. Table 4—4 shows the percent of hospital vacancies for selected allied health personnel.

Podiatrists

The podiatrist is a Doctor of Podiatric Medicine (D.P.M.). Podiatrists diagnose and treat diseases and deformities of the feet. Though they can perform surgical procedures on the foot, prescribe corrective devices and drugs, and administer physiotherapy, the large majority of visits to podiatrists are for soft tissue complaints (e.g., corns and warts) by patients who are seeking relief from discomfort. Most podiatrists are in private practice, and they are often called upon to treat patients in hospitals and nursing homes.

Training normally entails three or four years of prepodiatry study in a college or university (more than 90 percent of the students hold a baccalaureate degree when they begin professional studies), followed by four years of professional training in one of the nation's five accredited colleges of podiatry. Schools are accredited by the Council on Podiatry Education. The national examination, prepared by the National Board of Podiatry, is accepted for licensure by a growing number of states. There are over 10,000 active podiatrists in the U.S.

Chiropractors

Chiropractic is a branch of the healing arts that is concerned with human health and the prevention of disease. Doctors of chiropractic consider man as an integrated being, but give special attention to spinal biomechanics and musculoskeletal, neurological, vascular, and nutritional relationships (8). The word "chiropractic" is derived from Greek words which mean "done by hand." The profession of chiropractic evolved in the United States in the late 1800s and focuses on the treatment of illnesses by chiropractic manipulation, physiotherapy, and dietary counseling. The most characteristic aspect of chiropractic practice is the adjustment of the spinal column and extremities to relieve neurological, muscular, and vascular disturbances. Neuromusculoskeletal conditions account for 85 percent of all conditions treated (8). Sports and back injuries are an important part of chiropractic practice. Chiropractors use standard procedures and tests to diagnose conditions, but rely heavily on roentgenology (x-ray) of the skeletal system as a diagnostic tool.

Chiropractic education consists of a minimum of two years of college with courses in basic sciences and four years of study at a chiropractic college. The first two years of chiropractic college emphasize the biological sciences and clinical disciplines. The last two years emphasize practical studies with about half of the time being spent in college clinics. Upon graduation a Doctor of Chiropractic (DC) degree is awarded, but in order to practice graduates must obtain a license by passing an examination given by state chiropractic boards. The Council on Chiropractic Education is the accrediting agency for chiropractic colleges. There are 14 accredited colleges in the United States and one in Canada. Almost all state boards require graduation from an accredited college for licensure.

There are about 47,500 chiropractors in active practice. The majority are in solo practice; about 25 percent practice in groups. Approximately 30 percent of chiropractors are women. Reimbursement for chiropractic services is authorized for Medicare, Medicaid, state workers' compensation programs, and most private health and accident policies.

The AMA, AHA, and JCAH previously opposed insurance coverage, hospital admitting privileges, and physician referrals to chiropractors, maintaining that there was no scientific evidence of chiropractic's curative powers. Policies have changed and these organizations, although still skeptical, no longer oppose hospital privileges, insurance coverage, and physician referral of patients if the physician is unable to successfully treat certain back problems.

Health Administrators and Health Planners

The health sector is large and complex. It is labor intensive, a heavy user of people, and requires a large amount of money to fuel its operations. Skilled health administrators are much in demand to run the hospitals, nursing homes, primary care centers, health departments, mental health centers and hospitals, home care agencies, and so on. "To run" means to plan the activities, to assemble or secure the resources, and to manage the use of those resources so that the purposes of the organization are fulfilled. Planning is, of course, an essential part of every administrative job, but in the larger organizations, the planning function is frequently delegated to someone whose planning skills are well developed, to allow that person to focus on planning only, and to advise the administrator of what he or she should adopt as the planned course of action for the agency. In recent years, because of the complex interrelationships and dependencies between health agencies and government, specialized health agencies have developed whose principal purpose has been to plan.

Historically, the top administrator in most large health institutions was a physician or a nurse. Few were trained for their administrative roles. Even today, one finds health administrators and health planners who grew or fell into their jobs, whose academic preparation was not geared to either of these roles. In recent years, however, health agencies have turned increasingly to people who have academic training in health administration or health planning. The necessity for specially trained health-oriented people and not just any business administration or planning program graduate stems from the complex nature of the health sector and the historical context within which the agencies and health professions operate. People are needed who understand not only planning and administration but also the special aspects as they apply to the health field—the importance of knowing, in other words, the sociology of medicine and of the various health professions, of knowing about health and sickness and how the professions deal with them, and of understanding the constraints under which the health professionals operate—because the administrator and planner have to apply their skills and adjust to a milieu that is professionally dominated, indeed, professionally controlled. This finds expression in the time-honored doctrine of the doctor-patient relationship, into which there should be no interference. Increasingly there *is* interfer-

ence, some of it necessary because of the growing complexity of medical practice, but the good health administrator and health planner must know how to orchestrate that intercession without prejudicing the confidentiality of the doctor-patient relationship and without prejudicing the ability of the physician to render the best care for the patient. Well-trained health administrators and health planners are sensitive to these special circumstances and are able to apply their administrative or planning skills in that context so that the aims of the agency are achieved in terms of seeing that the highest-quality service is delivered.

The academic training of health administrators and health planners takes place in a number of settings. Until recently, most were trained and awarded a master's degree by a school of public health or a school of health administration. The course of study usually lasted one or two years, depending on the school. Initially, the *schools of public health* were geared to train a variety of public health workers, public health administrators being only one type. Most of the public health administration graduates went to work in public health departments, though in the last few decades graduates have been moving into other health administration areas, also. The *schools of health administration* were primarily geared to the training of hospital administrators. In fact, until about 1970, most of these schools were known as schools of hospital administration. The name change was designed to reflect the recognition by the schools that they were training not only hospital administrators but also administrators for other kinds of health agencies. Some of the schools of health administration were administratively part of schools of public health. Others were associated with schools of business administration. Some were in other organizational units of a university.

The late 1960s witnessed the development of a number of baccalaureate programs in health administration and health planning, and during the 1970s the number of programs grew rapidly. Some programs were geared to hospitals, some to long-term care, some to training generalist health administrators or health planners. During the early development period of the baccalaureate movement, the undergraduate and graduate programs clashed but, over time, worked out most of their differences. Most baccalaureate programs at this time are free standing in that they are baccalaureate programs only, and the faculty do not teach in a graduate program. There are a number of exceptions to this. There is no accrediting process for baccalaureate programs at this time.

A small number of associate degree programs in health administration have developed. The academic setting for these efforts is limited by the nature of professional resources available to these programs. They are too few in number and too small in student body for anyone to determine, at this time, what their future role will be. These programs have the potential for making a significant, positive contribution to the pool of health administrators.

SUMMARY

Nurses

The nursing profession is undergoing significant changes in its educational and training programs, in its nursing responsibilities, and in its relationship to the medical profession.

Historically nurses were trained in nursing schools associated with hospitals. Typically these schools had a three-year program with a large amount of on-the-job training, nursing patients in the hospital. Upon successful completion of the program, graduates were awarded a diploma and became registered nurses (RNs) after they passed the state licensing examination. Forty percent of RNs today are graduates of hospital/diploma schools.

Nursing education programs began to be offered at a few universities during World War I. They awarded a baccalaureate degree instead of a diploma. Baccalaureate graduates had to pass the same state licensing examination taken by diploma graduates to become RNs. Baccalaureate programs are increasing rapidly and their graduates now make up about 30 percent of all RNs.

Community colleges introduced two to two-and-a-half-year programs during the 1950s. Upon completion of those programs, students are awarded an associate degree; on passing the same state licensing examination as taken by the diploma school and college or university graduate, students become RNs. About 25 percent of practicing RNs hold associate degrees.

There are, therefore, three basic pathways to becoming a registered nurse. Each has an academic component; each uses hospital facilities for clinical training; and each graduate becomes an RN by taking the same state examination. There is considerable debate over the comparative operational competencies of the graduates of the different types of programs, but conclusions are difficult to draw because of the great variability among programs within each of the three pathways.

Diploma schools are decreasing primarily because of their cost to hospitals and the difficulty of absorbing those costs when they are not covered by insurance payments. Also, some nurse leaders believe nurses' training should be a part of an educational system and not under the control of a hospital or any other profession. The National Commission of Nursing endorsed the trend toward baccalaureate degrees in 1980. Nursing is also reexamining its role in the medical care system. Some nurse leaders see the associate degree nurse as a technical nurse who would perform those aspects of patient care not delegated to the licensed practical nurse (LPN) and the nurse's aide, while the baccalaureate nurse assumes the role of leader and teacher. Part of the tension arising from modifying nurses' roles involves the nurses' relationship to physicians. Although in the past physicians have dominated nurses, in today's medical world nurses are taking more responsibility for patients' care as new procedures and techniques evolve. However, many nurses want to be more involved along with physicians in decisions affecting patient care.

There has been specialization in nursing, just as in medicine. Public health nursing focuses on preventing disease and promoting health in the community. It also renders home nursing care to the sick along with other community nurses. The nurse practitioners are trained to provide extended nursing services in primary care such as history taking, physical examinations, ordering laboratory tests, and assuming responsibility for the medical management of selected cases, with emphasis on primary care. The majority are employed in ambulatory clinical practices, largely community-based clinics or centers. Some are employed in physicians' offices, hospitals, and at long-term care facilities.

Nurse-midwives are increasing in the United States. Most work in hospitals where they provide maternity and gynecologic care to women who do not have private physicians. Some enter private practice and work in collaboration with physicians to whom they refer high-risk patients and those with complications.

Licensed practical nurses (LPNs) are trained for about 12 months, mostly at public vocational schools. They are prepared to provide a variety of nursing services to nonacutely ill patients and to assist registered nurses with seriously ill patients. There has been a continuing shortage of nurses fluctuating from a slight shortage to a critical shortage depending upon the geographic area and the type of nurse needed.

Physician Assistants

Physician assistants (PAs) have been trained since the mid-1960s to extend the physicians' services by performing comprehensive physical examinations and simple laboratory procedures, providing basic treatment for people with common illnesses, and offering clinical care for routine emergency needs. The typical PA program consists of two years of training in the medical sciences and in clinical skills. To be certified to practice, the PA must graduate from an accredited program and pass a written examination developed by the National Commission on Certification of Physician Assistants. To retain certification, PAs must take continuing education courses, reregister every two

years, and pass a recertification examination every six years. Almost 75 percent of all PAs work with physicians in primary care specialties. Unlike the situation with nurses, when PAs are involved in patient care, the supervising physician is responsible for the PA's performance of duties.

Pharmacists

Pharmacists are the third largest group of health care professionals, exceeded only by nurses and physicians. Most practice in community pharmacies dispensing prescriptions, managing pharmacies, and making available to the public a wide range of items used in health care. They are increasingly involved in patient care functions such as clarifying the patient's understanding of dosage and potential drug-related conditions and referring patients to other health care resources.

The hospital pharmacy is an expanding area in which pharmacists along with hospitals are responsible for drug distribution procedures, ensuring that each patient receives the appropriate medication in the correct form at the correct time. There are two first professional degrees programs that usually qualify graduates for the licensure examination. About 90 percent enroll in a five-year baccalaureate degree program that awards a Bachelor of Science in Pharmacy (BS Pharmacy). About 10 percent enroll in a six-year doctor of pharmacy program and are awarded the Doctor of Pharmacy (PharmD) degree.

Dentists

Predental education and the first two years of the four-year dental school training are very similar to that for medical doctors. Graduates from dental schools are awarded either a Doctor of Dental Surgery (DDS) or a Doctor of Dental Medicine (DMD), depending on the school. Most of the nation's dentists are in private practice, and are general practitioners. Most are in solo practice. Approximately 17 percent of private dentists are specialists, which requires advanced education, experience, and examination to be certified. As tooth decay in American children is declining, dentists are spending more time on other dental problems such as management of periodontal (gum) disease and cosmetic dental procedures.

Optometrists

Optometrists are trained, and licensed by the state, to examine eyes to determine the presence of vision problems and to prescribe and fit eyeglasses. They serve as a major point of entry into the vision care system and may refer patients to ophthalmologists or other physicians for ocular or systemic diseases. Seventy percent of the optometrists are self-employed, mostly in solo practices.

Allied Health Workers

There are 28 allied health training occupations for which there is AMA program accreditation. Hospitals, clinics, blood banks, and junior/community colleges sponsor most allied health programs. There are other allied health programs, such as medical dietetics, dental hygiene, health education, and graduate programs in health administration, which are accredited by other bodies.

Podiatrists

The podiatrist diagnoses and treats diseases and deformities of the feet. Training usually entails three or four years of prepodiatry study at a college or university, followed by four years of training at one of the nation's five accredited colleges of podiatry. Upon successful completion of the program, a Doctor of Podiatric Medicine (DPM) is awarded. The national examination, prepared by the National Board of Podiatry, is accepted for licensure by a growing number of states.

Chiropractors

Chiropractors are health professionals who emphasize the adjustment of the spinal column and extremities to relieve neuromuscular and vascular problems. They are trained at chiropractic colleges and must pass a state licensing examination in order to practice. Payment for their services is covered by government and most private insurance companies. Although the AMA and AHA have opposed chiropractic treatment in the past, their relationship has become more cordial in recent years.

Health Administrators and Health Planners

Skilled health administrators are in demand to manage and plan the resources and activities of hospitals, nursing homes, primary care centers, health departments, and mental health facilities. The need for specially trained health-oriented people and not just any business administration or planning program specialist stems from the complex nature of the health sector and the historical context within which agencies and health professions operate. Academic training for health administrators and health planners takes place at the graduate level in schools of public health, health administration, business administration, and other units of universities. Since the 1960s, a growing number of programs in health administration and health planning have been offered at the baccalaureate level.

DISCUSSION QUESTIONS

1. What are some of the differences in nursing functions and training over the years, and why did they occur?
2. What, in your opinion, caused the tension in the relationship between nurses and physicians, and what solutions can you offer?
3. Is the nurse-midwife a viable part of our present-day health delivery system? Give reasons for your answers.
4. How will physician extenders and allied health workers be viewed by physicians and hospitals in the 1990s?
5. Compare nursing to other professions that require a baccalaureate degree, associate degree, and a high school diploma.

6. What role should nurses play on the health care team in hospitals?

REFERENCES

1. Friedman, E.: Nursing: Breaking the Bonds? *JAMA*, Vol. 264, No. 24, December 26, 1991.
2. National Commission on Nursing: *Summary Report and Recommendations*. Chicago, The Hospital Research and Educational Trust, April 1983.
3. Aiken, L.H., Mullinix, C.F.: The Nurse Shortage, Myth or Reality. *N Engl J Med*, Sept. 3, 1987.
4. Iglehart, J.K.: Problems Facing the Nursing Profession. *N Engl J Med*, Sept. 3, 1987.
5. Public Health Nursing Section, American Public Health Association: *The Definition and Role of Public Health Nursing in the Delivery of Health Care*. Washington, D.C., American Public Health Association, 1981.
6. Hearings before the Subcommittee on Health of the Ways and Means, House of Representatives, 95th Congress, First Session: *Medicare Reimbursement for Physician Extenders, Practicing in Rural Health Clinics*. Serial 95-8, February 28, 1977.
7. American Academy of Physician Assistants: *Physician Assistants: A Quarter Century of Care*. Alexandria, VA, May 1991.
8. American Chiropractic Association: *Chiropractic State of the Art*. Alexandria, VA, 1991.

Chapter 5

History of Hospitals

Religions and wars have had a great influence on the development of hospitals. In earliest times, sickness and disease were thought to be caused by an act against the gods or by an enemy's spell. Curing those affected focused on appeasing the gods, casting out the evil, or lifting the spell. It was only natural, then, that places caring for the sick would be close to religious structures. Attached to Egyptian temples there was often a "house of life" where the sick could stay to be healed or receive comfort from the gods. Priests looked after the patients and prayed with them. Physicians and attendants who had some training also cared for the patients.

In Greece there were temples known as *asclepieia* that would accept the sick, even the lower classes and the poor. There, assistant priests cared for the sick and prepared sacrifices for the gods. It seems probable that there were also hospital-like institutions in large cities where patients paid for their stay and where there was a physician in charge. In the third century B.C., the Romans began to dominate the Mediterranean region and brought Greek concepts of temple medicine and treatments of Greek physicians to Rome. As the Roman armies fought throughout the Mediterranean world, wounded soldiers were nursed in Roman homes near the fields of battle. When the armies began to spread farther and farther from Rome, a series of military hospitals developed. At first they consisted of a series of tents, but later buildings were located at strategic places. Excavation of some of these hospitals revealed that some accommodated up to 200 patients. They had wards, recreation areas, baths, pharmacies, and attendants' rooms. It is thought that similar buildings were provided by the Romans for gladiators and by large plantation owners for their slaves—people who had no homes in which to be cared for when they became ill and who were too valuable to be left to die. There is some evidence that others used these accommodations on plantations from time to time. Thus, in the Roman world there were three types of hospitals: the military/plantation type, the city hospital/dispensary run by physicians, and the temples of Asclepios, the latter two of Greek origin.

In the early Christian era accommodations for pilgrims, wanderers, paupers, the aged, and orphans, as well as the sick, disabled, and insane were combined into one establishment; however, it was not until the twelfth century that the word *hospital* was used. The early establishments were under the supervision of the bishop and managed by deacons. There are records of hospitals being established during the fourth century. For example, Helena, the mother of the Emperor Constantine, built a hospital in Constantinople; St. Ephram founded a hospital in Edessa during an epidemic; and Fabiola, a Christian matron, established the first hospital in Rome. In 325, the Ecumenical Council at Nicaea directed that houses for strangers to service the poor, sick, and travelers be established in each diocese. These charitable endeavors were based on the biblical text that speaks of giving meat to the hungry, drink to the thirsty, lodging to the stranger, and clothes to the naked, as well as visiting the sick and imprisoned. Christianity made the poor and the sick representatives of Jesus. Giving social assistance to these people was an act of mercy that enhanced the religious merit of the provider. Therefore, the Christian charitable establishments combined some or all of the groups in need of help.

It should be emphasized that only those people who had no homes or other means of care were found in these institutions. For all others, the best place for the sick was their own home, where family or servants cared for them.

The combination of an inn for pilgrims and sick care made sense, because many traveled by foot over strange routes, eating strange food that often made them sick along the way. Nursing care thus became an integral part of hospitality for pilgrims.

Usually the hospitality-infirmary units were part of monasteries where monks and nuns cared for sick members of their own community and the destitute who were sick. In general, members of religious orders were better educated than the lay population and received some training in care of the sick.

The Crusades, a series of military expeditions by Christians to free the Holy Land from the Muslims, which began in the eleventh century and lasted until the thirteenth century, prompted the expansion of hospitals and hospices along the routes taken by the Crusaders. Religious orders were established whose main functions were the care of the sick and the defense of the Holy Land. The Knights of St. John, also known as the Hospitalers, established hospitals in Jerusalem, Syria, Cyprus, Rhodes, and Malta. Many other hospitals in Europe were either established or taken over by them. The Hospitalers were forced to leave Jerusalem when the Muslims recaptured the city in 1187. The hospital in Jerusalem was reported to have had around 2,000 patients, both men and women. Other military nursing orders were the Teutonic Knights and Knights of St. Lazarus (originally designated to care for lepers). There were also nursing orders established among regular monks and nuns. As mentioned earlier, most of the hospitals served the traveler, pilgrim, poor, and orphaned in addition to the sick. By the end of the thirteenth century there were approximately 19,000 hospitals scattered throughout Europe.

During the Middle Ages (500–1500) the usual country hospital could accommodate about 25 patients and served the poor in the surrounding area as well as pilgrims and travelers. Most had one or two brothers, perhaps one or two sisters, and a master in charge. They tended the hospital lands, fed the travelers, and cared for the sick.

Urban hospitals were often built of stone and had long halls called wards, with special smaller wards for the very sick. The beds in these hospitals varied in size; some were large enough to accommodate three or four patients and were usually given to pilgrims, travelers, or the poor. According to law, the seriously sick had to have individual beds. Beds had straw mattresses that were seldom changed despite their attractiveness to lice, fleas, and other vermin. The mattresses were covered with linen sheets, and grey quilts were used for warmth. Pillows were made of feathers.

Both male and female patients slept naked except for a nightcap to prevent chills. However, clothes or cloaks were provided when they left the bed. During the winter, the typical hospital was heated by a large fire in each ward, and often iron tubs filled with hot coals were placed in the central aisle. Because of inadequate heating, beds were usually surrounded by curtains to keep out drafts.

Kitchens were often in separate buildings because of fire risks. Usually there were two main meals a day. Bread was the staple food, and meat, mostly mutton, was served when available. Very sick patients were given meat almost every meal if possible. Fish, fresh or salted, was sometimes served. Because many hospitals had some attached land that was cultivated, fruits and vegetables in season, as well as eggs and cheeses, were sometimes on the menu. Milk was seldom served, but most patients were allowed beer or wine.

Very few physicians were attached to hospitals until the beginning of the fourteenth century. Nurses, both men and women, being members of religious orders, had religious duties in addition to their nursing duties. The nursing monks and nuns were as much concerned with the soul as with the body, and religious feelings were also heightened among the sick, particularly those about to die (Fig. 5–1). Therefore, chapels were attached to most hospitals, often in a position so that patients could view the altar and hear the words of the Mass. As the wards became crowded, rather than lengthen them or build separate ones, cross wards became popular. In this arrangement, the altar was in the middle of the cross and each arm of the cross was a ward. Thus, four times as many patients could see and hear the same Mass. The cross form of hospitals was advantageous for religious purposes, but it also improved ventilation and supervision. Nurses could watch four times as many patients in the crossing area as on the single long wards.

The sixteenth century saw the rise of Protestantism with its emphasis on secular, rather than mo-

nastic, living, which resulted in the closing of some monastic hospitals and the dissolution of some nursing orders. Even in Catholic countries, less money was allocated to hospitals and monasteries. During this period, institutional care for the sick suffered a major setback.

With the closing of the monastic hospitals, the care of the sick, poor, and handicapped was provided by secular hospitals. In these cases the monarchs, nobility, and wealthy citizens, rather than the church, were the sponsors, and the costs were paid by citizens. However, during the transitional period, many of the poor and sick suffered from lack of facilities.

An example of this transition is St. Bartholomew's Hospital in London. It was founded in 1123 as a monastic hospital, but during the Reformation, when Henry VIII confiscated church lands, St. Bartholomew's was damaged and abandoned as were other hospitals in the city. From 1536 to 1544 paupers, beggars, cripples, the poor sick, and other destitutes roamed the streets of London with no place to go. The lord mayor of London headed a committee of citizens in petitioning the king to reopen the hospitals. They agreed to pay the operating expenses out of their own pockets. The hospital, along with several others, including one for the poor and insane (Bethlem Hospital, also known as Bedlam) were restored and opened as "Royal Hospitals," which were supported by donations and taxes.

In Catholic countries the long halls and the cross wards remained popular, but hospitals built during the Reformation by wealthy donors resembled country houses or palaces, buildings the donors found comfortable. The designs typically found were medium-sized wards accommodating 12 to 20 patients in a two- or three-story structure. Kitchens, offices, service units, morgues, and sometimes a chapel were on the ground floor. Wards and some private rooms were on the second and third floors. Fireplaces drew off foul air and provided heat. If there were no fireplaces, ventilating shafts were installed. Windows were high above the beds and latrines were placed on each floor.

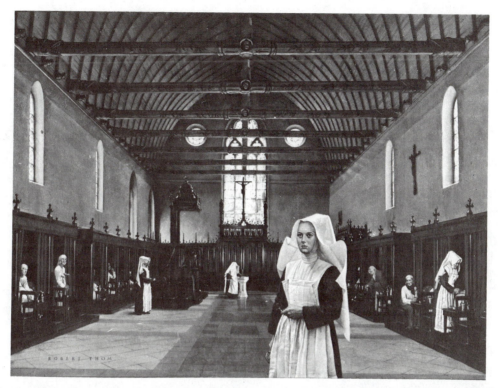

Figure 5–1. Medieval hospitals. The Great Room of the Poor (La Grand Chambre des Povres) is believed to be the world's oldest edifice to have been in continuous use as a hospital. Representative of medieval hospitals, it is part of the Hôtel-Dieu of Beaune, France, founded in 1443. Combined with modern professional hospital service, it carefully preserves the atmosphere of the fifteenth century. A small chapel is located at the end of the room. Sisters of the Congregation of Sainte Marthe, garbed in habits traditional to their ancient order, have cared for the sick, the aged, and the indigent in this hospital for more than 500 years, uninterrupted by wars, economic upheavals, or political changes. (Courtesy, Parke-Davis, Division of Warner-Lambert Company, Morris Plains, NJ.)

From the outside, it was hard to tell a hospital from a wealthy gentleman's home. Still these hospitals were mainly for the impoverished sick, who had no other place to be cared for, and for some travelers.

As the hospitals changed, so did the nursing services. Nursing orders remained in Catholic countries, but Catholic nursing orders organized after 1510 were for women, and in Protestant countries nursing also became women's work. In secular hospitals the matron was in charge, and

nurses were usually illiterate women who were also often alcoholics.

Hospitals in North America

Hospitals came to North America with the Spanish conqueror of Mexico, Hernando Cortez. He established the Hospital of the Immaculate Conception in Mexico City in 1527. The name was later changed to the Hospital of Jesus of Nazareth and still exists today. Soon hospitals were established in most of the major towns of Mexico (then called New Spain).

In 1635 the Hôtel-Dieu, the first hospital in Canada (then New France), was founded in Sillery in Quebec by the Duchess d'Aiguillon. It was staffed by the Augustinian Sisters of Mercy. They also set up an emergency hospital in a cottage to care for victims of a smallpox epidemic and thus established the second hospital in North America. Soon after, in 1644, the Hôtel-Dieu at Montreal was started by the nun Jeanne Mance, and was staffed by three nursing sisters of the St. Joseph de la Fleche order.

One of the earliest hospitals in what was to become the continental United States was established in 1658 in New Amsterdam, now New York City. It consisted of several houses, and it accepted soldiers and black slaves; civilians were not accepted until 1791. The first hospitals in the continental United States that were built specifically to care for the sick in the general population were voluntary hospitals. They were based on the British voluntary hospitals that flourished in the provincial centers outside of London in the eighteenth century. They differed from the earlier Royal Hospitals in Britain in that they were maintained by voluntary contributions, and the consulting physicians served without pay; the Royal Hospitals were maintained by both municipal governments and voluntary contributions, and their physicians were salaried.

The initiative in founding voluntary hospitals came largely from laymen and depended on gifts and subscriptions from donors who, for religious or humanitarian reasons, felt some responsibility for those less fortunate. These hospitals were governed by the wealthy and social elite. Their success depended on the willingness of the wealthy to help the poor because poor sick people were virtually all of the hospital's patients. It was still preferable to endure illnesses at home, if possible, and this the wealthy were better able to do. Britain's first voluntary hospital was established in 1720; numerous reports of success of this and similar hospitals made their way to America and influenced

development and administration of American hospitals.

Pennsylvania Hospital

The Pennsylvania Hospital, in Philadelphia, was the first permanent hospital for civilians in the continental United States and was a voluntary hospital.

During the 1700s, Philadelphia was the largest and most influential city in America. It was the third largest city in the British Empire and was famous for the Quakers (Society of Friends), who were noted for their leadership in humanitarian and scientific undertakings. Because of the number of immigrants who came through the city, there was an increasing number of poor people. It was in this city that Dr. Thomas Bond, a Quaker physician who had studied medicine in London and at the famous French hospital in Paris, Hôtel-Dieu, worked as a port inspector for contagious diseases and saw the need for an institution to care for the city's sick who were destitute. Philadelphia had an almshouse for paupers that gave some medical aid to those who were ill, but its resources were limited and its primary function was not the care of the sick. Also, Philadelphia, like other seaports, had quarantine hospitals to keep victims of smallpox, yellow fever, and other epidemic diseases isolated. These hospitals were closed when epidemics subsided and opened again with the next outbreak. But there were no facilities for the sick poor of the city. Dr. Bond had been involved in several efforts to bring about social improvements through voluntary organizations. Therefore, it seemed natural to establish a hospital in the same way. Around 1750, Dr. Bond began soliciting financial contributions to support the proposed hospital. He was fortunate to have as a friend and advisor Benjamin Franklin, whose strong support convinced others of the need for a hospital for the destitute sick and the mentally ill. A bill to establish a provincial hospital was introduced in the Pennsylvania Assembly. It passed largely because Franklin promised to demonstrate the public's support for a hospital by raising £ 2,000 by voluntary subscriptions. If that amount was raised, the Assembly agreed to allocate an equal amount. Thus, Franklin is thought to be the originator of the concept of "matching money" in government projects. The required amount was raised, and the Governor of Pennsylvania signed the hospital bill in May 1751. The Pennsylvania Hospital was patterned after the British voluntary hospitals.

The charter of the Pennsylvania Hospital stated that the contributors to the hospital had the right to make all laws and regulations relating to the hospital and that they should meet annually and elect 12 of their group to be the board of managers. An important feature of governing the hospitals by laymen was that it limited the physicians' control. Although in most cases the board of managers deferred to the judgment of competent physicians, they could and did overrule the physicians on some occasions.

The board of managers adopted specific rules concerning the admission of patients. It decided to refuse admission to incurables (except "lunatics") and smallpox or "other infectious distemper" victims until proper accommodations were available. It also excluded women whose young children were not cared for elsewhere. Those admitted had to make a travel or burial deposit, so they would not become a charge to the city if they survived and the hospital would not incur a burial expense if they died. Actually, local authorities, philanthropists, or others often provided travel or burial deposits for the sick poor. Also, if there was insufficient accommodation for several equally urgent cases, preference was given to those recommended by contributors to the hospital.

Although it would appear that the Pennsylvania Hospital intended to serve all of the sick poor who suffered from a curable, noncontagious illness, closer examination reveals that it was more concerned with providing for the "useful and laborious" poor rather than those who could work but would not. Both the British and Philadelphians endorsed the value of Christian charity and the potential of hospitals to increase medical knowledge and training, but they were equally concerned

with how to deal with the significant increase in the number of poor people. For many, keeping the poor content and getting poor workers back on the job before their families became a public burden were major reasons for a voluntary hospital. To ensure that the "useful and laborious" poor were admitted, each prospective patient was required to have a letter describing his or her case, signed by an influential person. The sick poor who were turned away from the hospital were forced to go to the local almshouse.

The managers also made provisions to admit paying patients if there was space. Paying patients were usually servants or slaves whose masters paid the bills, paupers whose bills were paid by "overseers of the poor," and the mentally ill from middle- and upper-class families. As a result, the relatives of the insane and masters of servants or slaves often became concerned with conditions at the hospital. This concern resulted in higher standards than were likely to be found in institutions serving only the poor. Usually, paying patients were charged more than the costs they incurred, and the excess money was used to subsidize the sick poor.

The hospital opened in 1752 in a rented private home. It could accommodate 20 patients at a time with a paid matron (to take care of the house and the sick) and three part-time physicians who agreed to serve for three years without pay. It took four years before a building site several blocks beyond Philadelphia's urban population was obtained and before the first wing of the new Pennsylvania Hospital was built and ready for patients. The new building was T-shaped. There was a long hall with a consultation room, apothecary shop, and apartments for the matron and other staff. Perpendicular to the middle of this hall was the men's ward, a hall 80 feet long and 27 feet wide with windows on both sides to provide ventilation. There were rows of beds on each side of the room and a wide aisle down the center. The female ward of the same basic design was on the second floor directly over the men's ward. The second floor also contained several private rooms for paying patients and for those who, because of their condition, were not admitted to the wards. In the basement of the building, below the men's ward, were cells for the insane, baths, the kitchen, and a pantry. Apart from the main building there were a wash house, stable, and garden. The new hospital building was the east wing of a plan for a larger H-shaped building, which would have a central building in the middle of the connecting wing. The total structure was not completed until 1804 (Figs. 5–2 and 5–3).

The building was financed by the subscriptions raised of £2,000 plus the Assembly's matching grant of £2,000, which was restricted to building and furnishing the hospital. Subscriptions in excess of £2,000 constituted the capital stock, which was not to be used but would generate interest to pay for the care of the sick poor.

At first the interest from the capital stock could not fully support the operations of the hospital. Private parties contributed to increase the capital stock, and in 1772 the Pennsylvania Assembly made a grant of £300 to the capital stock of the hospital.

Physicians for the new hospital were selected by the board of managers according to specific regulations. The six physicians (increased from the original three) selected had impressive qualifications (most had some medical training abroad) and served twice a week or a year without pay. Although there was no formal specialization, certain physicians tended to do the surgery, and others took a special interest in the mentally ill.

The administrator of the hospital was the ma-

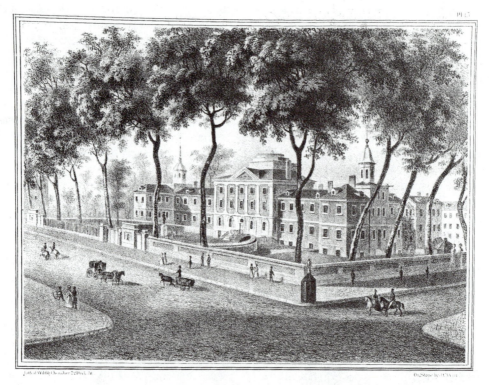

Figure 5–2. Pennsylvania Hospital—an early view. (Courtesy, Pennsylvania Hospital, Philadelphia, PA.)

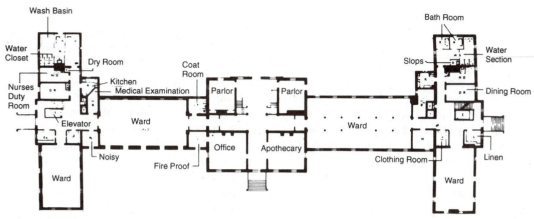

Figure 5–3. Pennsylvania Hospital—original first floor plan, 1775. (From *Report of the Board of Managers of the Pennsylvania Hospital,* 1897.)

tron, who was responsible for the purchasing, bookkeeping, and supervision of all staff except the apothecary. The hospital also hired a steward to assist the matron. Also hired were a male cell keeper to handle the insane, two or three nurses, and several maids. The new hospital also employed a cook, laundress, and gardener.

The hospital could support about 70 free beds, but at times the number of inpatients exceeded 100, about one third of them mentally ill. The number of paying patients varied from 22 percent during the first 10 years to about 13 percent during the second decade. Most of the paying patients were classified as "lunatics." Because paying patients were charged more than their cost of care, every three paying patients supported one poor patient. Although the master of a slave paid for the slave's hospitalization, free blacks were admitted as poor patients on the same basis as whites. Another category of paying patients included those with venereal disease. Venereal disease patients were sometimes required to pay extra fees in Great Britain because of the social implications of the disease. The board of managers in 1763 tried to keep the number of these patients to a minimum by not admitting them unless they were in danger of dying and could not be accommodated elsewhere. The percentage of both paying and non-

paying venereal disease patients was about 11 percent.

The hospital also ran an outpatient department, which, in the middle of the 1770s, was treating almost 200 patients a year.

The Pennsylvania Hospital offered an important opportunity in the training of physicians. In the early years, apprentices of hospital physicians were allowed to visit patients with their mentors without charge, and those apprenticed to nonhospital physicians were charged a fee for visiting the wards. Although students followed the physicians as they attended patients and discussed individual cases, no formal lectures were offered until 1763, when the hospital acquired a series of anatomical drawings and initiated lectures on anatomy for which all students paid a fee. Later, cadavers were used in the classes. The hospital also taught courses required by the College of Philadelphia's medical school (later known as the University of Pennsylvania School of Medicine). From 1762 on, the hospital had a medical library.

Between 1775 and 1783, the Pennsylvania Hospital endured a very difficult period because of the impact of the American Revolution. From its inception and through the Revolution, the board of managers had been composed predominantly of Quakers. Most of the Quakers were either neutral or passive loyalists during the Revolution. These leanings created hostile feelings from the revolutionary government in Pennsylvania and much of the public. This hostility, combined with the unsettled financial situation during that period and with the necessity of caring at different times for both Continental and British soldiers, resulted in decreased funding for the hospital. Conditions at the hospital deteriorated, and the mortality rate climbed from 13 percent during the Colonial period to almost 18 percent.

After the Revolution, conditions at the hospital improved and the mortality rate declined, but the hospital for many years could not afford to support the same number of sick poor as it had cared for in 1775. For one thing, the public seemed to be less interested in supporting public welfare institutions than it had been before the Revolution. Another change was that the board of managers was no longer composed mainly of Philadelphia's wealthiest and most distinguished citizens, but increasingly of merchants who were wealthy but who were not part of the political leadership of the city or the state. Rising costs were another factor that slowed the recovery of the hospital. Between the early 1770s and 1790s, the cost of caring for a patient rose 83 percent, which put a tremendous burden on the hospital's capital stock. Almost 57 percent more funds were needed in capital stock in 1793 to produce the income to support one poor patient. Maintenance work on the hospital, which had been neglected during the war, was also needed.

Despite these difficulties the board decided to complete the hospital by erecting a west wing and a central building. This decision was influenced by the fact that although the number of sick poor patients declined, the number of insane patients continued to increase, to the point that they were often housed in the wards with other patients. Most of the building funds were obtained from the Pennsylvania legislature, the rest from private donations. By 1798 the west wing was completed and by 1801 the center building was essentially completed. The west wing was used almost exclusively

for the insane. The center building buffered the physically ill from the mentally ill and housed the administrative offices, library, apothecary shop, and the living quarters for some of the staff. The operating room on the third floor of the center building was not ready for use until 1804. A skylight provided light for all but the most delicate operations. It also had an amphitheater that could accommodate 300 persons. The surgery at that time was very limited, because anesthesia had not yet been developed and infection was almost certain to occur because its cause and prevention were unknown at that time. Therefore, operations in the thoracic or abdominal cavities were rare. Most surgery was related to fractures and dislocations, and suturing muscles and tendons. Other surgical procedures were amputations and the removal of tumors. Lithotomies (surgical incision of the urinary bladder for removal of a stone) were also performed.

The number of sick poor seeking medical care at the hospital decreased somewhat with the opening of the Philadelphia Dispensary (an outpatient facility) in 1786, but the hospital still could not accommodate all of the sick poor who applied, not for lack of space, but for lack of money to provide food and services. By 1796, the board limited the number of nonpaying patients to 30 at one time, plus emergencies, because of limited financial resources. During that period there were twice as many mentally as physically ill patients at the hospital.

The practice of curious and sadistic visitors amusing themselves by watching and taunting the insane had begun in the Colonial period and continued to be condoned by the board of managers. They charged an admission fee for such visits. The cells for the insane were damp and cold, and attempts to heat them were unsatisfactory. As the number of insane inmates increased, a two-story brick building was built in 1825 for female patients on the corner of the hospital grounds. When the number of patients with mental disorders continued to increase, the board of managers decided to separate the physically ill from the mentally ill.

In 1841, all the insane patients were moved to a new building capable of accommodating 170 patients. The building was erected on nine and a half acres of land in west Philadelphia.

The main forms of therapy for the insane, as well as for many of the physically ill in the late 1700s, were bleeding and purging. At that time, physicians had little beyond their five senses and their experience to aid them in the diagnosis and treatment of medical conditions. The stethoscope and x-rays had not been discovered, the clinical thermometer was not in use, and the microscope was not used for medical diagnoses.

The first specialty officially recognized by the board of managers was obstetrics. In 1803 a "lying-in" ward was opened in the east wing of the hospital. However, those were the days before aseptic procedures; puerperal, or childbed, fever occurred repeatedly and forced the permanent closing of the maternity department in 1854.

During the nineteenth century the United States experienced dramatic growth in territory, population, and industry. New York became the largest and most influential city. Municipal and state hospitals were becoming permanent, and the role of hospital leadership passed from Pennsylvania Hospital to hospitals in New York and Boston.

The New York Hospital

The New York Hospital was the second of the three most important voluntary hospitals. It was chartered in 1771 by King George III at the request of a group of citizens headed by Dr. Samuel Bard. It was to provide care for the sick poor and instruction to medical students of the Columbia Medical School. The hospital was completed in 1775, but it was almost completely destroyed by fire before any patients could be admitted. By the time it was repaired, the Revolution had begun and the British used the building as a barracks. The first civilian patients were not admitted until 1791. The three-story hospital was built in an H shape. By 1811, the hospital accommodated about 300 patients; approximately 16 patients occupied each of the 14

wards. Although the hospital's main purpose was to accommodate the sick poor, those patients who were able were expected to pay some portion of their expenses. Ambulatory patients who were unable to pay donated services such as cleaning rooms, doing laundry, or nursing others. Incurables and people with contagious diseases such as smallpox or measles were not admitted.

A separate brick building was built to house the mentally ill. All of the insane were paying patients and were for the most part housed in private rooms. By this time the notion that the insane were insensitive to cold had been abandoned, and the rooms were heated by stoves in the basement and pipes running between the rooms. The number of patients soon exceeded the capacity of the facility. A grant from the state legislature enabled the governors of the New York Hospital to build a new, larger building to house the insane.

The New York Hospital received regular, substantial grants from the state which in large part paid for the buildings and allowed the hospital to care for a large number of charity patients (68 percent were charity patients in 1819). Again, only the poorest members of society used the hospital. Although the hospital was dependent on state funds, there was no evidence of state control. The board of governors of the New York Hospital functioned in much the same way as the Pennsylvania Hospital. The visiting governors spent much time deciding on the rate reductions and free admissions for people in special circumstances.

Massachusetts General Hospital

The need for a general hospital had long been recognized in Boston. Being an important seaport, and confronted with many sick and injured seamen with no homes or families to care for them, the city opened the Boston Marine Hospital in 1804 to accommodate about 30 patients. This was possible because Congress, in 1778, enacted a law requiring that 20¢ a month be withheld from the wages of each seaman on American ships to support seamen's hospitals in seaports. This was the first American compulsory health insurance law. Also, Boston, like many other American cities, had an almshouse whose main function was to give food and shelter to the poor, but which also provided a few beds for the poor who were sick. In addition to the lack of facilities for the sick poor, there was a lack of training opportunities for physicians in New England. In a period when medicine was beginning to make relatively significant advances, hospitals were important centers for the dissemination of new knowledge. It was there that a variety of cases with similar clinical symptoms could be studied. Hospital experience was becoming indispensable for the training of new physicians, but few of them could afford to study in Philadelphia. Fewer yet could study in the great hospital systems of London and Paris.

These facts were very much on the minds of a number of the distinguished Bostonians who met in 1810 to consider the establishment of a general hospital for the sick poor, needy pregnant women, and the insane. People who could afford it still preferred to be cared for at home. Supporters of the hospital petitioned the General Court (Massachusetts legislature) for a hospital charter. The problems of the poor and insane were described, but the concluding paragraphs emphasized the need for medical students in New England to have hospital training. They cited the advantages physicians from Philadelphia or New York had where hospital training was available. As in the founding of the Pennsylvania and New York hospitals, a training opportunity for physicians was thus a major factor in establishing the hospital in Boston.

The hospital was incorporated as the Massachusetts General Hospital in 1811. This voluntary hospital was a corporation composed of contributors with 12 trustees, four of whom were to be appointed by a board composed of the governor, lieutenant governor, president of the senate, speaker of the house, and the chaplains of both houses. Thus, the state had a share of control from the beginning. The legislation also granted, as an endowment, the Province House (an unproductive

estate that was initially considered and then rejected as a possible temporary hospital), on the condition that the corporation raise an additional $100 thousand in private subscriptions—again, the concept of matching funds for the establishment of a hospital.

Much like a fundraising drive today, the $100 thousand was raised by dividing the city into small districts, each with solicitors who lived there; organizations were contacted; the clergy supported the solicitation; the power of the press was used. Thus, funds for the hospital were donated not only by the wealthy merchants and upperclass, but also by schoolmasters, grocers, tailors, charitable and humane societies, churches, and others. The legal owner of the hospital was the corporation, which met once a year, but the trustees managed the institution. Government regulation or interference was not a problem, because the trustees were all Federalists with many friends at the state capitol.

The trustees were all aware of the best contemporary designs for hospitals. One trustee visited the hospitals of New York and Philadelphia, and information was gathered on the design of hospitals in Europe. Also, Charles Bulfinch, one of Boston's leading architects, was asked to make recommendations. Finally, an architectural competition was held for the design of the hospital; Bulfinch easily won. The hospital design was rectangular. The first floor housed the kitchens, laundry, a small sick room for dying patients, morgue, storerooms, and ward furnaces that supplied heat by air flues and hot water pumped through pipes. The second and third stories were used to care for the sick. On these floors the wings were composed of a large ward, smaller rooms, water closets (lavatories), and accommodations for nurses and doctors. The water closets made the Massachusetts General Hospital the first U.S. hospital to have interior plumbing. The hospital, noted for its imposing structure and utility of interior design, was completed and ready for patients in 1821 (Fig. 5–4). At this time the structure of the American hospitals was superior to their European counterparts, mainly because

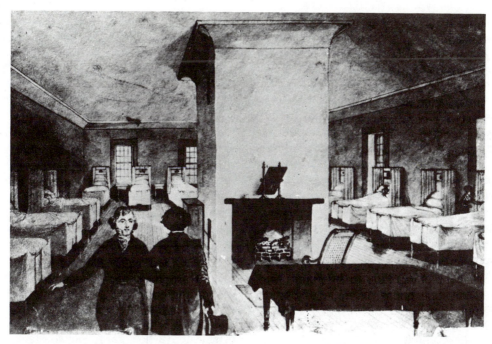

Figure 5–4. Massachusetts General Hospital—patient ward, 1845. (Courtesy, Massachusetts General Hospital, Boston, MA.)

American architects were able to design new buildings, not remodel old ones.

Finances were a major problem for the Massachusetts General Hospital. The operating expenses exceeded the income from endowments; thus, although only half of the hospital beds were occupied, many deserving persons were turned away because of lack of operating funds. In 1825 the Boston trustees proposed a successful method of increasing operating funds called the free bed subscription. People who contributed $100 would support one patient in the hospital free of expense during the following year. People and organizations responded well to the idea, and the drive for free bed subscriptions became an annual event. Because of these subscriptions, the hospital was able to give free care to about 40 percent of its patients, which was comparable to the percent of free beds at the Pennsylvania Hospital during the same period.

An important source of money for the hospital during the early 1800s was the Massachusetts Hospital Life Insurance Company, which, by an 1824 agreement, gave the hospital one third of all its profits over 6 percent and frequently lent money to the hospital. Also, as the reputation of the hospital increased, many citizens remembered it generously in their wills.

The board of trustees met monthly to deal with matters that ranged from ratifying the decisions of the superintendent concerning wages for attendants, building repairs, and purchase of supplies, to the selection of personnel and the investment of the corporation's capital. The admission policy of the hospital followed the precedent set by the Pennsylvania and New York hospitals in forbidding the admission of incurable patients. The reasoning was that the institution was intended to cure disease; if incurable patients were admitted or kept in free beds, there would soon be no room for treating and curing diseases. Therefore, those people with chronic or incurable diseases, except mental disorders, could not be admitted as free patients. If patients were classified as incurable after a reasonable period of time, they were discharged, to the almshouse if they had nowhere else to go. In case of accidents, patients were admitted immediately.

The visiting committee, one of the subcommittees of the board, inspected the hospital routinely and had the power to adjust rates and extend free care. The demand for free beds was so great that the trustees limited the free patient's hospital stay to four weeks unless the attending physician or assistant authorized additional time. In certain instances, the visiting committee would reduce or eliminate patient charges. For example, if the patient was progressing well but had depleted his or her resources, the committee might transfer the patient to a free bed for a few weeks. Sometimes they cancelled small debts of poor patients and even occasionally paid their fares home. On the other hand, the committee, after consulting with the physician or surgeon, sometimes ordered incurable patients to be taken to the almshouse.

One very persuasive reason for establishing a hospital was to provide care for the mentally ill. The care of the insane had been studied in Pennsylvania and New York. In contrast to the Pennsylvania Hospital, insane patients at the Massachusetts General Hospital were housed in a separate building from the beginning. One of the first activities of the board was to purchase an estate overlooking the Charles River, which was designated for the insane and named the McLean Asylum. The patients came from towns and villages throughout New England. The asylum was under the direction of the hospital trustees, but the financial accounting was separate. By this time bleeding and purging were no longer used in the treatment of the insane, and there was an emphasis on keeping the patient usefully occupied in a strict routine. The asylum had both a resident and attending physician.

The Massachusetts General Hospital, like the Pennsylvania and New York hospitals, was a teaching hospital. It provided practical clinical instruction

for the students of the Harvard Medical School. Lecturers in surgery and medicine at the medical school were supplemented with classes at the hospital. In time, the hospital also became the leading New England center for medical research, largely because it had an adequate number of patients to study.

Hospitals in the Western United States

Hospitals moved westward with the population. They appeared along the Mississippi River as navigation increased. In New Orleans, St. John's Hospital (later known as Charity Hospital) was founded in 1736 from an endowment left by a French sailor. It began serving about 24 people, but today Charity Hospital has 3,500 beds. The increased navigation along the Ohio River prompted the township trustees of Cincinnati to rent a house to care for the sick and indigent. In 1821, the Ohio legislature established a hospital to provide facilities for the sick poor, boatmen, and the insane, and to train medical students. At first the hospital was also used as an orphanage and almshouse. Later, the orphans, insane, and paupers were transferred, and the hospital today is known as the Cincinnati General Hospital.

The first hospital west of the Mississippi River was established because of the efforts of the Catholic Bishop of St. Louis. John Mullanphy, an Irish-American trader and merchant in St. Louis, gave some land and had a three-room log cabin built on it. Four Sisters of Charity journeyed from Emmitsburg, Maryland to St. Louis to run the hospital. The sisters used one corner of the kitchen for sleeping; the other two rooms were used for patients. The hospital opened on November 28, 1828 and the cabin was used for four years. As the number of patients increased, old dilapidated wooden houses nearby were also used. By 1832, John Mullanphy and other citizens provided a two-story brick building. That same year, the Asiatic cholera epidemic struck and, because there were no nurses to take charge of the hospital that cared for victims of epidemics, the Sisters of Charity opened their hospital to cholera patients. Because of the heroic part played by the sisters during the epidemic, the Mayor of St. Louis made their hospital the official City Hospital of St. Louis.

In 1845, St. Louis built a new hospital that became the official City Hospital, and the old St. Louis Hospital operated by the Sisters of Charity was renamed the Mullanphy Hospital.

Another cholera epidemic, even more severe than the preceding one, struck St. Louis in 1849 and killed more than 8 percent of the city's population. More than half of the Mullanphy Hospital's patients that year were cholera victims (1,331, of whom 519 died, including two of the sisters). In May 1856 when the City Hospital was destroyed by fire, the patients were transferred to the Mullanphy Hospital. During the Civil War, the Mullanphy Hospital took in the sick and wounded. The need for a larger hospital had been apparent for some time, and by 1874 the Daughters of Charity of St. Vincent de Paul (formerly the Sisters of Charity) took possession of a new and larger building, financed in part by the sale of the property given to the Sisters of Charity by John Mullanphy.

Mullanphy Hospital was the first private institution in the west to establish a regular nursing school, and the first hospital in the United States to establish a maternity hospital and foundling asylum. Mullanphy Hospital was also a teaching hospital for the Washington University Medical School. After a tornado virtually destroyed the hospital in 1927, a larger institution was built at a new site and was named De Paul Hospital to honor St. Vincent de Paul, who was instrumental in establishing the Daughters of Charity of St. Vincent de Paul.

Nightingale Hospitals

Florence Nightingale had a significant impact on the history of hospitals. Although Florence Nightingale is widely known for her reforms in the nursing profession, she also made a far-reaching contribution to the design and management of hospitals. During the Crimean War she took 38 nurses to the British Army military hospital at Scutari. She led an official government expedition, which was formed in response to public awareness of the lack of care and horrible suffering that wounded British soldiers were enduring. Until then, there were no nursing services for British soldiers. When she and her nurses arrived at Scutari in Turkey with supplies and equipment, she found a filthy, rat-ridden hospital in a converted Turkish barracks. It had no equipment or procedures to feed patients even at a subsistence level. The injured lay on floors in bloody blankets, were barely fed, and most wounds were untreated because of a severe shortage of surgeons. The mortality rate was 43 percent, due more to hospital fever (probably typhus) and dysentery than to war injuries. Even under these circumstances, the Nightingale nurses were refused access to the wards by the understaffed, overworked surgeons, who were disturbed mainly because they were women. The place where the surgeons least resented their influence was in the kitchen, so rather than nursing, the female group set up a kitchen. Only with the near collapse of the British Army were the nurses allowed in the wards. Once there, they cleaned up the hospital, paying particular attention to the useless overflowing lavatories, established laundry facilities, and began to attend the injured. By default, Nightingale also found herself managing and procuring supplies for the hospital.

After her return to England she wrote two important works: *Notes on Hospitals* (1858) and *Notes on Nursing* (1859). In her *Notes on Hospitals,* she brought together her vast experience and knowledge of hospital conditions. She did not limit herself to military hospitals, but advised on the construction of general hospitals as well. Her experience included visiting virtually all the hospitals in London, Dublin, and Edinburgh; country, naval, and military hospitals in England; and hospitals in France, Germany, Italy, and Belgium.

In the 1850s, the relationship between filth and disease was recognized, and sanitary measures for preventing disease were accepted. At that time, the prevalent theory of disease was that a vaporous emanation from humans could "enter into the putrefactive condition," causing disease. The germ theory of disease was yet to come.

In Nightingale's design, the dangerous emanations were quickly and continually removed by proper ventilation. The dominating theme of the Nightingale ward was pure air. To deprive the sick of pure air "is nothing but manslaughter under the garb of benevolence," according to her.

Her ideal ward, described in *Notes on Hospitals,* was oblong with windows on each side extending from two feet from the floor to one foot from the ceiling. Windows should make up one third of wall space, and there should be one window for every two beds. The wards should be 111 to 128 feet long, 30 feet wide, and 16 to 17 feet high. These dimensions were all calculated to provide the optimal flow of air. There should be 30 to 32 patients in the ward, each bed with 8×12 feet of "territory to itself." The water closets, lavatory, and baths, independently ventilated, should be located at the far end of the ward. The head nurse's room should be at the entrance to the ward with a window onto the ward so she could see all of the patients. Behind the nurse's room she called for a room for cleaning and storing dishes, washing vegetables, and the like. Fireplaces in the center of the ward would serve for both heating and further ventilation. Each ward should open onto a long corridor. This was the basic design for a pavilion hospital (Fig. 5–5).

Nightingale consulted and advised on the construction of hospitals both in England and America. Wards designed on these principles were used in the United States and Britain until recently.

Scientific Advances Influencing Hospital Care

Advances in science and medicine during the mid-nineteenth century revolutionized medicine and had a great impact on hospitals. Hospitals became important centers for disseminating new knowledge and places where all classes of society could benefit from treatment.

Surgery was radically changed with improved ways to deaden pain during operations. Until the mid-1800s, operations were limited mainly to amputations, repairing wounds, setting fractures, reducing dislocations, suturing muscles and tendons, and removing kidney stones and some tumors. Pain was somewhat lessened by giving large doses of brandy, wine, opium, henbane (a plant extract resembling belladonna), by constricting the limb above the portion to be amputated, and by hypnotism. Morphine was not introduced into general practice until 1844. In 1846, ether was first used for an operation at the Massachusetts General Hospital. From that date, operations could be performed on the inner cavities of the body without pain, but most patients died nonetheless from subsequent infection.

In 1865, an English surgeon, Joseph Lister, dramatically reduced surgical infections by using carbolic acid sprays during surgery. Lister postulated that microorganisms in the air caused infection. Later he realized that the organisms were also present on hands and instruments and insisted on the use of antiseptics on hands, instruments, and dressings. His introduction of antiseptic procedures was based on the work of the French chemist, Louis Pasteur, who, in opposing the theory of spontaneous generation, showed that organisms found in putrefying materials originated from the organisms found in the air. The introduction of antiseptics so revolutionized surgery that the history of surgery can be divided into two periods, pre-Listerian and post-Listerian.

Before Lister, Oliver Wendell Holmes, a physician at Harvard, observed that puerperal (childbed) fever was a contagious disease that was transmitted by the unclean hands and clothing of doctors and midwives (from other women having the disease or from patients with infections) to women undergoing childbirth. During the same period Ignaz Semmelweis, a Hungarian doctor, also concluded that unclean hands and clothing, as well as unsanitary hospital conditions, transmitted childbed fever, which killed 12 mothers out of every 100 in the Vienna General Hospital where he worked. By

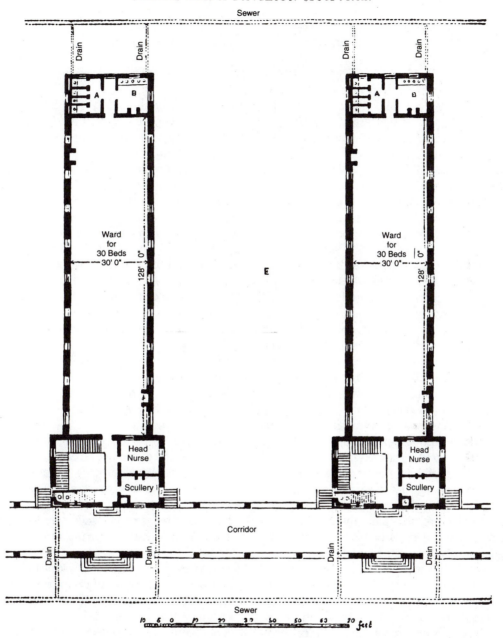

DESIGN FOR A PAVILION HOSPITAL.

A. Ward Closets.
B. Bath and Lavatory.
C. Lift in Scullery.

D. Private Closet.
E. Ornamental Ground.
Ward Windows to be 4 ft. 8 in. in the clear.

Figure 5–5. Pavilion Hospital—plan of the Nightingale ward. (From Nightingale, *Notes on Hospitals,* 1859.)

introducing antiseptic methods, he was able to reduce the maternal mortality resulting from childbed fever to only 1 to 2 percent. He was ridiculed for his work, and it was not until Lister's work that Holmes' and Semmelweis' work was given professional recognition.

The work of Semmelweis, Lister, and Holmes provided some evidence that microorganisms caused human diseases, but it was Robert Koch, a German physician, who firmly established the germ theory of disease in 1876. Since the sixteenth century it was thought that something could be transmitted from a sick person to a well person that caused the well person to become sick. After microorganisms were discovered, it was generally believed that they caused disease, but there was no proof. Koch studied anthrax, a disease of cattle that occasionally occurs in humans. He established that anthrax bacteria were always present in the blood of animals with the disease, and that if blood from an infected animal was injected into a well animal, the well animal would develop anthrax. Koch also grew the bacteria in nutrients outside the animal's body and found that, when those cultured bacteria were injected into a well animal, the animal also developed anthrax. Based on this and other experiments, Koch proved that specific bacteria produce specific diseases.

Using Koch's methods, bacteria that caused a wide variety of contagious diseases were isolated and identified. Once the causative agents were identified, cures were possible either by immunization, using killed bacteria or blood serum from recovered animals, or by other methods.

Koch used the microscope to identify disease-causing bacteria, and Rudolph Virchow used it to study diseased body tissue. In 1893, the first real hospital laboratory was set up in Paris, and laboratories soon became an integral part of every hospital. In the first part of the nineteenth century other instruments such as the stethoscope, clinical thermometer, and sphygmomanometer were introduced to aid in the diagnosis and treatment of disease, and toward the end of the century, Roent-

gen's discovery of the x-ray had an important impact on medical care.

The Johns Hopkins Hospital

The Johns Hopkins Hospital in Baltimore became world renowned because it incorporated many of the advances in hospital design and function, medical education, and medical care.

In 1867, a Baltimore businessman, Johns Hopkins, endowed the city with $7 million to be divided equally for the funding of a university and a hospital. The university and the hospital were to form two separate corporations with separate boards of trustees, but there was some liaison between the two, because several men sat on both boards.

Johns Hopkins purchased the 13-acre site for the hospital and pledged $100 thousand a year toward construction costs while he lived. He died within a year, and the income from the $2 million that he also willed the hospital amounted to approximately $120 thousand a year. The construction was to be financed only from the income; after the hospital was completed, the income was to be used for maintenance.

This was to be no ordinary hospital. Hopkins said it must "compare favorably with any other institution of like character in the country or in Europe." He stipulated that the hospital's staff should be surgeons and physicians of the highest character and greatest skill and that it be used as a teaching hospital for the university's medical school.

In a letter of instruction, Hopkins indicated to the trustees the nature of the hospital. It should be built to accommodate 400 patients, most of whom would be the indigent sick of the city and state. They should be received free of charge without regard to sex, age, or color. There should be space for a limited number of paying patients, and the income from their care should be applied to the care of the poor. Although the administration of the hospital was to be nonsectarian, a religious spirit should be apparent. A training school for female nurses should be established. Hopkins knew that the shape of hospital buildings influenced patient care, and that there was controversy over the best design for hospitals. Realizing the importance of the design to the usefulness of the hospital, he instructed the trustees to solicit the best advice from within this country and Europe concerning the construction and arrangement of the hospital. The hospital trustees interpreted Hopkins' mandate as meaning they should build the best hospital in the world.

In 1875, the trustees invited five eminent physicians, who were experts in hospital construction and management, to submit specific plans for the hospital incorporating the latest concepts of hygiene and treatment.

At this time, hospital designers were confronted with several alternatives. One of the main factors in the high mortality rate in hospitals was the spread of infection within the hospitals. During the Civil War, the use of tents had dramatically reduced the mortality due to infection. The barracks hospital plan had been endorsed by the English Sanitary Commission in 1864 and was used by both the North and the South during the Civil War. It consisted of detached buildings of a temporary nature, which could be destroyed when infection was rampant. Also, there was the pavilion type of hospital advocated by Florence Nightingale. Each of these alternatives could reduce the high rate of infection. It was known that some infective particles may emanate from the sick and cause the same sickness in another person who received the particles.

At that time it was generally felt that air was a major disinfectant, and thus a prime concern of hospitals was ventilation. Separation of patients or increasing the space between them was also recognized as a way to reduce infections. Filth was recognized as a factor in the transmission of disease, and there was also the problem of ridding the building of infection once it had occurred. In that respect the temporary barrack type of ward

with a life expectancy of 15 years was appealing. Nevertheless, all of the hospital planners opted for a permanent building. The plans of the five physicians were published and sent to many interested individuals and institutions for comment and criticism. Because of this and its large endowment, The Johns Hopkins Hospital attracted the interest of hospitals in the United States and Europe.

Dr. John S. Billings, assistant surgeon of the U.S. Army, was selected as the consultant to the hospital. He, with the aid of an architect, drew up new plans, took them to Europe for evaluation, and when he returned, drew up the final set of plans with the architect and the building committee. In the final plans the buildings were built of brick. There was a four-story administration building flanked by two pay wards, one for men and one for women (Fig. 5–6). Behind the male pay ward and to the left was the kitchen building; behind the female pay ward and to the right was the nurses' home. Behind each of the pay wards was an octagonal ward, plus three common wards and an isolating ward which were rectangular. Behind the kitchen was the operating room (amphitheatre), which was connected to the dispensary. The wards and other buildings were connected by a covered corridor. The apothecary was directly behind the administration building, and in the back corners of the property were the pathological institute and the laundry. Much attention was paid to the ventilation of the hospital. On the rectangular and octagonal wards, two types of ventilation were used to see which was better.

The building began in 1877 with the construction of the administration building and the two pay wards and continued for 12 years, because only the income from the endowment could be used. When the income was expended, construction ceased until the income accumulated again. Finally, in 1885, the hospital was opened for patients.

An important function of the hospital was its integration with the medical school's curriculum.

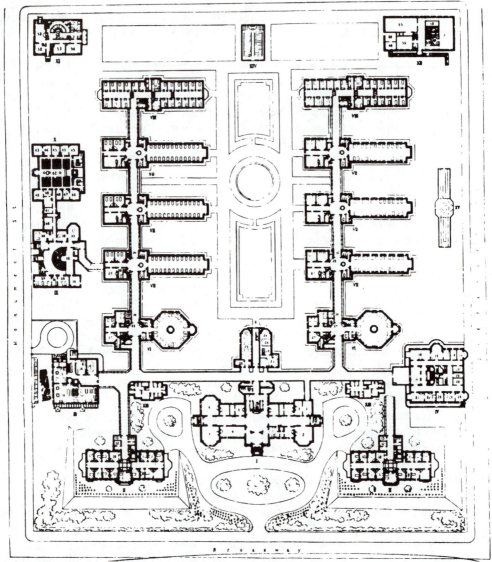

Figure 5–6. Johns Hopkins Hospital—final plan by John S. Billings, 1876. (From Ochsner and Sturm, *The Organization, Construction and Management of Hospitals,* 1907.)

The clinical methods established at the hospital enhanced research and promoted improved teaching of future physicians.

The nurse training school introduced a two-year course of systematized instruction at the hospital rather than the usual practice of placing nursing students with private families during the second year.

A very generous endowment, international consultation, early recruitment of leading clinicians, and careful planning resulted in a hospital with a worldwide reputation for excellence to which others would look for many decades for the latest and best in medical care and training (Figs. 5–6 and 5–7).

Increased knowledge, new technology, and societal pressures caused hospitals to modify and develop as the decades advanced. Hospitals changed in many ways. For example, when the principle of the germ theory of disease became understood and aseptic techniques were practiced and hospital infections began to decrease, the type of patient changed. It became advantageous for sick people, regardless of their financial status, to be treated in hospitals. The number of separate paying patient wards and expensive private rooms increased, and this is turn altered the way in which hospitals were financed. Additionally, as the number of paying patients increased, there was an increasing patient demand for privacy, which led to the replacement of the large pay bed wards with semiprivate rooms accommodating two to four patients. This development forced changes in the nursing supervision of patients and also increased

construction and operating costs. Infection control also affected hospital planning. No longer was it necessary to have separate buildings or separate floors for certain conditions.

With the introduction of iron and steel for construction, along with the development of elevators, hospitals could be built with multiple stories and occupy less ground space, a most fortunate development as city populations grew and land prices rose.

Changes in the American hospital in the past 50 years have been dramatic. "Nevertheless, the modern hospital's basic shape had been established by 1920. It had become central to medical education and was well integrated into the career patterns of regular physicians; in urban areas it had already replaced the family as the site for treating serious illness and managing death. Perhaps most important, it had already been clothed with a legitimizing aura of science and almost boundless social expectation" (12).

Hospitals are still evolving in response to tech-

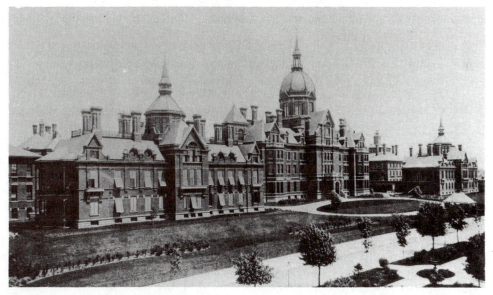

Figure 5–7. The Johns Hopkins Hospital. The building behind the oval in this old photograph still stands and continues to serve as the main entrance to the hospital. (Courtesy, The Johns Hopkins Medical Institutions, Baltimore, MD.)

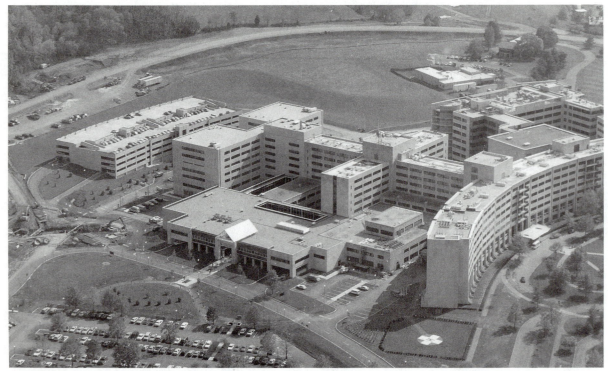

Figure 5–8. Penn State's Milton S. Hershey Medical Center is the home of Penn State University Children's Hospital, University Hospital, and the College of Medicine. (Courtesy, The Milton S. Hershey Medical Center, Hershey, PA.)

nological developments, societal needs, and pressures from special interest groups (Fig. 5–8).

SUMMARY

Early hospital development in western Europe was the result of Christian concern for the poor and the sick. The churches established and ran institutions that not only took care of the sick, but also helped paupers, travelers, and others in need of care. Only the destitute sick were cared for in these institutions, because it was far more desirable to be cared for at home by family or servants. With the rise of Protestantism in the sixteenth century many monastic hospitals closed and monastic nursing orders declined. The care of the sick, poor, and handicapped was taken over to a large extent by secular hospitals that were supported by donations and taxes.

Voluntary hospitals developed in Great Britain during the eighteenth century. These hospitals were governed by the wealthy and social elite and were maintained by voluntary contributions from people who felt an obligation to aid the poor sick. The British voluntary hospital greatly influenced the development of hospitals in America. The first three permanent hospitals built specifically for sick civilians in America were voluntary hospitals. They were governed by an elected or appointed board of laymen which adopted specific rules concerning the admission of patients, patient charges, and the administration of the hospital. Buildings were financed by a combination of state government grants and voluntary contributions. In the case of the Pennsylvania Hospital, the Pennsylvania Assembly allocated funds for the hospital on the condition that an equal amount be raised by voluntary contributions. Thus, the concept of "matching money" in government projects originated. The three voluntary hospitals accumulated capital stock from voluntary donations and in some cases by government grants, and the interest was used for operating costs. Matrons were the administrators of the hospitals; physicians considered it a prestigious event to be selected by the board to serve the hospital, and they served part-time without pay. The principal reasons for establishing these hospitals were the desire to accommodate the sick poor and the mentally ill, and to train physicians. All three of the hospitals were associated with medical schools.

Although the majority of the patients were the destitute sick, it was still preferable to care for the sick at home; there were some paying patients (i.e., the mentally ill, servants, or slaves). The paying patients were often charged more than the cost of care, and the excess money helped to support the free patients, a practice that still exists today.

The spread of infection within hospitals was a major factor in the high mortality rate of patients. Before the infectious process was thoroughly understood, the primary method of attempting to control infections was "proper" ventilation and adequate space between patients. This influenced the design of hospitals and, based on ventilation considerations, the pavilion type of hospital emerged and was popular in Europe and in America. The typical pavilion hospital was a series of separate wards, each opening onto a long corridor.

An understanding of the infectious process, the introduction of aseptic procedures, and the use of anesthesia, as well as other scientific advances, changed the nature of hospitals. Surgery was no longer limited to minor or heroic procedures; operations could be performed on the thoracic and abdominal cavities of the body. Hospitals, with reduced rates of infection and up-to-date medical equipment, became a desirable place for sick people who could afford to pay, as well as for the poor.

The Johns Hopkins Hospital incorporated the latest advances in nineteenth century hospital design into a pavilion-type structure and integrated the function of the hospital with a medical school curriculum.

Iron and steel construction materials, elevators, the acquisition of advanced technological equipment, desire for privacy, current societal needs, pressure from special interest groups, and changes in types of funding are all factors in the continuing modification and development of hospitals.

REFERENCES

1. Abel-Smith, B.: *The Hospitals in England and Wales, 1800–1948.* Cambridge, Harvard University Press, 1964.
2. Castiglioni, A.: *A History of Medicine.* New York, Alfred Knopf, 1947.
3. Chesney, A.M.: *The Johns Hopkins Hospital and The Johns Hopkins School of Medicine,* Vols. 1–3. Baltimore, The Johns Hopkins Press, 1943.
4. Eaton, L.K.: *New England Hospitals, 1790–1833.* Ann Arbor, University of Michigan Press, 1957.
5. Franklin, B.: *Some Account of the Pennsylvania Hospital.* Baltimore, The Johns Hopkins Press, 1954.
6. Owens, L.M.: *The St. Louis Hospital—1828.* St. Louis, St. Louis Medical Society, 1965.
7. Packard, F.R.: *The Pennsylvania Hospital from 1751 to 1938.* Philadelphia, Engle Press, 1938.
8. Sigerist, H.: *A History of Medicine,* Vol. 2. New York, Oxford University Press, 1961.
9. Thompson, J.D., Goldin, G.: *The Hospital: A Social and Architectural History.* New York and London, Yale University Press, 1975.
10. Walker, K.: *The Story of Medicine.* New York, Oxford University Press, 1955.
11. Williams, W.H.: *America's First Hospital: The Pennsylvania Hospital 1751–1841.* Wayne, Pennsylvania, Haverford Press, 1976.
12. Rosenberg, C.E.: *The Care of Strangers—The Rise of America's Hospital System.* New York, Basic Books, 1987.

Chapter 6

Hospitals

The environment in which hospitals function is changing dramatically, and this is forcing them to make significant changes in the ways in which they are organized and in which they operate. Following World War II the federal government encouraged the construction, expansion, and renovation of hospitals by providing grants under the Hill-Burton construction act, and the results were impressive. New hospitals were built, and existing institutions were expanded and upgraded. Simultaneously, the rapid growth of health insurance, followed by the introduction of Medicare and Medicaid, increased the demand for health care (1, p. 228). Government also facilitated growth by allowing nonprofit hospitals to issue tax-exempt bonds for construction and acquisition of capital intensive new technologies. These developments were in large measure dictated by the development of antibiotics and other new drugs, new anesthetics, new instrumentation, and new knowledge that permitted physicians to treat what was previously untreatable, as well as to treat other patients more effectively.

By the late 1960s and early 1970s, concern began to mount over the rapidly rising cost of health care. Many states passed certificate-of-need (CON) legislation to prohibit the construction or expansion of hospitals unless they could prove more beds were actually needed. As health care costs continued their dramatic climb, government and others encouraged shorter hospital stays and more outpatient services. Corporations, seeking to contain costs incurred by their employees, began to require second opinions about the necessity for surgery before the surgery would be covered by insurance, and they modified their health insurance policies by requiring higher copayments and deductibles. They began to review the length of and necessity for inpatient hospital stays, and encouraged their employees to join cost-effective health maintenance organizations (HMOs) and other alternative delivery systems. A number of state governments started to control the rates charged by hospitals. Then, in 1983, the federal government tried to slow the cost spiral by changing the way it paid hospitals for Medicare patients. These patients accounted for about 40 percent of hospital revenues.

As government and businesses moved to control health costs, hospitals were transformed from expanding institutions with little regard for costs (because they were largely reimbursed for them) into institutions with a declining number of patients situated in an environment that had become very competitive, and in which the payers were questioning the efficiency and quality of their services.

To understand this shift in emphasis one first needs to describe the basic structure of the hospital field, that is, the types of hospitals, the monitoring and accreditation of hospitals, and the finance of hospitals.

Community Hospitals

Community hospitals provide short-term general care and are owned by groups other than the federal government. They constitute 81 percent of the total number of hospitals in the United States and account for 92 percent of all hospital admissions each year. They may be owned by not-for-profit groups, for-profit, or investor-owned groups, or state and local governments. The number of community hospitals, the number of admissions to them, the occupancy rate, and the length of stay at community hospitals have all declined during the past decade (Table 6–1).

The community hospital is the hospital with

TABLE 6–1. Community Hospital Data, 1980 and 1990

	1980	1990	Percent Change
Community hospitals	5,830	5,384	−7.7
Beds (in thousands)	988	927	−6.2
Admissions (in thousands)	36,143	31,181	−13.7
Average length of stay (in days)	7.6	7.2	−4.1
Occupancy rate (%)	75.6	66.8	−11.6
Outpatient visits (in thousands)	202,310	301,329	+48.9

SOURCE: American Hospital Association: *Hospital Trends*. Chicago, 1991.

which we are most familiar. It provides a variety of diagnostic and therapeutic services for both medical and surgical cases. It is usually thought of as an acute, short-term (30 days or less) institution. At its most advanced development, it handles almost every kind of case; it is truly a *general* hospital. But there are, and have always been, compromises of this ideal. In the early part of this century, it was easier for a hospital to approach the ideal, as the ideal was then defined, because the limits of our knowledge and technology did not suggest or permit the sophisticated differentiation that we now find. In those days, there were no antibiotics, no open heart surgery, and much less sophisticated radiologic and pathologic technology, nor were there any of the monitoring devices that one finds today in an intensive-care or coronary-care unit. In those days, the general hospital did do virtually everything, except where tradition, clinical considerations, and/or chronicity dictated that it not handle certain types of cases. For example, with few exceptions, mental patients were relegated to special hospitals. By tradition, they were outside the mainstream of medical care, in large part because the problems those cases presented were beyond clinical competence; the medical doctors simply did not know enough about the problem to know how their skills could be effectively applied. As a result, the problem of mental illness was essentially a chronic disease, although the symptoms were often acute.

Tuberculosis (TB) patients were also separated, and if one goes back far enough, one finds other contagious diseases isolated in special hospitals such as isolation hospitals, fever hospitals, or contagious disease hospitals. In some communities, obstetric and gynecologic cases were reserved for special women's hospitals, and eye, ear, nose, and throat (EENT) cases went to EENT hospitals; nor should one forget the chronic disease hospitals for children with their special services for severe cardiac and orthopedic problems. Frequently, these special hospitals were started by individual physicians who needed a few beds for their own convenience or to minimize risk of infection from other

kinds of cases. Maternity (lying-in) hospitals and
EENT hospitals are examples of these. As we shall
see, many of these private hospitals evolved, over
time, into larger for-profit (proprietary) hospitals
and, in some cases, into community not-for-profit
hospitals.

The compromises today on the ideal model of
a general hospital are very different. No longer is
there the need or justification for separate hospitals
for TB and contagious disease cases. These can
now be prevented or handled on an ambulatory
basis; when hospital care is needed, the services
of a general hospital are usually more appropriate.
Nor is there need for short-term segregation of the
mentally ill, though tradition and limited knowledge
still keep these patients out of most general hospitals. Today the differentiation and the compromises on the ideal model of a general hospital are
dictated largely by technology and cost. Some
kinds of cases require highly trained clinicians
whose skills cannot be maintained unless they are
employed in a large hospital with a high volume
of cases. Open heart surgery would be one example. One would hardly want to be operated on
by a cardiac surgeon whose skill is maintained
solely in a rural 25-bed general hospital. But cost
is another issue, and a related one, for highly
specialized services typically require extensive support from other hospital services. An open heart
surgery team requires, among other things, a good
kidney service and sophisticated laboratory support. Neither of these could be justified clinically
or economically in a 25-bed general hospital. Thus,
general hospitals today are almost always compromises on the ideal, with the smaller hospitals tending to compromise more than the larger ones.
Table 6–2 shows the increasing percentage of
community hospitals that provide sophisticated
medical technology not available generally 20 years
ago.

The typical community hospital is nonprofit and
voluntary. It is nonprofit (some use the phrase not-
for-profit), in that it is not required to pay taxes on
its income or property, nor does it distribute any
leftover monies to any individual as profit. It is

**TABLE 6–2. Trends in Selected Medical
Technologies Provided by Community Hospitals,
1985 and 1990**

	Percentage of Hospitals with Technology	
	1985	1990
Angioplasty	0	20.6
Cardiac catheterization	18.4	27.5
Cardiac rehabilitation	0	40.0
CT scanner	55.5	70.1
Lithotripsy	.9	6.3
Magnetic resonance imaging (MRI)	0	18.2
Open heart surgery	12.2	16.8
Organ transplantation	4.9	10.4

SOURCE: American Hospital Association: *Hospital Trends.* Chicago, 1991.

voluntary, because the development and financial
backing of the institution is done voluntarily by
citizens without government coercion.

Responsibility for a community general hospital
rests with a board of trustees, often called a hospital governing board, whose members are elected.
Trustees typically receive no pay for their services
as trustees.

Election methods for trustees vary. Some boards
are highly restrictive and almost self-perpetuating.
In many cases, the trustees are elected by voting
members of the hospital corporation, voting members typically securing the privilege of the ballot by
having contributed to the hospital. The hospital's
charter defines the manner of election. Though
the electorate may be nonrepresentative of the total
community because the eligible voters may be
nonrepresentative (trustees tend to be drawn from
the business, banking, industrial, and professional
leaders in the community), the general view is that
the trustees are nonetheless trustees for the total
community served by the hospital.

The reliance on community business, industrial,
and professional leaders on hospital boards has
longstanding historical roots. These people were
the very ones who could provide leadership in
raising funds to support the hospital, and in a great

many cases they underwrote hospital deficits with personal checks. Though the latter practice has declined sharply, these community leaders still tend to dominate the boards because of their ability to exercise influence on behalf of the hospital, because of their valued entrepreneurial skills that they apply to hospital work without cost to the hospital, and because of their positions, in which they can readily allocate some of their working time to hospital activities.

In recent years court decisions and federal regulations caused hospital boards of trustees to become more active in their oversight role. They are responsible for:

- Developing and monitoring the implementation of policies.
- Hiring and evaluating the performance of the hospital administrator (often called the chief executive officer, or CEO).
- Assessing the hospital's financial status.
- Appointing physicians to the medical staff.
- Assessing the quality of care delivered.
- Developing short- and long-term plans.

The majority of the board's time is spent on financial matters. Although the health professionals decide patient treatment, hospital boards have the legal responsibility for the quality of patient care.

The community general hospital, like most general hospitals, may be large or small, teaching or nonteaching. The size of the hospital, typically indicated by the number of beds, depends on the size of the population served, the range of services provided, and whether it is used as a referral hospital. A small community may only be able to justify a small general hospital, just large enough to support the general run of cases. Depending on the community, this may mean only 6, 20, 75, or 100 beds. Smaller communities must also limit the range of services provided, because the volume of patients may be so small in a specialized area of medicine that not enough patients would use the service to justify the expense of developing and maintaining it. Similarly, in such cases, there would

not be enough cases to enable the specialist to maintain his or her skills. In these instances, the more specialized services needed by a patient would be secured by referring the patient to another facility that has been able to put together and maintain that service. As one looks around the country, one can find a number of large community hospitals in relatively small communities; their size and complexity are justified by the fact that they are referral hospitals. Generally speaking, however, the larger the community served, the larger the hospital, in terms of number of beds, range of specialists, and range of supporting equipment and services.

A community hospital may also be a *teaching hospital*. Teaching hospitals are those hospitals that have an approved residency program. It should be emphasized that the presence of nursing or other health professional programs in a hospital does not define it as a teaching hospital.

It might be noted that historically most teaching hospitals were either public general hospitals for the poor or other types of general hospitals with a large number of indigent patients. These indigent patients were the ones on whom the medical students, interns, and residents learned. The patients, in a sense, paid for their care by allowing their bodies to be used for medical training purposes. The poor frequently resented this form of payment, and they often looked upon the hospital as the place where "they" experimented on patients. It was, in part, this perception by the poor that contributed to the development of Medicaid, under which all people were entitled to private care, but by that time (1966), teaching hospital practice had changed, and all patients, paying as well as indigent, were teaching patients. Medical school hospitals are teaching hospitals that train undergraduate medical students in addition to having residency programs.

Church community general hospitals may be small or large, teaching or nonteaching, or affiliated with medical schools. They are different only in that they are owned or heavily influenced by the churches or church groups that sponsor them. A large number of Protestant denominations and Catholic orders and dioceses own and operate hospitals. Their roles in this field have deep historical roots. Though rooted in a religious denomination, none is discriminatory in terms of access to care (save the limitation dictated by whether or not one's physician has admitting privileges), although a church hospital may be sensitive to the special spiritual or dietary needs of the denomination that sponsors it. Whereas a Lutheran or Catholic hospital may make heroic efforts to meet the dietary needs, for example, of an Orthodox Jew, a Jewish hospital would be geared to meet such needs routinely. It might be noted, with regard to Jewish-sponsored hospitals, that the sponsorship is not by the synagogue or other official body but by the Jewish community.

As suggested earlier, there is a tendency for the churches to lessen the extent of their control of the hospitals. This is reflected in the makeup of their boards, on which nonchurch members serve and fewer church officials and ministers serve. This may be a reflection of the increased secularization in American society as well as recognition of the need for many other talents for the successful direction of a hospital.

State government general hospitals are of three types. First are hospitals owned and operated by the state as part of the state university medical school operations. These hospitals are more or less under the control of the university medical school. The second type of state general hospital is part of the state penal system. The third type, found in some states, are general hospitals to serve poorer sections of the state.

County and city community general hospitals exist in many parts of the country. In the large urban areas, these tend to be indigent hospitals, although since the advent of Medicare and Medicaid and the growth of private health insurance, some of the predominantly indigent hospitals take private patients. The governance of these hospitals by local government varies from the highly political to the highly professional, depending on the style or pattern of political practice in that area. In the

larger cities, these are frequently teaching hospitals and also hospitals with strong medical school ties. Some famous hospitals are in this group, including Bellevue in New York, Cook County in Illinois, and Boston City Hospital.

One other type of governmental general hospital is one established by a special government hospital district or authority. Like school districts, these special governmental authorities typically have certain taxing powers as well as authority to establish and run the hospital. These hospitals tend to be similar to community general hospitals.

University general hospitals are mostly controlled by university medical schools. State universities usually have *de facto* control of the university medical school hospital, although ultimate ownership is by the state government. Other medical schools control their hospitals in similar ways, except that ultimate control may rest with the university board of trustees. There are, of course, many variations and gradations vis-à-vis ownership and control. Some medical schools do not have their own hospitals but rely, instead, on affiliated institutions. Tradition, along with the affiliation agreements, may give the medical school considerable control of the institution even though it does not own or manage it.

Cooperative community hospitals are very similar to community general hospitals, except that they are generally organized with strong consumer control, and medical services are provided by physicians in group practice.

All the above hospitals are nonprofit by virtue of their governmental status or their having met the state's requirements for nonprofit standing.

About 15 percent of community hospitals are *for-profit* or *investor-owned* institutions. They are owned by one person, a group in a partnership, or a corporation. In the United States, these hospitals are often called private hospitals. The word "private," however, can be misleading, for in many other countries "private" refers to nongovernmental, and a private hospital in those countries can be either nonprofit or for-profit.

Over the decades, the situation of these hospitals

has changed considerably. At the time of Flexner, it was estimated that 56 percent of the hospitals in the nation were proprietary (2). There was a steady decline to 25 percent in 1941, and 11 percent in 1968. In recent years, the number of acute investor-owned hospitals and their beds has increased.

Most of the investor-owned hospitals were originally set up by physicians to meet local needs. As one leafs through the *AHA Guide* (3), which is issued annually and lists all hospitals, one can hypothesize that those very small 10- and 13-bed general hospitals that exist today and are owned by individual physicians continue in that tradition. Generally, however, the individual physician-owned hospital has given way to the larger institutions because of population shifts, increased costs, and the necessities of modern clinical practice. Some of the very small institutions that continue to exist undoubtedly have a very limited range of services; in many cases they may be nothing more than facilities for relatively minor cases or holding beds for the eventual transfer of the more acutely ill patient.

Among the investor-owned general hospitals are a number that are controlled by a partnership. These are very similar to the single-ownership hospitals. One finds the partnership arrangement relatively common among the proprietary, nongeneral, or specialized hospitals.

It might be noted here that *doctors'* hospitals, in which the words *doctor* or *doctors* appear, may be for-profit or nonprofit. Some were established, as noted above, to meet community needs, there being no alternative. Some were established as a result of professional conflicts within an existing hospital, one group breaking off to establish its own institution. Some were established by physicians who were unable to secure hospital privileges at existing institutions. Some, as noted with EENT hospitals, may have developed as institutions in which specialized therapy could be administered in what the physician felt was a more controlled environment. Some came about because of physician frustration with lay administration—how the institution was run and what was and was not

purchased. Some were developed as a vehicle for making money over and above the income from professional practice. These reasons apply, of course, to all physician-owned hospitals whether they use the word *doctors* or not. There is a tendency for all of these hospitals to evolve into nonprofit institutions, though this is not without its problems. In mid-1978, in northern Virginia, one such hospital wanted to become a nonprofit institution, but the move was opposed by local government because of the adverse effect this would have on the tax base of local government.

Among the investor-owned hospitals, the corporately owned hospital is perhaps the most important. There have developed a number of corporations that build, own, and/or operate general and special hospitals in the United States and overseas. Most of the firms are small, but some are quite large. The Hospital Corporation of America, for example, which is based in Nashville, owns 74 hospitals in the United States. It manages under contract 200 others. Humana, Inc. of Louisville is another of the large corporations, owning 81 hospitals in the United States. Most of the investor-owned hospitals are members of the American Hospital Association (AHA) and are accredited by the Joint Commission on Accreditation of Healthcare Organizations (JCAHO). Not all investor-owned hospitals are community general hospitals; many are specialized institutions—psychiatric, drug dependency, rehabilitation, and so on.

Some of the community hospitals pay corporations for management services. Some, as we noted from the data cited above, have turned to these corporations to build their hospitals as well.

The investor-owned hospitals are controversial. To appreciate the controversy, one needs to recognize that they still labor under the shadow cast by the very large number of proprietary hospitals that existed before the national hospital accreditation program began in 1952, a shadow that raised many questions about quality of care in proprietary hospitals in terms of the qualifications of the doctors and nurses and the appropriateness of their services, the cleanliness and overall safety of the facility, and so on. The situation is different today in that most of the hospitals are accredited by JCAHO and are further monitored by the Peer Review Organizations (PROs). There are, in other words, no data to support the assertion that quality of care or efficiency of care is below the average standard of the other hospitals.

The investor-owned hospitals suggest that it is possible to provide efficient quality care at costs comparable to or below those of other general hospitals and to make a profit as well. The non-profit hospitals contend, on the other hand, that the proprietary hospitals tend to be small and are thus able to handle the easy cases, leaving the tougher and more expensive kinds of care to the nonprofit institutions. This, the nonprofits argue, forces their average costs up. They also argue that the investor-owned hospitals make a profit on the easy cases, which "profit" in the nonprofit hospitals would be an offset against the more expensive cases. The economics of the health field dictate that the small hospitals can only handle a limited range of clinical cases and cannot justify much of the very sophisticated equipment and services. Significantly, most of these hospitals are located in four states: California, Florida, Tennessee, and Texas.

Carefully controlled studies have been reported (4–6), and their results, as summarized by the editor of *The New England Journal of Medicine,* suggest "that the claims of greater efficiency for the investor-owned chain hospitals cannot be substantiated from their record to date in the three states covered by these studies. Despite their centralized management, the investor-owned chain hospitals have not reduced their operating expenses below those of comparable not-for-profit hospitals, and they have been more costly to those who pay for their services (7)." The editor goes on to conclude that "as businesses, the investor-owned hospital may have been more successful at generating net income (before taxes) for their owners, but only by virtue of charging more per admission, not by operating less expensively. Judged not as businesses but as hospitals . . . they have been *less* cost-effective than their not-for-profit counterparts." In one of the studies (by Pattison and Katz)

it was found that the investor-owned hospitals used more tests and supplies per admission, and charged more for them, which contributed to their increased costs (6).

The description of community general hospitals applies to both *allopathic* and *osteopathic* institutions. Although the allopathic (MD)-oriented institutions predominate in this country, the same types of hospital standards apply also to the hospitals that were established to serve osteopaths. The separation has historical roots that go back to the time when neither would relate to the other school of medicine. But times have changed, and now osteopaths (DOs) serve on the staffs of allopathic institutions and MDs on the staffs of osteopathic hospitals. In some communities, mergers of the institutions have been consummated.

Maternity hospitals, women's hospitals, and EENT hospitals are declining in number and many of them have merged or affiliated with other institutions.

Children's hospitals are community hospitals that typically have special facilities dealing mainly but not exclusively with chronic and congenital cardiac and orthopedic pediatric problems. Whether needed surgical care is performed in these hospitals or in other institutions varies. Advances in technology and scientific medicine generally dictate a close affiliation with other hospitals in order to benefit from the latest instrumentation and the now essential supporting specialties and services. Typically, these hospitals have a strong service in rehabilitation medicine.

Before considering the organization of the community hospital and factors affecting its operation, we might digress briefly to describe some of the other kinds of hospitals that exist. We should note that the American Hospital Association (AHA) classifies obstetric and pediatric hospitals as community hospitals even though each serves a special clientele.

Noncommunity Hospitals

Noncommunity hospitals are defined by the AHA as those hospitals that, in general, care for patients requiring hospital stays longer than 30 days. These include psychiatric hospitals, hospitals for tuberculosis and other respiratory diseases, chronic disease hospitals, institutions for the mentally retarded, alcoholism and chemical dependency hospitals, and other long-term hospitals and hospital units of institutions, including armed services hospitals, veteran's hospitals and Indian Health Service facilities.

Except for the number of nonfederal, for-profit psychiatric hospitals, which has increased almost 30 percent, the number of noncommunity hospital beds decreased in all categories from 1980 to 1990 (Table 6–3). The average length of stay also decreased.

Sponsorship of noncommunity hospitals varies from community to church to government to investor-owned to university. Government control, as we shall note, is particularly prominent in the areas of mental illness and mental retardation.

State governments and, in some instances, local governments have been primarily responsible for establishing facilities for the care of the mentally ill. The *state psychiatric hospitals* have tended to be remote facilities in the countryside, and underfinanced. Patients were frequently there for extended periods of time, sometimes for decades. In recent years, governments have sought to close these facilities, because current theory holds that most of the mentally ill can be dealt with in community settings, either in community facilities or on an outpatient basis. The psychiatric hospital in the United States, as in many other countries, has been called on not only to deal with the mentally ill but also to shelter many aged persons for whom there is no appropriate community facility or home. In government psychiatric hospitals, moreover, one frequently finds mentally retarded patients who were inappropriately placed and sometimes other patients who suffer primarily from chronic physical illnesses.

As large institutions, the need exists for full medical and surgical services as well as psychiatric services. In some hospitals, the surgical services are on the grounds; in other hospitals, the patients are transferred to a community hospital for surgery and, as necessary, for more specialized medical consultation and testing. Because these institutions are underfinanced and consequently understaffed, they have attracted a large number of international medical graduates (IMGs) whose native language is not English and who are not fully licensed. Because care of the mentally ill requires extensive verbal interaction with the patient and understanding of the patient's values and social milieu, the IMG staffing patterns are cause for considerable concern. The concern is heightened when so few of the IMGs pass the state licensing examinations.

TABLE 6–3. Trends in Noncommunity Hospitals, 1980 and 1990

	Number of Hospitals		Number of Beds (in thousands)		Average Length of Stay (in days)	
	1980	1990	1980	1990	1980	1990
Psychiatric hospitals (nonfederal)	534	757	215	160	118	66
Federal hospitals (all types)	361	337	117	98	17	15
TB-respiratory disease hospitals	11	4	2	0	48	62
Long-term hospitals	157	131	39	25	160	88
Hospital units of institutions (e.g., prisons, universities)	74	36	4	2	10	19

SOURCE: American Hospital Association: *Hospital Trends.* Chicago, 1991.

The understaffing of these hospitals has frequently led to a backup of patients in the admission wards with resulting delays in diagnostic workups, delays sometimes lasting more than a month. The understaffing has also led many hospitals to "warehouse" patients, to store them without providing an active treatment program. This has been the subject of some litigation, and courts have been ordering states either to provide treatment or to release the patients. In the 1960s and 1970s with the introduction of new medications for the mentally ill, there was a strong movement to move patients out of psychiatric hospitals and treat them at community mental health centers. The number of patients in state psychiatric hospitals dropped dramatically, but states have been unable to close psychiatric hospitals because they were often located in areas where they were the major source of employment and the political pressure to keep them open was successful despite the small number of inpatients. Unfortunately, deinstitutionalization was often a disaster. Because there were few community treatment facilities, many of the mentally ill were not treated and lived on the streets. The problem has not been corrected.

Nongovernmental psychiatric hospitals have been developed by church groups, by the community, and by investor-owned groups. As mentioned earlier, the investor-owned, or for-profit, hospitals account for the increase in the number of nonfederal hospitals. The nongovernmental hospitals are generally better staffed, providing prompt diagnostic workups and active treatment programs for all patients. The cost is much more than in government institutions.

There is a slight nomenclature issue that ought to be noted. In the general hospital setting, "private" hospitals in the United States are usually equated with "investor-owned" or "for-profit." Although this use of "private" is imprecise, it is still commonly used. In other countries, "private" typically refers to nongovernmental institutions that may be nonprofit or for-profit. The word "private," when applied to mental hospitals in the United States, conforms to the foreign practice and refers

to "nongovernmental," that is, church, voluntary, and investor-owned.

Turning from the mentally ill to the mentally retarded, we find a similar situation; that is, most hospital care is provided in government institutions that tend to be located in remote settings and to be understaffed and underfinanced. Many of these institutions are typically known as *state schools and hospitals*. Training and education are an important part of the work with the mentally retarded; hence the coupling of "state school" with "hospital."

Tuberculosis and other respiratory disease hospitals declined by almost 60 percent between 1980 and 1990 (Table 6–3) and it appeared they would disappear; a new drug-resistant strain of tuberculosis bacteria identified in the early 1990s has been spreading rapidly, however, and may make TB hospitals necessary once again.

There are many kinds of special hospitals for special diseases or conditions such as cancer, leprosy, alcoholism, orthopedics, burns, epilepsy, cardiac ailments, and geriatrics. There are also research hospitals such as the Rockefeller University Hospital (40 beds) in New York City, the Clinical Center (504 beds) of the National Institutes of Health (NIH) in Bethesda, Maryland, or St. Jude Children's Research Hospital (48 beds) in Memphis. One should not forget the college and university infirmaries. Leafing though the *AHA Guide* can be an educational experience in terms of the variety of institutions, their origins (as indicated by their names as well as by type of control), their sizes, their services, and their mergers.

The *federal government* owns and operates general hospitals for clientele for whom it is responsible. Specifically, the federal government, through the Department of Defense, has a large number of army, navy, and air force hospitals. Though some of these hospitals specialize, most are general hospitals. The Veterans Administration (VA) also has a large number of hospitals throughout the country to care for veterans with service-connected disabilities as well as nonservice-connected disabilities when the veteran cannot afford private care. Some of its hospitals are psychiatric, but most are general, with strong rehabilitation medicine services. The Indian Health Service in the Department of Health and Human Services (HSS) has 45 hospitals located on various Indian reservations. General hospital services are also provided by the U.S. Department of Justice for inmates of federal prisons.

One should bear in mind that the definitions that apply to the various hospitals are not rigid. As noted at the outset, all hospitals are in a sense compromises on the concept of the total hospital. Not only do hospitals in each category differ from each other in scope of services, but they also differ in patient mix. Whereas a special hospital may exist in one community, the same kind of hospital in another community may be part of a broader-based institution. Specialized hospitals sometimes developed because of the presence of a benefactor, or because a physician had a unique therapeutic approach that could best or easily be handled separately. What is clear, however, is that rising costs, coupled with new technology and the interdependency of the various specialties, are dictating affiliations and mergers. Completely free-standing institutions, including the very small community general hospitals, are a dying breed.

Regionalization and Multihospital Systems

The future of many community hospitals (especially small, rural hospitals) may well depend in large part on the concept of regionalization whereby small hospitals affiliate with larger, more urban hospitals. Under regionalization, each level of hospital (small rural hospitals, moderate-sized hospitals, and large regional referral centers) would provide only those services that they are able to provide efficiently and effectively. Thus, the small rural hospital would provide basic general care; the moderate-sized hospital, more specialized care and equipment; and the regional hospital, the most sophisticated and expensive special types of care. Patients would have access to a full range of ser-

vices and would be admitted or transferred to the appropriate level of hospital according to their medical needs. With this type of arrangement, hospitals would not have to duplicate expensive services, could obtain consultation assistance from medical personnel in larger hospitals, and would have the advantages of sharing personnel and joint purchasing. The affiliation could range from an informal regional working agreement to a merger of institutions into multihospital or multi-institutional systems with a single, coordinated management structure. Many European countries have regionalized their hospital systems to provide hospital services more efficiently. The occasional hesitancy of small institutions in this country to enter into the more formal regional agreements stems from a longstanding desire for local control, coupled with a fear that the arrangements would serve the financial and occupancy rate needs of the higher-level institution at the expense of the smaller institution.

A recent nationwide survey found that more than one third were affiliated with some type of regional arrangement or multihospital system, either not-for-profit or investor-owned. Hospitals affiliated with multihospital systems charged more, incurred higher expenses per admission, and profited more than freestanding hospitals.

Hospital Statistics

The most reliable source for data about hospitals is the AHA. Each year the AHA conducts a survey of all hospitals that are registered with the association. Not all registered hospitals are accredited institutions or members of the AHA. All registered general hospitals do have, however, at least six inpatient beds, an organized medical staff, continuous nursing services, a pharmacy service supervised by a registered pharmacist, a governing authority and chief executive, up-to-date and complete medical records on each patient, food service, clinical laboratory and diagnostic X-ray services, an operating room, and control of patient admission by the medical staff. Though anatomical pathology services need not be present, they must be regularly and conveniently available (3). Comparable requirements are listed by the AHA for registration of special hospitals. The listings are as complete as one can find. (They include both allopathic and osteopathic facilities.)

The results of the AHA annual survey are published in two volumes each year. One volume, the *AHA Guide* lists all registered hospitals, their addresses and telephone numbers, the names of the administrators, and for each hospital, information about its control, type of services and specific services, whether it is a long-term or short-term stay hospital, as well as data on its admissions, expenses, and personnel. The *Guide* also lists the names, addresses, telephone numbers, and chief executives of a large number of international, national, and state health organizations and agencies. It also lists many of the educational programs in the health field.

The companion volume to the *AHA Guide* is *Hospital Trends* (8), which provides a composite statistical profile of all registered institutions. It does this nationally, by region, and by state. It does it by hospital size and hospital sponsorship. One can quickly ascertain how many hospitals of all types there are in the United States, how many beds they had, and the average occupancy. One can find information on births, the number of bassinets, the number of employees, payroll expenses, costs, revenues, total assets, and average length of stay. There are data on the number of nurses, physicians, dentists, and licensed practical nurses employed by the hospitals; the number of residents and other trainees; the number of surgical operations; and a breakdown of the outpatient visits in categories of emergency, clinic, and referred. There are data on the number of postoperative recovery rooms, intensive care units for cardiac care only, intensive care units for mixed patients, open heart surgery facilities, pharmacies and their staff, X-ray therapy, cobalt therapy, radium therapy, diagnostic radioisotope facilities, therapeutic radioisotope facilities, histopathology laboratories, organ banks, blood banks, electroencephalographic services, re-

spiratory therapy departments, premature nurseries, neonatal intensive care units, self-care units, skilled nursing or long-term care units (many general hospitals have or are developing these units as part of their complexes), hemodialysis services, burn care units, physicotherapy departments, occupational therapy departments, rehabilitation services, psychiatric services (including inpatient, outpatient, partial hospitalization, emergency, foster care and/or home care, consultation, and educational), clinical psychology services, outpatient departments, emergency departments, social work departments, family planning services, genetic counseling services, abortion services, home care departments, dental services, pediatric services, speech pathology services, hospital auxiliaries, volunteer services departments, patient representative services, alcoholism/chemical dependency services, and TB and other respiratory disease units.

Other useful reports are issued periodically by HHS. Among these is *Health•United States,* an annual report by the secretary to the Congress. The National Center for Health Statistics within HHS publishes a large number of reports throughout the year. The Health Care Financing Administration publishes the *Health Care Financing Review* quarterly. These reports and publications relate not only to hospitals but also to other components of the health field. Another useful source of data is the *Source Book of Health Insurance Data,* published annually by the Health Insurance Association of America.

Hospital Organization and Administration

The governing board of a hospital not only establishes policies for the institution but also hires the administrator. The board also grants admitting privileges to physicians and dentists and others, usually on recommendation of the medical staff.

The administrator of a hospital may have been trained for that role with a masters or baccalaureate degree in health administration. Some administrators have no formal academic training in the health field. Many hospitals, however, have as their administrator a nurse; some of these are small rural hospitals; many are Catholic hospitals run by the various nursing orders. The rationale for the nurse as administrator in the smaller hospitals is based on the fact that nurses constitute the largest body of specialized personnel in the institution. These hospitals, moreover, because of their relatively small size, have a limited range of services, and the complexities of management may not require specialized training. Many of the very large hospitals have physicians as administrators, only some of whom have special training. Psychiatric hospitals characteristically have a psychiatrist as administrator.

The word *administrator* is used in a generic sense. Some hospitals designate the top administrative person as *president, chief executive officer* (CEO), *executive director,* or, in many psychiatric hospitals, *superintendent.*

The organizational functioning of a hospital is not as clear-cut as it is in business and industry. The lines of authority are not precise. The board appoints the administrator. The board also appoints the medical staff. Membership on the medical staff allows physicians to admit patients and continue to treat them and call in specialists as needed. Though the medical staff is technically accountable to the board, it has a daily functional relationship with the administrator. Nursing service is administratively accountable to the administrator but professionally accountable to the medical staff. Other personnel, such as the pharmacists, lab and X-ray technicians, and dietitians, are also administratively accountable to the administrator but professionally accountable to the medical staff.

The hospital is really the physician's workshop, although some argue that it is also the center for meeting all community health needs. However, it is only the physician who can admit a patient (except in a few circumscribed areas in which admitting and treatment privileges are held by other health professionals), and all others must act on the physician's orders. But the physician typically does not hire or fire unless, as a member of the medical staff, the physician is an employee of

Sample Corporate Structure for Hospitals

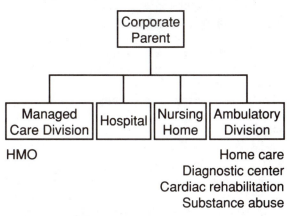

HMO

Home care
Diagnostic center
Cardiac rehabilitation
Substance abuse

Figure 6–1. Sample corporate structure for hospitals.

the hospital. Even then the physician's authority is circumscribed by a certain administrative accountability to the administrator.

Physicians are the driving force in hospitals. They ask that certain procedures be done for the patient and that certain supplies or equipment be purchased. It is up to the administrator and the nurses and others working with the administrator to cooperate to the greatest extent possible with the physician. As one might guess, conflicts occur: personality clashes, misunderstandings, and insufficient funds create problems. The various parties try to resolve differences, figure out ways to get the needed funds, and reach agreement on outstanding issues. When the medical staff and administrator cannot resolve differences, then the board must enter to decide.

Most hospitals minimize tensions between hospital governing boards and the medical staff by having a physician representing the medical staff as a member of the board. Hospitals depend on physicians to refer patients to them and fill their hospital beds. An individual physician may have admitting privileges at several hospitals and choose among them to which hospital they will admit their patients so hospitals try to make theirs the most attractive to the doctor by making his or her dealings with them convenient and pleasant. It sometimes means obtaining equipment the physicians want or prefer. At times physicians and hospitals compete with each other as both develop and expand outpatient services such as freestanding ambulatory and diagnostic centers to improve their financial status.

Hospitals are changing their organizational structure to a corporate model and calling themselves *medical centers* to create fiscal flexibility at a time when there are greater constraints placed upon hospitals by government programs (Fig. 6–1). The corporate model permits a hospital to set up profit-making operations, such as a medical office building or a freestanding clinic, with the profits kept completely separate from hospital operations and thus not taken into account by government, insurance companies, and business coalitions as they identify hospital costs in determining how much the hospital should be paid for care. The profit operations, in other words, cannot be counted as an offset against losses in hospital operations, such as in care of the poor who have no insurance or Medicaid protection. The profits are then free for use as the overall governing body sees fit. Corporate restructuring is a rapidly developing phenomenon, although in 1988 the Congress was considering legislation to curtail such profit-making activities by nonprofit organizations, with much opposition from the AHA.

Despite the varieties and complexities of hospital organization, in practice the hospital tends to function reasonably well; over the years, accepted patterns of functioning have been agreed to so that each group knows what its role is, what its responsibilities are, and what its authority is. The medical staff, in particular, has delegated to it by the board certain professional responsibilities, and these are typically described by the medical staff bylaws, which the board has approved. More importantly, however, the smooth functioning can be attributed to improved quality of administration, which came with the introduction of sound management practices and appropriately trained administrators.

Medical Staff Privileges

Physicians apply to a hospital for staff privileges.* If the hospital is a closed group practice hospital, then the only way to become part of the hospital staff is to be accepted by the medical group. Hospital bylaws define how a physician may secure admitting privileges. Typically, in community general hospitals, the physician who seeks privileges makes application to the board. The board typically seeks the advice of its medical staff, which judges the applicant's qualifications and character and makes a recommendation. The decision about appointment to the medical staff is based on a variety of factors and not just whether the physician is licensed and of good character. Specific questions include the following: What kinds of admitting privileges are sought? Does the physician seek surgical privileges? If so, what kind? Is the applicant qualified for that kind of surgery? Do the qualifications warrant authority to read electrocardiograms? Is the applicant qualified to treat the kinds of patients for whom admitting privileges are sought? Does the hospital have the needed support services for this physician? Are there enough beds to accommodate his or her patients?

The larger and more complex the hospital, the more precisely defined the admitting privileges are. In some remote rural hospitals, a family practitioner may be doing general medical care, reading electrocardiograms, handling obstetrics, and performing a variety of surgical operations. The same physician in a large urban teaching hospital might be restricted to carefully circumscribed family practice privileges with no reading of electrocardiograms, no obstetrics, and no surgery.

Staff privileges also fall into several categories. The *active medical staff* consists of those physicians accorded all rights and privileges and re-

---

*Although dentists, podiatrists, and others may have staff privileges, and though more may be securing privileges in the future, the changes will be extremely slow. It is appropriate, therefore, to be concerned primarily with *physician* privileges, and to continue to refer to the body of admitted professionals as the *medical staff.*

sponsibilities; they provide most of the care, offer leadership in various committees, and may hold a variety of medical staff offices.

Associate medical staff are the more junior physicians or those who wish to become active staff when vacancies occur. Their access to beds for their patients may be limited.

Courtesy medical staff is the category for those physicians who seek the privilege of admitting only occasional patients and who do not wish to become part of the active staff, either because the bulk of their admissions are to other hospitals or because the physicians do not have practices that necessitate frequent admission of patients.

The *consulting medical staff* consists of those who serve primarily as specialty consultants to members of the active staff. In some types of cases, for example, the law or hospital or medical staff bylaws may require the attending physician to secure consultation, and this staff is available in the event an appropriate consultant is not on the active or associate staffs.

The *honorary medical staff* designation is reserved for distinguished physicians whom the hospital may wish to honor, as well as for those members of the active staff who have retired.

The bylaws, rules and regulations, and offices of the medical staff organization vary from hospital to hospital. Typically, however, each staff has what is usually called a *chief of staff.* This physician is usually elected by the medical staff for a fixed term and represents the staff's interests to the board and to the hospital administration. This is the formal line for communication, particularly on major issues, but hospitals also have a wide informal mechanism that functions as the rule. In some hospitals, the chief of staff is called the *medical director.* Usually, this signifies that the physician is fulltime, salaried, and appointed by the board. Fulltime salaried physicians, other than radiologists, pathologists, anesthesiologists, and emergency department physicians, are usually found in the larger teaching hospitals. When a hospital has divided its staff into clinical departments or services, there is

typically a chief of service for each clinical area, and each chief reports to the chief of staff.

Clinical and Supporting Departments

The clinical organization of the general hospital varies depending on its size (typically indicated by the number of beds), the pattern of patient mix among the various specialties, and the extent of specialization of the medical staff. Except in the very small hospitals, obstetrics tends to be segregated in a separate wing or on a separate floor of the hospital along with the newborn nursery. This is principally done to minimize the risk of infection to the newborn and mother. Pediatric cases also tend to be segregated. The assignment of other patients to clinical services or departments varies considerably. If there is any departmental breakdown in the smaller hospitals, it tends to be into medicine and surgery, with patient assignment as appropriate. As specialization increases in a hospital and the volume of patients increases within each specialty, there is a tendency for departments to be established with beds assigned to that specialty. When the volume of patients is sufficient to justify it, the specialty beds may be located in a separate wing or on a separate floor. The establishment of specialty services with assigned beds permits a more effective and efficient concentration of support services peculiar to that specialty— equipment, specially trained nurses, and other personnel—and contributes to the development of the specialty and its scientific work. In very large hospitals, one may find not only separate pediatric and obstetric units but also separate units or floors or wings for most of the medical specialties, and in some cases even for some of the subspecialties.

Though assignment of beds to a given specialty has clinical advantages, it decreases institutional flexibility in terms of bed use. There may be more patients needing admission in medicine, for example, than there are beds to accommodate them, yet there may be empty beds on one of the surgical floors that normally cannot be used for those medical patients. The surgical floor might not be staffed or supplied to handle medical cases, and the surgical specialists would be very upset to find the beds assigned to them used to service medical cases. The surgeons may find, if the beds are used to service medical cases, that they cannot admit their patients, and the delays may well cut into the surgeons' incomes and interfere with efforts to strengthen the surgical service. If a hospital wants to build or strengthen a clinical service, it usually has to give assurances to the specialists that they will have an appropriate environment in which to do their work. Part of that environment is beds.

To illustrate, a community was seeking a urologist for its hospital. One visited, was impressed, and then asked, "How many beds will I have?" He was told that he would have to queue up like the other physicians and get a bed if one was available. The urologist immediately replied, "I have five beds assigned to me in the community where I am presently located; I see no reason why I should move here."

There are several additional units of the general hospital that need to be identified because of the increased importance they have. The first of these is the *emergency department* (sometimes called *emergency room*), and the second is the *outpatient* or *ambulatory services* (or *care*) *department*.

Historically, the smaller hospitals handled emergencies by calling on a member of the medical staff who happened to be in the hospital at the time. Night coverage was frequently handled by members of the active staff taking turns sleeping in the hospital to handle any emergencies that arose. In teaching hospitals, the interns and residents handled the emergency department. In recent years, there has developed a trend whereby emergency departments are staffed by fulltime physicians 24 hours a day; more recently, these physicians have undergone special training in trauma medicine. The emergency department is not only for emergencies; it has also become the family physician at night and on weekends. One even hears of patients calling up at night to find out which of the emergency department physicians is

on duty in hopes of getting to see the one they prefer. Emergency department physicians are typically paid a salary and receive, in many hospitals, a percentage of the business over a certain amount. In some parts of the country, the use of hospital emergency departments is adversely affected by freestanding ambulatory care or emergency clinics.

The *outpatient* or *ambulatory care department* was a feature common to many of the larger general hospitals, particularly teaching hospitals. Generally speaking, it provided a wide range of specialty consultation services for physicians in the community and, in particular, for those patients who could not afford private consultation. Because these departments often duplicated the services available from private specialists in the community, the departments were largely for care of the poor except in those areas in which community-based specialists were not readily available. The recent increase in ambulatory (in and out on the same day) surgery, which previously required two- and three-day admissions, has prompted more general hospitals to develop and expand ambulatory care or outpatient departments. Further encouragement for this is the tendency for more specialists to enter salaried hospital practice. In some instances, ambulatory services may be provided in the emergency department. This is likely to occur in smaller hospitals in which space is at a premium. Ambulatory surgery is, of course, less costly than the surgery done on an inpatient basis, and it frees inpatient beds for other cases. In some hospitals, it may even cause the institution to be overbedded, that is, to have more beds than it needs. We might note here that whether or not a hospital has too many beds is normally determined by its *occupancy rate,* the average percentage of beds occupied over a fixed period of time. Most authorities suggest that the occupancy rate should be between 80 and 90 percent, which allows for room renovations, emergencies, and weekend and holiday drops in occupancy.

Some of the larger teaching hospitals are developing departments of *family medicine.* These departments serve as family physician to a community or to an enrolled group, and they ensure referral of patients needing hospitalization to that hospital.

Supporting patient care services are three medically supervised departments: *anesthesiology, radiology,* and *pathology.* In smaller hospitals, these may be supervised by part-time specialists; in larger hospitals, however, the specialists work fulltime and are paid by salary, salary plus a percentage of the business, or sometimes fee for service. Both radiology and pathology are rapidly expanding departments owing to rapidly developing technology (Figs. 6–2 to 6–5).

All hospitals have a number of other support services. Whether they have departmental status or not depends on the size of the institution and the rationale of those responsible for establishing the organizational arrangements. Some of these services are nursing, pharmacy, medical records, and dietary. Larger hospitals also have such services as inhalation therapy, physiotherapy, occupational therapy, and medical social work.

Increasingly, hospitals are seeking new ways to cope with rising costs.

Shared services—services shared with other hospitals—such as laundry, purchasing, and computers, is one such mechanism. Whether a hospital participates in a given shared service or purchases the service from an outside firm depends on whether its needs can be adequately met in this way and whether it is economically advantageous. Some hospitals find it advantageous to contract to outside firms for some needed services such as food,

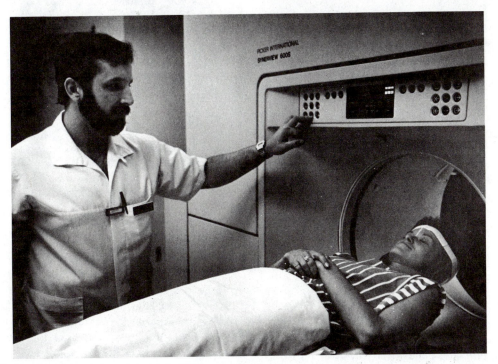

Figure 6–2. Computed tomography (CT) scanners offer radiologists opportunities to observe soft tissue damage. Major medical centers may have two or three such scanners. In 1992 each cost over $800,000. Magnetic resonance imaging (MRI) scanners, similar in appearance, provide even greater technological breakthrough without the danger of radiation exposure to the patient at a cost of $3 million per unit. (Courtesy, Geisinger Medical Center, Danville, PA.)

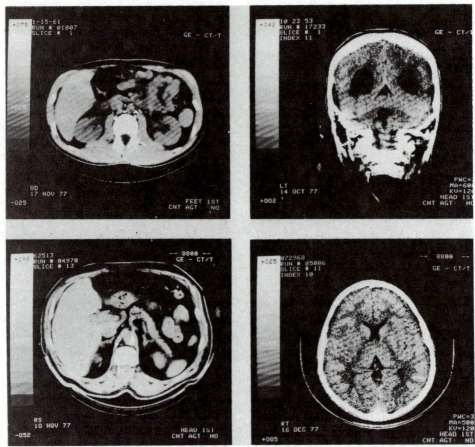

Figure 6–3. CT scans. The whole-body scanner is a versatile unit permitting patient scans feetfirst or headfirst. The two scans on the left are abdominal scans, and the scans on the right are head scans. (Courtesy, General Electric Company.)

security, housekeeping, and even for nurses and other personnel.

Private, Semiprivate, and Ward Beds

Most general hospital beds fall in one of three categories. *Private room* beds are for only one patient and provide a maximum amount of privacy. They cost more than *semiprivate rooms,* which have two or more beds. Most health insurance coverage is for care in a semiprivate room, with the patient paying an additional amount if he or she elects a private room. (Some health insurance policies pay for private room care if the private room is medically necessary.) *Ward beds* were historically for charity cases. They were usually in a large room with beds (sometimes as many as 100 or more), lined up on each side and down the middle of the ward. Although some such wards still exist, there is a tendency for these beds to be in smaller rooms of five to eight beds. The use of the word *ward* is perhaps becoming obsolete in the charity sense, because most patients are now covered by some form of insurance or government program.

The distribution in the number of beds between

private, semiprivate, and ward varies from hospital to hospital.

Hospital Licensure and Accreditation

Hospitals are licensed to operate by state governments, and each state has its own requirements. Generally, the various states have focused their attention for licensure on hospital physical plants, for example, fire safety, heating, space allocations, and sanitation. Very few states have moved beyond this to tie licensure to professional standards.

We noted in an earlier chapter that the American College of Surgeons (ACS) suppressed its 1919 hospital inspection report, because the conditions it found were so poor. The ACS and the American Medical Association (AMA), however, have worked consistently for reform of hospitals. Though they were concerned, as were the states, with physical plants, these professional bodies were also concerned with matters relating to quality of care.

Their efforts at reform culminated in 1952 with the initiation of a hospital accreditation program by the Joint Commission on Accreditation of Hospitals (JCAH).

Joint Commission on Accreditation of Healthcare Organizations

The Joint Commission on Accreditation of Hospitals (JCAH) changed its name to the Joint Commission on the Accreditation of Healthcare Organizations (JCAHO) in 1987 to describe more accurately the variety of health facilities it accredits. Referred to simply as the "Joint Commission" this private, not-for-profit organization sets standards and accredits 84 percent of the nation's general hospitals, as well as long-term care facilities, psychiatric hospitals, substance abuse programs, outpatient surgery centers, urgent care clinics, group practices, community health centers, hospices, and home care agencies. The Joint Commission is governed by a 28-member Board of Commission-

ers composed of three public members, an at-large nursing seat, and representatives from the American College of Physicians (ACP), the ACS, the American Dental Association (ADA), the AHA, and the AMA. In addition, nationally recognized health care professionals serve on advisory committees that provide input on accreditation standards and surveys. Seeking accreditation is voluntary; hospitals and other health care organizations apply for accreditation and request an on-site survey. Typically, a hospital accreditation survey team consists of a physician, an administrator, a nurse, a medical technologist, and perhaps other health professionals, depending on the services the hospital offers. The survey team assesses the extent of a hospital's compliance with the Joint Commission's standards by gathering data and by an on-site visit. Its standards, which cover the gamut of hospital activities from fire safety to sanitation to bed-space allocation to professional services, have been designed to ensure an optimal environment within which quality professional services can be provided. It also requires that the hospital see to it that physicians keep their patient medical records up to date, that there is a regular review of pathology reports on all tissues removed in surgery as a check on unnecessary surgery, that medical audits of patient medical records are made as a check on the quality and appropriateness of medical care, and that there is a regular review of utilization as a check on the necessity or appropriateness for admission and length of stay. The findings are reported to the Board of Commissioners, which makes the accreditation decision. After three years the hospital must undergo another survey to renew its accreditation.

Accreditation is important for the hospital in many ways. First, the Joint Commission has agreements with about 42 states in which accreditation may fulfill all or part of the state licensing requirements. Second, most health insurance policies only pay for care in accredited hospitals. Also, accredited hospitals are considered to meet Medicare and Medicaid standards for payment without undergoing a federal inspection. Additionally, voluntary accreditation demonstrates to the public that a hospital meets certain national standards. Finally, the accreditation process provides an opportunity for hospitals to assess their strong and weak features and make improvements.

The basic question accreditation has answered is, "*Can* this organization provide quality health care?" The accreditation process has traditionally focused primarily on organizational structure, processes, and equipment. Now the Joint Commission is moving beyond determining an institution's capability of providing quality care to answer the question "*Does* this organization provide quality health care?" It is developing more precise and objective quality assurance indicators that include, for the first time, clinical indicators to track clinical processes and outcomes in order to evaluate the diagnosis and treatment of patients.

The public is increasingly aware that there is a wide variation in medical practice patterns and clinical results, and consequently it has questions about quality of care. Furthermore, government, business, and insurers want objective information on the quality of care in hospitals. Against this background, the Joint Commission has made assessment of the quality of hospital care a top priority. The president of the Joint Commission, Dr. Dennis O'Leary, stated, "To the present time, neither the available data management technology nor, quite frankly, the will of the profession have provided a foundation for exploring the potential applications of patient outcome information." He goes on to say, "Truly effective quality assurance systems are rare indeed. But the need to develop and implement these systems is now a matter of self-interest for hospitals and physicians. Happily, the necessary technology, including sound software packages, and demonstrably effective quality assurance methods are rapidly becoming available, and the resurgent interest of professional specialty organizations in establishing national clinical performance standards criteria is a reflection of the fact that our professional will is very much alive and steadily strengthening." (9, p. 570). According to O'Leary, quality control and quality assurance activities with internal monitoring systems are necessary in hospitals, as in business, to cope with competition and to respond to outside data on hospitals. They may even save money by avoiding complications and adverse clinical outcomes, as well as by decreasing professional liability costs (9, p. 572).

Performance indicators (standards) have been developed for anesthesia, obstetrics, trauma, cardiovascular, and oncology care and are expected to be used in accreditation evaluations. Other indicators such as medication usage and infection control are scheduled for development (10).

Although the Joint Commission has contributed much to the improved quality of care in hospitals, many have been critical of its activities, claiming that the organization, whose board mainly consists of leading medical associations, is not inclined to publicize poor medical care or disaccredit hospitals. In fact, only 8 of the 1,750 hospitals inspected in 1991 lost accreditation. The Joint Commission sees its inspections as an educational device for improving performance rather than for removing accreditation. However, Medicare and Medicaid reimbursements depend on accreditation and the federal government expects certain standards to be fulfilled if hospitals are accredited. It monitored accreditation inspections and found that one third of the hospitals accredited by the Joint Commission did not meet Medicare conditions of participation (11). In New York State, state investigators found significant deficiencies in the Joint Commission inspections and now does its own. These and other criticisms caused the Joint Commission to create an additional category of "conditional accreditation" and impose stricter timetables for improvement and the release of limited information to the federal government about those hospitals that do not meet the standards.

The history of the Joint Commission goes back to 1913, when the ACS was formed. Almost immediately the ACS embarked upon a hospital standardization program, when it found that more than half of the applicants for fellowship in the ACS had to be rejected because the case records they were required to submit were inadequate. In the first field trials only 12 percent of hospitals with 100 beds or more met the standards the ACS had established to ensure that patients received proper care. The ACS developed the Minimum Standard for approval, and by 1950 more than half of the hospitals in the United States met the Minimum Standard. However, it soon became apparent that the ACS could not cope with accreditation alone in light of the increasing sophistication of medical care, the rapid emergence of nonsurgical specialties, and the constant need for standards to be expanded and updated. Therefore, in 1951 the ACP, the AHA, the AMA, and the Canadian Medical Association joined the ACS to form the Joint Commission on Accreditation of Hospitals, which offered accreditation to hospitals that applied and complied with its standards. In 1959 the Canadian Medical Association withdrew to participate in its own program, and in 1979 the American Dental Association became a member of the Board of Commissioners. In 1966 the Joint Commission, in a major policy decision, changed the standards it used for accreditation from the *minimal essential* standards for proper patient care to the *optimal achievable* standards. As other health organizations developed, the Joint Commission became the accreditation body for them. By 1987 it changed its name to include other organized health facilities and programs.

Other Performance Evaluators

Hospitals have been interested in their efficiency, quality of care, and performance in relation to other hospitals for many years. In 1955 the Commission on Professional and Hospital Activities (CPHA) was established to assist them in evaluating such issues. It was sponsored by the ACP, the ACS, the AHA, and the Southwestern Michigan Hospital Council. The presence of this substate regional council among national organizations stems from the council's pioneering work, beginning in 1950 under a Kellogg Foundation grant for the study of professional activities in hospitals through inter-

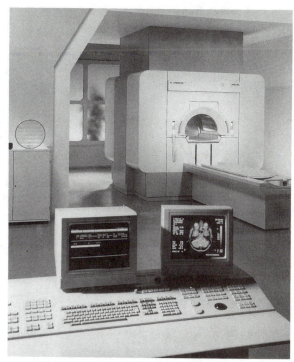

Figure 6–4. MRI unit. (Courtesy, Philips Medical Systems.)

hospital comparisons of hospital statistical reports. The 1950 project was known as the Professional Activity Study (PAS), and it continues as the largest program under CPHA. At the heart of PAS and of other studies carried out by CPHA are the medical abstracts of all hospitalized patients in participating hospitals, which permit a hospital to review its performance over a period of time by such factors as the type of hospital service to which the patient was admitted, final diagnosis, length of stay, type of surgery, and name of physician. Reports are prepared for hospitals monthly, semiannually, and annually.

The Hospital Utilization Project (HUP) is a program similar to CPHA that contracts with hospitals throughout the United States to collect performance data for hospitals. The events that led to its formation illustrate an important point: when organizations are challenged, there is usually much

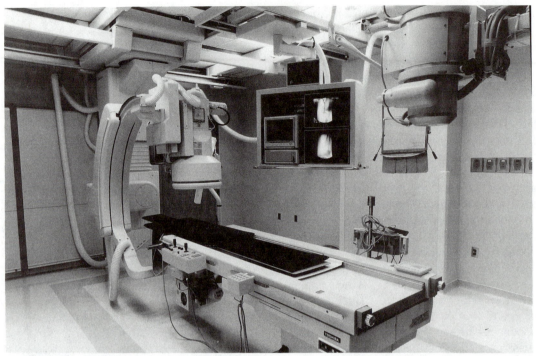

Figure 6–5. Diagnostic angiography, a field of specialty in radiology, uses small catheters to direct and inject radiopaque contrast into specific areas of the body to diagnose aneurysms, tumors, and blood vessel occlusions and narrowings. Angiography can also be used to treat a wide variety of diseases, including tissue abscess and clots in the arteries. Units such as this cost $1.5 million in 1992. (Courtesy, Crozier-Chester Medical Center, Upland, PA, a member of the Crozier-Keystone Health System.)

defensive behavior, but changes often emerge; it is the way change comes about.

During the late 1950s, Blue Cross and Blue Shield plans in many parts of the country were experiencing high utilization and increased costs, and they made applications to the various state insurance commissioners, which regulated them, for rate increases. Generally, insurance commissioners had little data to work with other than that provided by the applicants. There was concern, however, because of frequent charges about unnecessary surgery, unnecessary admissions, and unnecessary lengths of stay. For example, one hospital administrator in upstate New York had put a notice on the doctor's bulletin board urging the

physicians to admit patients and keep them in a little longer in order to maintain the hospital's occupancy rate. Most Blue Cross plans were, moreover, well aware of those two-day admissions for acute medical problems, many of which turned out to be admissions for costly diagnostic examinations that the plans did not cover.

In some states, the insurance commissioners commissioned studies to ascertain the extent of need for rate increases and the extent and nature of the problems. The studies were informative, but, in many instances, the data were inconclusive. This was often the case, for example, with regard to necessity for surgery, which is frequently a highly judgmental matter about which doctors may disagree. In Pennsylvania, in 1958, the insurance commissioner leveled his charge against the physicians in the Pittsburgh area, stating that they used hospital services unnecessarily and that patient stays were prolonged beyond the point of need. The physicians were taken aback and had no data with which to refute the charges. But they began to collect the data by reviewing the medical records. The process was slow and difficult, so they turned for help to the Allegheny County Medical Society and the Hospital Council of Western Pennsylvania. More than 30 local corporations contributed start-up money, and in 1963 HUP was operational. Though the physicians reacted defensively to the insurance commissioner's charges, his charges led to the creation of a new process for strengthening the peer-review process in hospitals.

With the recent advances in data collection, hospital performance can be measured and compared more objectively than ever before. One example is a state council in Pennsylvania that collects and distributes information on quality indicators as well as cost data. It is described toward the end of the chapter.

Hospital Costs

We hear a great deal about rising health costs, and in particular about rising hospital costs—and not without cause. In 1950, for example, the average cost of hospital care was about $15.62 per day, and the average cost of hospital stay amounted to $126.52. For 1966, the first year of Medicare, the cost was $48.15 and $380.39, respectively. In 1981, the figures stood at $245 and $1,851. For 1990, the costs were $756 and $5,021 (8). The bulk of these increased costs have been borne by industry and government, the former through the phenomenal growth of private (voluntary) health insurance that industry has increasingly paid for as an employee fringe benefit, the latter since the introduction of Medicare and Medicaid (Fig. 6–6). Both industry and government have fretted over these

Who Pays the Hospital, 1990

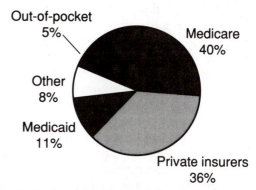

Figure 6–6. Who pays the hospital, 1990.

rises, industry because it forces price increases in industrial products, government because it forces politically unpopular tax increases.

Three factors account for most of the rise in hospital costs and in health costs generally. The first major factor is the increase in population. We simply have more people today than we did in 1950 (239 million versus 203 million). This population is, moreover, an aging population that requires more, longer, and costlier types of care.

The second major factor is inflation. Everything costs more—drugs, linens, food, fuel, and personnel. More than half of a hospital's budget is consumed by its payroll, and as a heavy employer of unskilled labor when the federally mandated minimum wage goes up, hospital labor costs jump accordingly. Similarly, hospital payroll costs overall have risen in recent years as mandated contributions to the Social Security system have risen.

The third major factor in hospital and health care cost increases is new technology and new services. As a result of scientific advances, we are able to do more things to help people than heretofore. But the price of new technology is high. Not only is the equipment expensive, but the personnel needed to operate it is also costly.

Of the major factors accounting for most of the

rising hospital costs, the introduction and diffusion of new technology appear to be the easiest to control. However, the record is not promising.

Every few years, there is a new controversy in the health field, a controversy that arises from new technology. The new technology permits the management of cases in new ways: lifesaving, more effective clinical management, better diagnosis. Cobalt therapy, coronary care, renal dialysis, open heart surgery, and computed tomography (CT) each occupied center stage because of its high cost and the alleged desire of all hospitals to develop the new service. Now that the CT scanner is considered an essential unit for most hospitals and is accepted as commonplace, magnetic resonance imaging (MRI) is taking the preeminent position as a costly item that many argue should be found in only a few hospitals. MRI units cost about $3 million, depending on the magnetic field strength and options that can go with them. In addition to the purchase price, one must also bear in mind that it is costly to maintain and operate and may require modifications to the building in which it is housed. If history is any guide, we can anticipate that efforts to prevent its spread will give way as some new item of technology comes on the scene.

Those who are most concerned about rising health costs are quick to bemoan the "duplication" of very costly equipment and services, and they are most critical of what they perceive to be competition among hospitals to be the first with the new technology, and the desire of other institutions to keep up with the hospital that is first. This free-wheeling rhetoric fails to recognize some very important points and does a disservice to hospitals.

First, what is perceived as duplication may well be the simple recognition by the hospital that the quality of patient care and physician efficiency can be enhanced by acquiring new technology. The CT scanner is an excellent case in point: government and health planning agencies tried very hard to slow their acquisition by hospitals because of the costs involved. It is difficult to determine the number of CT scanners needed in an area to provide high-quality medical care if they are used too often. Despite efforts to limit their distribution, 70 percent of U.S. hospitals have them, far more than Canada or western Europe. Do they have too few or we too many? Is there an optimal number somewhere between? MRI scanners were not available in 1985, but are already in 18 percent of hospitals and there are a number of independently owned ones.

In some cases hospitals share costly medical equipment such as an MRI scanner by installing them in mobile vans that move from one hospital to another in order to use it efficiently, have the technology available locally, and to contain costs.

Even when it is feasible to share facilities and high-technology equipment, a very good case can be made for duplication and the resulting excess capacity.

Let us assume, for example, that a large hospital decides to develop an open heart surgery unit. Physicians on the staff may want such a service available to their patients when necessary. Let us also assume that other open heart surgery units in the community are not operating at full capacity. For the sake of efficiency, should the new unit develop? If it does develop, the cost of care in the community may indeed be higher because of the inefficiencies resulting from unused capacity.* But what would be the salutary effect on the hospital that seeks to develop the service? Not only would the physicians have greater pride in their institution and a new resource, but the very presence of the open heart surgery unit would cause other associated units to be strengthened, which would have the effect of an overall strengthening of the hospital clinically. If the hospital is denied the opportunity to develop the service, one can safely say that the quality of care in that hospital may not be the best because of the weaker associated services; also,

---

*Our assumption here is that the caseload at both hospitals would be sufficient for the heart surgery teams to maintain their surgical competence.

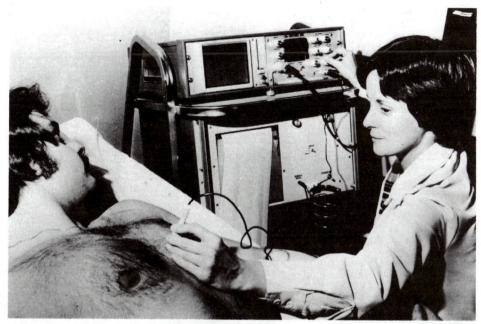

Figure 6-7. Echocardiograph. This unit uses ultrasound to test for abnormalities in the valves, muscles, and chambers of the heart. The unit cost in 1992 was approximately $200,000. (Courtesy, Hamot Medical Center, Erie, PA.)

the hospital might lose some of its clinicians, who would feel frustrated about the inability to see an optimal professional environment developed. This would further weaken the hospital clinically. The same "rats leaving a sinking ship" syndrome could also develop if hospitals are forced to close some units because of low occupancy. This is no idle supposition; we have considerable evidence of physicians leaving other countries because of what they feel were unsatisfactory professional environments.

Technology has spread despite the efforts of government and the health planning agencies. These bodies slowed the process somewhat, but eventually the technology spread basically because the public wanted it, and its acquisition was facilitated both because hospitals were paid close to cost or charges by most health insurance policies and because it was relatively easy for them to borrow

money since they were good credit risks. Another facilitating element was the hospital administrator, a frequent genius at knowing how to manipulate the system for the good of the community.

As stated by the Hospital Association of Pennsylvania:

Increasing hospital costs have been, and will continue to be, significantly related to the inflationary economy of recent years. The industry's highly trained professional personnel and wide range of services and supplies sharply reduce its ability to control costs without curtailing necessary community services and/or reducing the quality of patient care. Although hospitals must buy, build, and hire in the same marketplace, they cannot offset costs by increasing production, as can industry, or by levying additional taxes, as can government.

Notwithstanding, it is fashionable to place the blame for rising costs on physicians, who are ac-

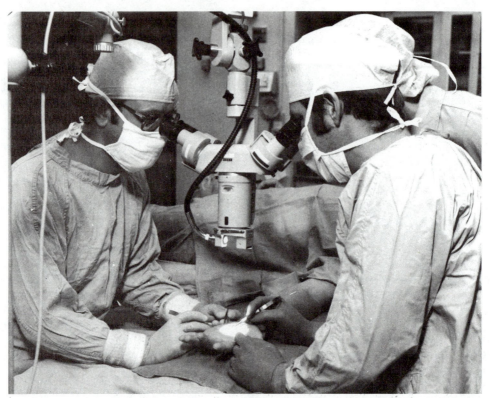

Figure 6–8. Surgical microscopes are used in eye, neurosurgery, and reconstructive surgery. Units such as this cost $60,000 to $100,000 in 1992. (Courtesy, York Hospital, York, PA.)

cused of prescribing medications and tests indiscriminately, and on hospitals, for their overall inefficiencies. Both groups also stand charged for wanting the very latest in technology regardless of cost and need. To some extent, the blame is valid and the charges appropriate. Physicians have not been trained to consider the cost implications of what they do, and to some extent they are reacting to the growing number of malpractice suits. To some extent, also, they may have been helping the hospital meet its losses caused by less-than-cost payments by Medicaid and by care to the poor who either were not eligible for Medicaid or were dropped from the Medicaid rolls because they earned too much to qualify but were still too poor to be able to pay for hospital care.

As to acquiring the latest item of technology,

having it available in the hospital where one practices, rather than having to schedule its use in the hospital across the street, is very convenient. The critic may argue that this is wasteful, but it can, as suggested earlier, contribute to institutional pride, which, in turn, can contribute to an institutional concern for excellence in medical care. Hospitals, like all organizations in all sectors and like governments, have their share of inefficiency and waste, but the extent to which it exists is not known. It is probably much less than what the critics claim, because what to the critic is inefficient, wasteful, or unnecessary may be important to the hospital, to the physician, and to the patient in terms of improved quality of care.

Also bear in mind that physicians and hospitals, in their expansive efforts, have been reacting to pressures in the environment. Until about 1970, practically everyone, including federal elected and appointed officials, were touting all of the advantages to be derived from new technology, new drugs, and new hospitals, and awarding grants to facilitate their development. The appetite of the public was whetted by a steady stream of newspaper and magazine articles about the new developments, and television programming contributed its share to the public's euphoria. It was only when the Medicare and Medicaid bills came in that government began to have second thoughts, leading some critics to argue that government had become interested in the cost of everything and the value of nothing. Blame was heaped on physicians and hospitals when in fact the accusers were equally, or perhaps even largely, at fault.

Unnecessary Surgery

Surgeons are among the most highly paid physicians. Drama surrounds them, and the more dramatic the procedure, the more it costs, not only in terms of the surgeon's fee but also in terms of the hospital support system needed to back up whatever the surgeon does.

We are told often about unnecessary coronary bypass operations, unnecessary tonsillectomies, and so on. We know, also, that in Canada and Britain the surgical rate for some procedures is far less than in the United States. The reports make good news, but, typically, the full story is much more complicated.

A favorite whipping post is surgery for hysterectomy. One of the best discussions of the clinical indications for elective hysterectomy appeared in *The New England Journal of Medicine* on July 29, 1976, under the heading of "Public Health Rounds at the Harvard School of Public Health." The discussants described what were in their judgment the clinical indications for elective hysterectomy. The indications extended far beyond benign and malignant lesions, and they included birth control and improvement of the quality of life. It is clear from that discussion that the medical profes-

sion is not in agreement about the indications for elective hysterectomy.

In an assessment of the costs, risks, and benefits to be derived from elective hysterectomy, Bunker et. al. concluded (12, p. 270):

The principal benefits of elective hysterectomy, it is assumed, are improvements in the quality of life. Menstrual discomfort and inconvenience will be relieved, but these benefits may be offset by a variety of unpleasant sequelae associated with hysterectomy and castration. There are no data on what proportion of women, on the balance, are benefited by elective hysterectomy. While the benefits are unmeasured and uncertain, the costs are large. These costs are rarely paid by the patient. Society, if it is to pay the costs, must decide whether to allocate public funds for a procedure if it appears to be more of a convenience or luxury than a necessity.

They also noted that "the individual patient may consider that the quality of life benefits of hysterectomy are sufficient to offset attendant risks; indeed, based on the extremely high hysterectomy rates reported for physicians' wives, who should be reasonably well informed 'consumers,' it seems likely that many women will make this choice" (12, p. 269).

Quality of life may well account for some of the surgical rate differences between countries. In Canada and Britain, surgical care is rationed by use of a surgical waiting list for elective and nonemergency surgery. The rationing is dictated by the inability of the government to provide sufficient beds and professional and support services to eliminate the backlog of cases and to deal with new cases as they come along. Depending on one's condition, a patient may have to wait six months, a year, or longer unless the patient chooses to incur the cost of private care. By the time the hospital gets around to the elective surgical case, the patient may well have decided to live with it or may even have died from some other condition. Varicose veins will not kill a person, but they can be discomforting and painful. Many people with gallstones can keep them and bear with the occasional attack. So, too, with many inguinal her-

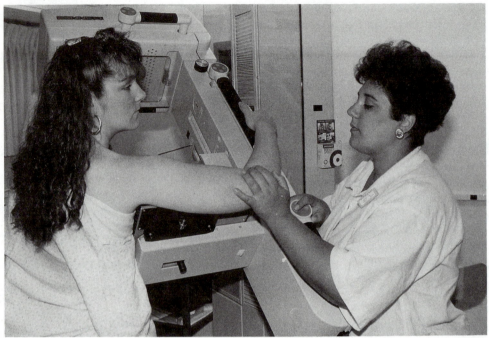

Figure 6–9. A technologist positions a patient for a mammogram. Mammograms can detect breast tumors too small to be detected by self-examination. The unit shown cost over $50,000 in 1992. (Courtesy, Centre Community Hospital, State College, PA.)

nias. The sociology of the society may also have a bearing on these cross-national differences and merits study. Is the American patient, for example, a more decision-oriented person, more desirous of a quick, radical solution, unwilling to live with whatever life or the authorities serve?

This is not to say that there is no unnecessary surgery, but rather to suggest that the extent to which it exists is not easily determined, nor is the cause. Professional judgments and patient choices all play a role. It should be emphasized, moreover, that once a professional consensus emerges, there is invariably a time lag before all physicians get the message, reflecting the slowness by which new knowledge is disseminated. One needs also to remember that what might have been medically indicated yesterday might become contraindicated today because of new knowledge. Whether the surgery is necessary or not may thus reflect when

it was done, whether there were any special clinical considerations, and whether the information about need had been disseminated.

Caesarean sections (C-sections) are less controversial when unnecessary surgery is discussed. C-section births have continued to increase even though a 1980 NIH panel and a 1982 American College of Obstetricians and Gynecologists study recommended that the trend be halted. Most physicians agree that the C-section rate should be about 8 to 10 percent, but despite the increased risk of mortality and morbidity and a longer recovery rate, the national rate has continued to increase to nearly 25 percent in 1991—an increase of 450 percent since 1965! Although fear of lawsuits sometimes causes physicians to do a C-section at the first sign of risk or a problem, the difference in hospital and physician remuneration is also suspected to be an important factor. At least 10 stud-

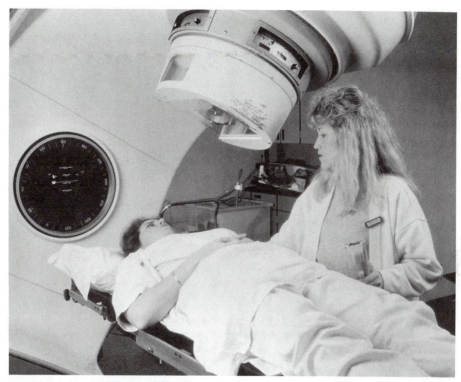

Figure 6–10. Linear accelerator. The linear accelerator saves healthy tissue by destroying only cancerous cells with radiation. This $1.1 million high-energy accelerator uses dual proton and electron beams in the treatment of deep-seated tumors, which are the hardest to treat as they lie closer to vital organs. (Courtesy, Crozier-Chester Medical Center, Upland, PA, a member of the Crozier-Keystone Health System.)

ies have shown that private patients with insurance have substantially higher rates of C-section deliveries than underinsured clinic patients. In 1989 the total cost of a normal delivery in a hospital averaged $4,334, while the cost of an uncomplicated C-section was $7,186. Some insurance companies eliminate the profit motive by reimbursing doctors at a single rate regardless of the type of delivery. Hospitals with clear clinical guidelines for when a C-section is justified, a second opinion requirement, and peer review have reduced their C-section rate significantly (13). However, many obstetricians believe that major reductions in the C-section rate will not occur without major malpractice reforms.

The extent to which unnecessary surgery stems from sloppy diagnosis and avarice is simply not known, though it is probably slight (with the possible exception of C-sections), because the various peer checks [JCAHO review; residency training programs; tissue committees; Professional Activity Study (PAS), HUP, and Professional Review Organizational (PRO) reviews; family physician referrals, and second opinions before surgery] and the risk of malpractice suits serve as regulatory devices. Certainly, unnecessary surgery resulting from sloppy diagnosis and avarice is much less frequent today than in years past and is becoming less of a problem as peer review mechanisms are strengthened.

Oversupply of Hospital Beds

The number of hospital beds set up and staffed for use has declined as a result of a decline in the number of hospitals, a reduction in admissions and the average length of hospital stays. Significant decline began in 1986 and affected mostly rural hospitals with less than 100 beds.

Occupancy rates in both urban and rural hospitals declined about 10 percent between 1980 and 1990. By 1990 small rural hospitals with 6–24 beds had an occupancy rate of only 32 percent while large hospitals with 500 or more beds had an occupancy rate of 77 percent (8). According to the AHA, the total average occupancy rate for all community hospitals was 66.8 percent (see Table 6–1). Government and others maintain that there are still too many hospital beds in the nation. One area in which excess bed capacity appears is in obstetrics. It is generally acknowledged that as a result of a declining birth rate, we have more obstetric beds than we need. Pediatric units also typically have low occupancy: children simply no longer are afflicted with conditions requiring hospitalization to the extent they were when the hospitals were built. Conversion of pediatric and obstetric beds for other uses sometimes poses problems because of structural features of the units and the desire to maintain segregated units. Is it advisable, for example, to place adult medical and surgical cases within pediatric or obstetric units? What would be the costs of conversion designed to maintain separate sections? Are the costs so great as to make construction of new beds elsewhere more desirable, particularly since the pediatric and obstetric bed needs could change if either the population served by the community or the birth rate changes?

It is argued that we cannot afford to maintain excess capacity. Typically, proponents of this view cite the cost of maintaining an empty hospital bed, but figures are often misleading. If the costs they cite are based on the average cost per patient day when the hospital is operating at optimal capacity, it does not follow that it costs the hospital the same

if beds are not occupied, yet this is frequently what is implied.

The average cost per patient day is determined by dividing the total cost of running the hospital by the number of patient days during a fixed time period. If occupancy drops, the hospital may still incur some expenses for those empty beds with regard to heating, electricity, and cleaning, though even these items are not necessarily continuing expenses if the construction permits turning down the heat and closing off the rooms. Empty beds would not draw upon drugs, food, linens, laboratory and radiology services, nursing services, and so on, so some of the variable hospital costs would drop, and over time fewer items would be purchased and fewer nurses hired. However, fixed costs that are part of the average cost would not be affected by the elimination of beds, such as bond obligations, the cost of laboratory and radiology equipment, and the basic maintenance of those services by personnel who could not be cut back without jeopardizing the service for the remaining beds. Moreover, while reducing overall costs somewhat, eliminating beds would create a higher average cost, because the fixed costs would have to be spread over the remaining beds. What then, would be the cost of an empty bed? Certainly not the average cost per patient day.

The issue of excess beds is muddied by the fact that hospital administrators are loathe to close beds the state has given them license to operate. If the unused beds are officially closed and the license for them is given up, the hospital would have to secure the state's permission to reopen them if it later needed those additional beds. The state, because of its desire to hold down costs, might not permit this to occur. Alternatively, the state might drag the matter out over a prolonged period of time simply to slow down the overall cost of care. In 1988 this became a real issue in New York State. Hospitals there had been forced to close beds, and when the AIDS epidemic hit, there was a marked shortage of available beds. AIDS patients and others were backed up in the emergency departments or were denied admission altogether. The moral of the story is, according to one hospital administrator: "A licensed bed is a licensed bed, and never give it up!"

The real issue here is that government is now paying a heavy proportion of total hospital costs in the country, and it is searching for some quick way to control government outlays. When Bunker and colleagues, in their study of elective hysterectomies, concluded that "society, if it is to pay the costs, must decide whether to allocate public funds for a procedure if it appears to be more of a convenience or luxury than a necessity" (12, p. 270), they open a Pandora's box; the issue is not only payment of the physician's fee and hospital's bill but also whether we even want to allow the health system to have the capacity to handle such cases. Under current legislation we seem to be moving in the direction of a negative response. This raises some interesting questions regarding the rights of individuals in a free society, including the right to freely dispose of earned income.

Prolonged Hospital Stays

The average length of stay for patients in the United States has decreased less than half a day between 1980 and 1990. The decline coincides with the beginning of Medicare's use of diagnosis-related groups (DRGs) in the prospective payment system (PPS) and reflects hospitals' attempts to become more efficient. In 1990 the average length of stay was 7.2 days, far lower than in the rest of the world. There were considerable variations in the United States depending on the geographical area. Under the PPS the length of hospital stay is determined by medical necessity rather than what is desirable. Patients are discharged who are less able than before to cope independently, and sometimes without adequate support services.

The accepted practice in patient care changes as new knowledge and new technology are acquired. In recent decades, there has been a tendency to shorten the length of hospital stay. Since hospital care is so costly today, there is keen

interest in making certain that patients stay only as long as is necessary.

But not everyone shares such a view. The patient, for example, may prefer to stay in the hospital a few extra days rather than go to an intermediate care facility if that facility, in the patient's judgment, is not adequate or if it is not covered by insurance. Or, the patient or physician may feel it appropriate to keep a patient a few extra days if there is no one at home to assist the patient on discharge. The hospital administration may also be anxious to keep patients in longer, particularly if the hospital's occupancy is down, providing the patient's insurance policy pays. If the patient stays longer than necessary, the level of service required does not cost as much as normal because no definitive nursing or laboratory services may be necessary, and the only cost may be the cost of meals and laundry. But the hospital collects its usual amount from insurers. What an easy way for a hospital to make money to offset losses or high costs in other areas! It might be noted that if such prolonged lengths of stay are reduced, it does not mean that the overall cost of care will be reduced accordingly; in the long run, it may simply be redistributed, driving the remaining costs up, or it may mean the hospital will not be able to finance whatever purchases it feels are necessary or desirable. The increased use of utilization review is making prolonged stays less and less likely: not only are physicians and hospital personnel becoming more critical in their judgments regarding need to stay in the hospital, but also someone is watching to blow the whistle.

Unnecessary Hospital Admissions

Total hospital admissions decreased 14 percent between 1980 and 1990 despite a 10 percent increase in the U.S. population. This, like the decline in the length of stay, occurred after the introduction of the PPS. Also, utilization review has been making unnecessary admissions less and less of a problem. However, it is worth noting some of the factors that have gone into this alleged abuse of hospitals, because allegations tend to persist long after the disappearance or lessening of a problem.

During the 1970s, there was a marked shift in how physicians provided hospital care. Increasingly, physicians began to utilize outpatient services. Outpatient or ambulatory surgery is perhaps the most noteworthy advance: instead of admitting a patient for two or three days for certain types of surgery, the patient would go to the ambulatory or outpatient department, have the surgery done, and be sent home a few hours later. One has to be careful, however, in judging current inpatient care for what is now typically done on an outpatient basis. The physician may feel that there are clinical or other considerations that may make admission desirable. Unnecessary admissions are a little like unnecessary surgery; clinicians may disagree over the appropriateness for admission, and the disagreements may be pronounced as quality-of-life considerations are taken into account (such as there being no one at home to take care of the patient).

Another type of "unnecessary" admission develops from the way health insurance policies are written. Health insurance typically, but not always, does not cover tests for diagnosis. The basis for this exclusion is historical: there was no way the health insurance firm could predict what its utilization would be, and without an ability to predict utilization, there was no way to calculate a premium. Therefore, diagnostic tests were excluded, as were admissions to the hospital primarily for diagnosis. Many policies, however, did cover these diagnostic tests in hospital *if* they were part of or incidental to an admission primarily for treatment. Though this may seem like hairsplitting, it was very important for the solvency of the health insurance company, since the admission for treatment was calculated in the premium; therefore, all accompanying expenses were coverable. The "unnecessary" aspect of admission came when physicians admitted their patients for two or three days for purposes of diagnosis, claiming, however, that the admission was for treatment and the tests for diagnosis were incidental to or an integral part of

the treatment process. They did this mostly to help the patient receive coverage for tests that were felt necessary and that the patient might not otherwise be able to afford.

Controlling Hospital Costs

As hospital costs rise, they must be covered if the hospital is to continue to operate. One way or another the costs of personnel, equipment and supplies, utilities, insurance, debt obligations, drugs, and so on must be covered. It meets those costs with income from a variety of sources: gifts and endowment income, occasional government grants, but mostly from payments for care of patients. Some of the payments come from insurance companies such as Blue Cross and from government programs such as Medicare and Medicaid. Before DRGs these sources of payment tended to be on the basis of hospital *costs* for care, frequently less than cost, rarely, if ever, more than cost. Other insurance programs, commonly referred to as the commercial insurers as distinct from the nonprofit insurers like Blue Cross, have tended to pay hospital *charges* for care of their covered subscribers. Typically, charges are higher than costs, enabling a hospital to cover losses in other areas and to accumulate money for the purchase of needed equipment or for other expansions.

Government and the insurance companies have been hard pressed by the continuing upward spiral of hospital costs. Though sometimes sympathetic to the plight of the hospitals, government is faced with a dilemma: it can either raise taxes to pay for the increasing costs for which it is responsible or it can shift money from another source (such as defense or education) to health. Both choices are politically explosive, so a third alternative appears more practical—that is, trying to contain hospital costs. Insurance companies have a somewhat similar problem: unless some way can be found to contain costs, the rates they charge must go up, and raising the rates does not sit well with the major purchasers of their policies because it forces them to raise the price of their goods and services, which can have an adverse effect on their corporate profitability. Very few commercial insurance companies still pay hospital charges. Increasingly the rate of payment is negotiated or fixed at what the insurance company believes is appropriate. Thus, not only have government and the insurance companies been interested in containing the rise of hospital costs, but business and industry have also been interested because they are the principal purchasers of health insurance policies. In a growing number of urban centers this has led to the formation of *business coalitions* designed to develop coordinated strategies to contain costs through PROs, monitoring of physician and hospital charges, and other mechanisms. Certificate of need (CON) legislation, utilization review, and the shifting of more costs to the patient have also been employed; but the costs continue to rise. The federal government made the most dramatic attempt to slow the rise in hospital costs when it introduced its prospective payment system (PPS) for hospital patients covered by Medicare, with fixed payments based on assignment of each patient's diagnosis to a DRG. Efforts to control costs are described below.

Peer Review Organizations

Since the advent of Medicare and Medicaid, government has been assuming an increasing share of the costs of medical care, and the costs have been rising rapidly.

The initial legislation for Medicare in 1965 required utilization review; in 1967, this was extended to Medicaid. The 1971 amendments to the Social Security Act mandated the development of Professional Standards Review Organizations (PSROs) throughout the nation to give assurance that services paid for under Medicare, Medicaid, and under the Maternal and Child Health and Crippled Children's Programs are medically necessary, of high quality, and delivered at the lowest possible cost. The Health Care Financing Administration (HFCA) concluded that this gave the PSROs "responsibility for limiting the *cost* of care while assuring the

proper quality of care." HFCA went on to note that these objectives, though complementary, were sometimes in conflict because the medical profession tended to stress the quality assurance element, whereas the Congress seemed more interested in the cost control element.

More than 185 PSROs developed throughout the country. A major part of their work entailed preadmission review and concurrent review of hospital admissions: using physician-established criteria for hospital admission, admissions certified as appropriate were certified for a specific number of days, the number depending on the diagnosis and the norms for that area. The PSROs also reviewed admissions that went beyond the norm. The actual review of cases was delegated by the PSROs in 78 percent of the cases to the respective hospital utilization review committees. This would of course account for the emphasis by those committees, and in turn by the PSROs, on quality of care factors, and less sensitivity to cost control through control of utilization.

In addition to preadmission and concurrent review activities, PSROs carried out a variety of retrospective studies on quality of care, utilization, and patterns of care which served in part as a basis for the criteria employed in concurrent review. Because the rising costs of Medicare and Medicaid were a significant problem for both federal and state governments, the emphasis on cost efficiency was increasingly impressed upon the agencies, but the results of PSRO efforts were mixed. In early 1978, the President's Office of Management and Budget (OMB) proposed that PSRO funding be deleted from the budget request to the Congress because of a Department of Health, Education, and Welfare (HEW) study showing that PSROs did not have any significant effect on reducing costs and did not contribute significantly to increased quality of care. OMB's view did not prevail, but congressional dissatisfaction was also evident in that the appropriation for fiscal 1979 provided funds for hospital review activities but not enough for the reviews Congress had earlier directed for ambulatory and long-term care. In October 1978, the PSROs came under criticism from the General Accounting Office (GAO). The GAO criticized the salary schedules for PSRO executive directors that HEW had issued. The GAO also felt that there was room for PSRO efficiency in terms of combining some administrative staffs and functions, given the fact that in 21 states there was more than a single PSRO; in those 21 states, there were 164 PSROs. A month later, HEW's PSRO supervising office, HCFA, released a new evaluation which it felt demonstrated PSRO effectiveness in both cost containment and cost control. But costs were still going up, and the drive to abolish PSROs continued. In 1981, the funding for some agencies was cut off, and the administration sought again to abolish all PSROs. The Congress resisted and came forth with a compromise, agreeing to eliminate the large number of PSROs, but to replace them with a much smaller number of PROs that would be responsible for quality control but would also focus more vigorously on controlling hospital costs of Medicare patients. However, PROs still give primary attention to cost control rather than quality of care and their sanctioning process for more serious problems seems to be largely ineffective (14). Their unsuccessful performance is partly due to the same organization having conflicting responsibilities; monitoring costs and assuring quality of services and another reorganization is likely.

Each PRO is an organization that successfully bid for a contract with the HCFA to carry out the required peer review functions. Although physician-sponsored groups are preferred, other groups such as Blue Cross may qualify to become a PRO. Because Congress has been concerned with quality of care as well as cost, it has continually expanded the duties of PROs. By 1987 they were required to review quality of care in HMOs, nursing homes, ambulatory care setting, and hospitals. They are also now required to review care of all cases in which a Medicare patient is readmitted to a hospital less than 31 days after the most recent discharge, as well as to review all written complaints about poor-quality care provided to Medicare patients. Even though the quality of medical

care of Medicare patients is being assessed by PROs, few physicians have been sanctioned (see Chapter 3).

PROs' other responsibility is cost control, which essentially means utilization control, and which includes activities such as retroactive and concurrent reviews of cases for the appropriateness of care.

Certificate of Need

A number of steps have been taken by government to deal with the escalation in health care costs. The PROs were one such approach, but they have not been able to make an effective dent in this problem. This is not to suggest that PSROs and PROs have not served a useful purpose, but rather to say that they have not been effective. Another approach to rising health care costs has been to require health facilities to secure from state government a *certificate of need* (CON) for major capital expenditures and major expansions in services in order to be eligible for Medicare and Medicaid payment for use of those expanded services or facilities. As Blue Cross and other insurance programs faced cost pressures, many of them also sought shelter in CON legislation as a hoped-for way to control their spiraling health care costs, and tied their payments to it. The federal mandate to the states for CON laws set a dollar amount above which a facility had to secure a CON for new services, beds, or equipment.

In 1987 Congress repealed the CON requirement, but allowed the states to continue CON programs if they wished using their own criteria. Many states continued CON programs. However, many hospitals feel that the CON programs in some states need to be revised to eliminate bureaucratic red tape and delays, so that health care organizations can respond quickly in the current climate of increasing competition and eroding profits. Some health care organizations oppose CON as being politicized, poorly managed, costly, and ineffective; advocates believe that some regulation is necessary, especially in areas where the population is growing. Whatever its merits, it is clear the CON has not been effective in controlling costs.

CON may slow down expansion; in slowing down, it serves to contain costs somewhat. Whether the health needs of the population are served by this is open to some question. Whether there is a real cost saving is also open to question. Denial of a CON to a hospital in one community because of unused capacity at a hospital in another community to some extent hides some costs, that is, the costs incurred by patients who are now forced to go to the other community. These consumer-borne costs may include transportation, food, hotel, and lost time at work, as well as personal inconvenience. These costs are rarely, if ever, calculated. The dollar costs to a hospital of preparing a CON application, and of trying to justify it, are also very high. The history of regulatory agencies in the United States does not provide much assurance that the CON approach can be as effective as its advocates had hoped. Costs are still rising, and ingenious hospitals have often found ways to get what they want overtly or covertly.

State Rate Regulation

A growing number of state governments have adopted legislation to regulate hospital costs and charges, or at least to attempt to influence them. Apart from pressures from various forces in those states, each state government has a special interest in containing hospital costs, because it is their responsibility to pay a sizable share under Medicaid. In some states there are voluntary rate review programs under Blue Cross, hospital association, or some public body leadership. The scene around the country varies.

Most of the rate review programs rely on *prospective reimbursement* as the preferred method for setting a hospital's rate. Under prospective reimbursement, a hospital negotiates in advance the rate it will be paid by the government, health insurance companies, and/or paying patient. The laws vary concerning to whom and to what the negotiated rate applies.

Although the rate review statutes and CON laws seem to have slowed the rate of hospital expenditures and charges, more needed to be done.

Prospective Payment System

Hospitals have historically been paid by most insurance and government programs on a *retrospective* cost, or near cost basis, that is, they paid after the costs were incurred. Some private insurance programs even paid whatever the hospital charged, which could be higher than costs. These methods of payment did not encourage hospitals to operate efficiently or to economize. The very nature of these retrospective systems was an inducement to order extra tests and drugs, and to keep patients in the hospital longer than necessary. Though physicians made these clinical decisions there was no reason for them to exercise critical judgment because the patient was covered by insurance, and there was no reason for the hospital to be concerned. In fact, there were often good reasons for a hospital to encourage such clinical laxity. But, as the costs of Medicare continued to rise rapidly, there was serious concern about the solvency of the Medicare program, and the federal government sought new ways to contain costs and increase its control over hospital payments. For years, the federal government had been dissatisfied with retrospective cost-based reimbursement to hospitals because under it there was no incentive for hospitals to operate efficiently, and higher hospital costs generally resulted in accompanying larger hospital Medicare payments.

A fundamental change was needed and, beginning in 1972, several demonstrations were conducted to evaluate a wide variety of alternate payment systems. After 10 years of research and demonstrations a prospective payment system (PPS) was chosen as a viable alternative to the retrospective cost-based reimbursement for Medicare patients. Thus, in 1983 Congress amended the Social Security Act to provide Medicare payment for inpatient hospital services under a prospective payment system in which payment is made at a predetermined, specific rate for each discharge according to its classification in one of almost 500 DRGs. The legislation still provided for capital-related costs such as taxes, rent, depreciation, and direct medical education costs to be reimbursed on a reasonable cost basis. Indirect medical education costs are also covered. Excluded from the DRG-based PPS are psychiatric, rehabilitation, alcohol and drug, children's, and long-term care facilities, and Christian Science sanatoria. It is interesting to note that these facilities (except Christian Science sanatoria) are largely for-profit organizations. They are excluded from PPS reimbursement and are still paid on the basis of costs incurred. The number of these institutions have increased while the number of for-profit acute care hospitals that are under PPS for Medicare patients have remained the same. As the profits decline, for-profit investors in health care facilities shift to more profitable health facilities.

The transition to this PPS was made in a four-year phase-in period during which a decreasing portion of the total prospective payment rate for cases at each hospital was based on the hospital's own historical level of cost. By 1988, prospective payment was based entirely on the federal rate, which is a combination of urban and rural national rates per discharge, adjusted by an area wage index and a cost of living amount for Alaska and Hawaii. Also, hospitals may receive additional payments under this PPS for "outliers," which are atypical cases that require an exceptionally long inpatient stay or exceptionally high costs compared to the overall distribution of cases in the same DRG.

The primary objective of the PPS is to change the economic incentives of hospitals under the Medicare program by offering strong encouragement to reduce hospital costs. Under PPS, if a hospital can provide care at a lower cost than the DRG payment, the hospital profits by keeping the difference. If, on the other hand, the cost of care exceeds the DRG payment, the hospital must bear the additional cost except in "outlier" cases.

As predicted, the introduction of this system brought about important changes in hospitals, the medical profession, and the entire health care sector. For the first time in the history of Medicare, there was a decline in the number of discharges (which means that fewer people were hospitalized) and the length of stay (Table 6–4). The greatest decrease in both were between 1983 and 1985, but after 1988 the discharges began increasing and the length of stay, while still less than 1983, remained relatively constant. It is unlikely that the substantial cost savings that occurred in the early years of PPS will happen again.

There has been much concern that hospitals are sending Medicare patients home prematurely, but a Department of Health and Human Services (HHS) Inspector General's report using 1984–1985 data found that fewer than one of every 100 Medicare patients was discharged too early (15). The study reported that the premature discharges were more likely in small, rural hospitals and were frequently associated with poor-quality care and longer than average length of stays. The report was concerned only with medically premature discharges and did not take into account discharges made when appropriate post hospital care resources were not available.

There has been indirect evidence that Medicare patients are now sicker when they leave the hospital under the PPS. Medicare discharges to home (self-care) have decreased, whereas discharges to home health agencies and to other types of facilities have increased. This was expected because of the emphasis on shifting the site of care from the hospital to other settings. Discharges to home health agencies and skilled nursing facilities have increased, but Medicare patients are reported to experience difficulties in obtaining needed posthospital services. Most hospitals have employed discharge planners to facilitate the discharge of patients from acute care hospitals to appropriate posthospital services. Virtually all hospital discharge planners report difficulties in placing patients in skilled nursing facilities, primarily because of restrictions in Medicare rules and regulations regarding eligibility and coverage and because of

TABLE 6–4. Medicare Short-Stay Hospital Discharges and Average
Length of Stay, 1983–1990*

| Year | Discharges | | Average Length of Stay | |
	Number (in thousands)	Percent Change	Number (in days)	Percent Change
1983	11,547		9.8	
1985	10,335	−10.5	8.7	−11.2
1988	10,257	−0.8	8.9	2.3
1990	10,650	3.8	8.9	0
1991	10,797	1.4	8.6	−3.4

SOURCE: Health Care Financing Administration.

*Excludes psychiatric, children's, long-term care, and rehabilitation hospitals.

the shortage of skilled nursing beds (16). Over 85 percent of the discharge planners surveyed also reported problems with home health care placement because of Medicare rules and regulations. The major factor making posthospital placement more difficult is the incentives in PPS to discharge patients as soon as is medically appropriate. Thus, as the PPS reduces hospital costs, it exacerbates problems in other health care sectors.

Most hospitals continued to earn profits during the first years of PPS. The hospital profit margins on PPS cases averaged 14.5 percent during the first year of PPS owing to the ability of hospitals to keep their costs below the DRG rate of payment set under PPS. However, subsequent profits have not been as large. By 1989 the average profit from PPS vanished except for major teaching and urban hospitals. More than 50 percent of hospitals reported losses, especially small rural hospitals (17). The profits, we need to be reminded, are necessary to cover losses in other areas, e.g., the losses incurred from care of the uninsured and from low Medicaid payments, as well as the needed purchases a hospital may have to make to improve the quality of care. As profits decline, hospitals are improving their utilization review departments to minimize unnecessary procedures and practices without affecting the quality of care. Another way hospitals have increased their income is by manipulating the codes that are used to describe the

patient's condition and treatment so that cases are assigned to DRGs for which the payment is higher. According to the HHS Inspector General's report, the coding mistakes averaged 20 percent, but the errors mostly favored hospitals, creating the suspicion that some hospitals may be deliberately manipulating DRGs to increase their income. Whether or not this is the case, the errors cost Medicare about $300 million in overpayments to hospitals in 1987 (15).

There has been a great deal of concern that the quality of care might be adversely affected under PPS, but there is no evidence that the quality of care declined.

Medicare payments increased for outpatient and posthospital care since PPS was implemented. Hospital outpatient revenues have increased, primarily because more surgical procedures are now being done on an outpatient basis.

PPS has been successful in slowing the rate of growth in hospital costs. Before PPS hospital costs were growing 15 percent annually. Between 1983 and 1985 the rate dropped to 6 percent and after 1985 increased to 10 percent, suggesting that the reduction in cost growth may not be effective in the long run (18). PPS has not only slowed the increase in hospital costs for Medicare patients; it has also affected other payers for inpatient hospital services. Several state Medicaid programs are using Medicare's PPS as a model for controlling their hospital costs. Some Blue Cross and other private payers of hospital care are also implementing DRG-based payment systems to control their costs.

As mentioned earlier, the federal PPS only applies to inpatient hospital care for Medicare patients. Outpatient care such as emergency department treatment and same-day surgery are paid on a cost basis. Hospitals have been making a profit on these services, but that may soon end. Congress is considering establishing ambulatory patient groups similar to DRGs and paying a fixed rate according to the group. Outpatient care rose sharply after the introduction of DRG payments and half of all surgeries are now done on an outpatient basis. Fixed payments would save the federal government millions of dollars, but hospitals would have to find other ways to recover losses from increasingly less profitable inpatient care.

Hospital Competition

A competitive market in health care developed in the 1980s, in part because government and private purchasers of health care, concerned about the rapidly rising cost of care, became more aggressive in buying and paying for services. Another factor was an oversupply of physicians and hospital beds. Under these conditions, a buyers' market developed as demand for health services increased. Whenever there is a buyers' market, there are winners and losers among those who have something to sell. In this instance, the buyers were increasingly able to set the prices and the conditions under which they would pay hospitals. A third operative factor in this changing environment was an administration in Washington that wanted to deregulate the health sector, to let market forces prevail to a greater extent than before, and to shift responsibilities from the federal government to the states and the private sector (19, pp. 35–36).

In this environment, hospitals with their decreased occupancy rates were forced to compete for patients. They promoted amenities such as homelike delivery rooms and special meals for new parents; they provided medical services that were popular with the public. Hospitals advertised on radio, television, and on billboards. They affiliated with other hospitals (horizontal integration) to achieve economies of scale in supplies and services, and to secure a dependable flow of patient referrals.

They also contracted with large purchasers of health care to provide services at a discount rate. Employers, as major purchasers of health care for their employees, compare costs for hospital care, but they are also interested in the quality of the care provided. In order to make well-informed choices in the selection of hospitals, employers and labor groups in Pennsylvania, for example, encouraged the creation of an independent state council to collect and distribute cost and quality data on all acute care hospitals having over 100 beds in the state. Hospitals are now required by law to provide cost and quality data to the council, which issues hospital effectiveness reports on 60 DRGs. The reports include the cost of services for each DRG for each hospital as well as quality indicators such as the number of deaths, the expected number of deaths, the actual and expected number of patients who are unstable after one week. The expected numbers are adjusted for the severity of illness and ages of the patients. When the information is publicized, hospitals can see how they compare with others and take measures, if necessary, to improve their performance. Wide variations have been found in cost and quality. In one city the death rate for coronary artery bypass surgery was significantly higher and 50 percent more expensive than at a nearby hospital (20). Health care purchasers use this type of information when deciding which facilities to use. Many hospitals in Pennsylvania oppose the publication of this material, although the hospital association is in favor of continuing the agency. Other states are watching this approach rather than attempting to employ regulation to contain costs (21). Iowa has recently adopted the Pennsylvania system.

As profits from inpatient care decreased, hospitals expanded more profitable outpatient services into such areas as primary care, surgery, extended care, rehabilitation, home care, and occupational medicine (vertical integration) (Fig. 6–11). Although such diversification was necessary to survive and to provide a competitive price to purchasers of health care, it also frequently put the hospitals in the position of competing for patients with the physicians on their medical staffs, and with other health professionals and community health agencies. This has changed the traditional physician-hospital relationship and the hospital-community health agency relationship. In some cases in which physicians threatened to offer services on their own that would compete with those offered by the hospital outpatient department, such as in surgery and radiology, the hospitals went into

a business partnership with those specialists in their freestanding enterprises.

Diversification

The most successful diversification strategy has been freestanding outpatient surgical units, which have been profitable for almost 80 percent of hospitals that have established them. Other diversification strategies that have been financially successful for many of the hospitals are freestanding diagnostic centers, cardiac rehabilitation services, substance-abuse programs, inpatient rehabilitation units, industrial medicine clinics, sports medicine programs, home health services, and women's medicine programs (22, p. 36). There is a corre-

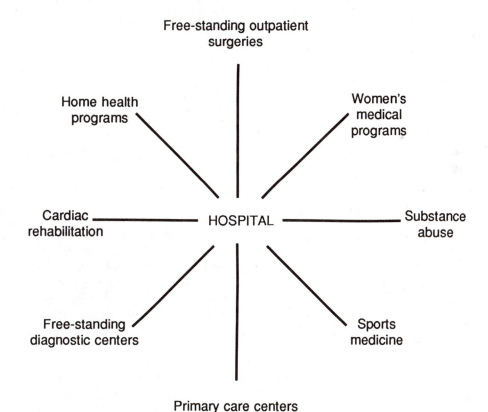

Figure 6–11. Diversification through vertical integration.

lation between the size of the hospital and profit-ability. For example, more than 77 percent of hospitals with 400 beds or more report they make money on outpatient surgery satellites, but only 40 percent of hospitals with fewer than 200 beds report a profit (22, p. 42). There is a similar correlation in cardiac rehabilitation programs and satellite outpatient diagnostic centers, probably because of the volume of patients needed to maintain profitability.

These new activities were undertaken so that hospitals could survive in a competitive environment. However, as mentioned earlier, maintaining quality of care in a competitive environment has become an important concern for health care providers, health care purchasers, and consumers.

Current Trends

Those concerned with health policy have identified some critical trends with which hospitals will have to contend in the coming years (23):

- An excess of acute care beds as the use of acute inpatient services continues to decline.
- Hospital rates continuing to increase at a greater rate than general inflation.
- Profits and reserves declining.
- Medical technology continuing its rapid development.
- Cost of capital increasing.
- Purchasers of health care becoming a more critical force in shaping future health policy and in determining the use of health care services.
- Competition increasing among hospitals, physicians, and other health care providers.
- Multihospital systems and alliances growing.
- Medicare and Medicaid annual expenditure increases being severely curtailed by government.
- Private health insurance coverage declining with the increase in service industries.
- Ambulatory, home health care, and outpatient surgery services increasing.
- Health care services for the elderly growing.
- Nursing and other staff shortages continuing and increasing.

SUMMARY

In 1990 there were 6,650 hospitals in the United States, with some 1,200,000 beds. These were hospitals of all sorts: psychiatric hospitals, TB hospitals, chronic disease and rehabilitation hospitals, mental retardation hospitals, federal government hospitals (VA, military, etc.), special hospitals, and short-term community general hospitals.

The community hospital is the hospital with which most of us are familiar, the community facility to which the physician admits his or her patients for short periods of acute care. Typically, most of the patients in these hospitals are in for less than 30 days, and most are also in for acute illnesses. These hospitals range in size from six beds to more than 1,000 beds. The tendency is for the smaller hospitals to close or to merge with other institutions because of rising costs and the need for expensive equipment.

The community hospital is most commonly a nonprofit institution. Governance is typically by a board of trustees or directors who appoint the medical staff and hire the administrator to carry out their policies and to manage the daily operations of the institution. In the nonprofit institutions at least, the board members receive no compensation for their services as board members. It is the responsibility of the board not only to set policy and oversee the institution's operations, but also to ensure the availability of money to maintain the institution. Members of the board of a hospital are typically elected or appointed by the group that sponsors the hospital.

Some community hospitals are also teaching hospitals, which means that they have responsibility for training medical specialists in one or more of the specialties. Some of the teaching hospitals are also medical school hospitals, which have the added responsibility of training people to become physicians. Teaching hospitals tend to be larger hospitals with more sophisticated services, and they tend to have a greater number of fulltime salaried medical staff. Most community hospitals have few, if any, fulltime salaried physicians, although a growing number are appointing fulltime emergency department physicians.

The community hospital is a general hospital. It handles the general run of cases. There are special hospitals for the mentally ill and the mentally retarded. Many of these are run by state governments, although some local government institutions and a considerable number of private institutions (both for profit and nonprofit) exist. Around many large cities one can find children's hospitals, orthopedic hospitals, women's hospitals, ENT hospitals, eye hospitals, and rehabilitation hospitals. Most of these are tending to merge or affiliate with other institutions for the same reasons that the smaller general hospitals are doing so. In particular, costs and scientific advances in the various specialties are forcing mergers because of the dependence of the specialties on sophisticated services that can only be supported by the larger institutions.

The operation of hospitals in any state, except for federal hospitals, is only with the approval of the state government. This is granted by the issuance of a license only after the state licensing body is assured that the institution meets the standards laid down by the state. Typically, the state inspects hospitals and focuses heavily on cleanliness, fire safety, and other physical plant matters.

Most hospitals, including many federal hospitals, voluntarily submit themselves to accreditation review by the Joint Commission on Accreditation of Healthcare Organization (JCAHO). This body looks at certain physical plant matters but mostly at matters relating to quality of care. Many health insurance companies and government programs only pay for care in an accredited institution.

Over the past decade hospitals have changed from expanding institutions with little regard for cost to institutions with reduced occupancy and a great interest in cost containment. They are now more business-like institutions that stress efficiency and they compete for patients. The changes were caused by the efforts of government and other large health care purchasers to slow the dramatic increases in health care spending. Medicare changed its method of paying for inpatient services to a prospective payment system based on DRGs, which encouraged cost savings. Since then the annual growth rate in hospital costs slowed for some years, but is beginning to rise again. Admissions and lengths of hospital stays decreased. As inpatient care became less profitable, hospitals increased and expanded their outpatient services.

There has been a decline in the number of acute hospitals and hospital beds, with most of the decline being in small rural hospitals. Quality of care became an increasingly important issue as data collection methods enabled hospitals and health care purchasers to compare hospital performance records. Hospitals continue to search for ways to maintain or improve their efficiency and effectiveness in a climate of increased competition and cost constraints.

DISCUSSION QUESTIONS

1. To what extent is competition healthy between non-profit and investor-owned hospitals? Among non-profit hospitals?
2. Should licensure and accreditation standards be optimal or minimal?
3. What kinds of people should serve on hospital boards, and why?
4. Should accreditation of hospitals continue to be voluntary? Should accreditation be carried out by a nongovernmental agency? What are the advantages of the voluntary process?
5. Does your community have too many, too few, or just the right number of acute hospital beds? What about for the next 10 years? Is any action necessary?
6. Should hospitals be encouraged to adopt the swing-bed approach if they have low occupancy?
7. What steps need to be taken to deal with the unnecessary surgery problem?
8. What advantages and disadvantages do you see in the DRG mechanism for paying hospitals?

REFERENCES

1. Custer, W.S., Musacchio, R.: Hospitals in Transition: A Perspective. *J Med Pract Manage*, Vol. 1, No. 4, 1986, pp. 228–233.

2. Stewart, D.A.: *The History and Status of Proprietary Hospitals.* Research Series #9, Chicago, Blue Cross Association, 1973.

3. American Hospital Association: *AHA Guide.* Chicago, 1991.

4. Lewin, L.S., Derzon, R.A., Margulies, R.: Investor-Owned and Nonprofits Differ in Their Economic Performance. *Hospitals,* July 1, 1981.

5. State of Florida, Hospital Cost Containment Board: *Annual Reports 1981–82, 1982–83.* Tallahassee, FL, 1982, 1983.

6. Pattison, R.V., Katz, H.M.: Investor-Owned Hospitals and Not-for-Profit Hospitals. N Engl J Med, Vol. 309, August 11, 1983, pp. 347–353.

7. Relman, A.S.: Investor-Owned Hospitals and Health Care Costs. *N Engl J Med,* Vol. 309, August 11, 1983, pp. 370–372.

8. American Hospital Association: *Hospital Trends.* Chicago, 1991.

9. O'Leary, D.S.: A Concept for Fulfillment. *J Med Assoc Georgia,* August 1987, pp. 569–572.

10. Joint Commission on the Accreditation of Healthcare Organizations: *Committed to Quality.* Chicago, 1990.

11. *New York Times,* May 17, 1992.

12. Bunker, J.P., Barnes, B.A., Monsteller, F.: *Costs, Risks, and Benefits of Surgery.* New York, Oxford University Press, 1979.

13. Myers, S.A., Gleicher, N.: A Successful Program to Lower Caesarean-Section Rates. *New England Journal of Medicine,* Vol. 319, 23, Dec. 8, 1988, pp. 1511–1516.

14. Lohr, K., Schroeder, S.: A Strategy for Quality Assurance in Medicare. *New England Journal of Medicine,* Vol. 322, 10, March 8, 1990, pp. 707–712.

15. *American Medical News,* February 19, 1988.

16. U.S. General Accounting Office: *Posthospital Care.* Washington, D.C., January 1987.

17. *Modern Healthcare,* June 17, 1991.

18. The Urban Institute: *Policy and Research Report,* Washington, D.C., Summer 1991.

19. McNerney, W.: "Competition in the Delivery of Health Care," in Raffel, M.W., Raffel, N.K. eds: *Perspectives on Health Policy: Australia, New Zealand, and United States.* Chichester, John Wiley & Sons, 1987.

20. *The Wall Street Journal,* January 22, 1992.

21. Sessa, E.: Information is Power: The Pennsylvania Experiment. *J Health Care Benefits,* January 1992, pp. 44–48.

22. Sabatino, F.G., Grayson, M.A.: Diversification: More Black Ink than Red Ink. *Hospitals,* January 5, 1988.

23. Hospital Association of Pennsylvania.

Chapter 7

Ambulatory Care and Mental Health Services

Ambulatory Care Services

Ambulatory care covers a wide range of services for the noninstitutionalized patient. The large majority of ambulatory care is provided by office-based physicians. It is estimated that about 705 million visits were made to doctors' offices in 1990, or about 2.9 visits per person (1). However, there are a number of other ways ambulatory care is delivered and they are described in this chapter.

In recent years the number and kinds of ambulatory or outpatient facilities have increased to allow more patients to receive treatment outside of expensive acute care hospitals. Many of the procedures formerly done in hospitals are now able to be performed on an outpatient basis. The usual types of ambulatory care facilities such as hospital outpatient departments and community health centers have expanded to include facilities such as surgery centers, diagnostic imaging centers, and even cardiac catheterization laboratories. Many of these new facilities are for-profit and are operated by chains, either independently owned (not affiliated with a hospital) or with hospital affiliation (Table 7–1). Also, many nonprofit health care systems with hospitals (e.g., Kaiser Permanente and other large health maintenance organizations [HMOs]) have expanded their ambulatory facilities as part of an integrated, cost-efficient way to provide care.

Hospital Outpatient Departments

Hospitals offer ambulatory care services in clinics where people with nonurgent medical problems can receive treatment. Clinics are separate from emergency department services, but the emergency department often handles nonurgent patients during hours the clinics are not open. Clinics may be general or specialized (e.g., a diabetes clinic). Historically, only hospitals with teaching programs or those in (usually urban) areas where patients could or would not go to doctors' offices had clinics, and they served mostly those with low incomes. The situation has changed since com-

TABLE 7−1. Ambulatory Care Facilities Operated by Chains, 1991

	Nonhospital Affiliated	Hospital Affiliated	Total	% Increase Since 1990
Primary/urgent care	56	913	969	4.0
Occupational health/ industrial medicine	42	297	339	14.5
Rehabilitation	43	267	310	22.0
Diagnostic imaging	791	220	1,011	22.0
Chemical dependency treatment	—	204		−7.7
Psychiatric clinics	—	201		1.5
Sports medicine	4	191	195	22.6
Surgery centers	9	115	124	14.8
Fitness/wellness centers	5	66	71	6.0
Cancer centers	8	63	71	9.2
Pain clinics	16	40	56	16.7
Cardiac catheterization	1	25	26	44.4

SOURCE: Modern Healthcare, May 18, 1992.

petition among hospitals has increased, and now hospitals are establishing and expanding clinics, some of them in the community away from the hospital (freestanding). These clinics are also attracting middle-income persons to provide the hospital with additional income and to "feed" patients to their hospitals for admission.

Community Health Centers

Community neighborhood health centers began to develop in the late 1960s, initially with funding from the Office of Economic Opportunity (OEO) and, later, the U.S. Department of Health, Education, and Welfare (HEW). These centers were primarily to provide comprehensive ambulatory services for a defined population of poor people. The poor had, of course, always received large amounts of care from health departments, indigent hospitals, and on charitable or government-financed bases in nongovernmental general hospitals. The larger hospitals, and particularly medical school hospitals, had long histories of care of the poor on both an inpatient and an outpatient basis. But the outpatient care was often demeaning; there were impersonal, crowded surroundings, and long waits on hard benches. The neighborhood health center

was designed to overcome these demeaning features not only by providing a broad range of primary and secondary ambulatory care services by salaried physicians and other health professionals but also by emphasizing prevention, having available a wide range of supporting nonmedical services, and providing these services in the neighborhoods in which the people lived. Important, too, was the concept that the people who were served, the consumers, should be involved in the control of their centers.

When possible, the centers were financed on a fee-for-services basis from Medicare and Medicaid and other vendor payments and from government grants. As with so many government programs, there comes a time when priorities shift and funding tapers off. In addition to decreased funding, community health centers face additional problems. The demand for services far exceeds their availability because they are the only source of medical care for the poor in many rural areas and in many inner-city neighborhoods. Sharply increasing malpractice insurance rates are consuming funds that used to be used for patient services. One important service these centers provide is prenatal and obstetric care for low-income women who are considered to be high risks by insurance companies. In order to keep insurance costs within a manageable cost, some centers have had to reduce services to pregnant women (2).

Primary Health Care Centers

Primary health care centers are community health centers that provide a more limited range of services. They also have major financial problems, and the rural centers have difficulty attracting and retaining professional staffs. Many of these centers have developed with support from one of several federal programs: National Health Service Corps (NHSC), Rural Health Initiative (RHI), Health Underserved Rural Areas (HURA), and the Appalachian Regional Commission (ARC). Such support augmented local organizational efforts and local building of the facilities. The typical federally supported center has two family practitioners and one dentist. The supporting services beyond nursing vary from center to center. Some have visiting consultant services, pharmacy services, nutrition services, or other services. The financial problems are varied. Some result from community overbuilding of the facility, incurring a debt that is difficult to pay off from center earnings. Some centers overextend themselves in terms of the supporting services they provide. A steady flow of patients who pay a fee for service is also a problem: in rural areas, there is a frequent turnover of professional staff, and with each turnover, the centers lose patients—people seek older practitioners who are likely to stay around, even though they may have to travel greater distances. Some centers also report a drop in patients due to the unaccustomed high cost of care; the newer and younger doctors who practice in these centers typically practice a type of care that employs more tests than the old-time practitioners used. The patients sometimes reject this more advanced type of care, preferring to find an older practitioner who is not as fancy, providing clinical judgment instead of tests and consequently delivering care that is not as costly. The long-term survival of these centers depends not only on attaining financial stability but also on finding a way to attract and retain professional personnel.

Community Mental Health Centers

Spurred by the introduction of psychotropic drugs and the assumption that the mentally ill could be treated more effectively in a community setting, support for community-based care grew steadily, and in 1963 Congress passed legislation to stimulate, by means of grants of money, the development of comprehensive mental health services through community mental health centers. The decline in federal monies and the concentration of centers in poverty areas highlight the major problem facing these centers: Despite all the good they may do, financial problems are major and inevitably must affect at least the comprehensiveness of service, let alone the survival of the centers. Community mental health centers are discussed in more detail later in this chapter under Mental Health Services.

Ambulatory Surgery Centers

In recent years, there has been a dramatic increase in the amount of surgery performed on an ambulatory basis. Hospitals all over the country are experiencing a rise in the number of surgical patients who come into the hospital and go home on the same day, cases that previously had required at least an overnight stay in the hospital if not a two- or three-day stay. One can appreciate how this can affect a hospital's use of beds and its overall organization.

Many surgeons, however, have been accustomed to performing a limited amount of ambulatory surgery in their offices, depending on their facilities, support services, and self-imposed limits. One of the major limits was anesthesia. The surgeon typically would employ a local anesthetic, not a general anesthetic, because the latter should be administered by board certified anesthesiologists.

Advances in anesthesiology as well as rapidly changing technology made it possible to perform an increasing number of operations on an outpatient basis. During the 1970s, a number of freestanding—that is, not hospital-based—surgical centers began to develop in several parts of the country.

After the American College of Surgeons began to approve freestanding surgical centers in 1981, the number of facilities increased rapidly throughout the country until, in 1991, there were about 1,500 facilities performing some 3 million surgical procedures. The number of procedures is expected to reach 4 million by 1994. The most common procedures performed at these ambulatory surgical centers are in ophthalmology (mostly cataracts), gynecology, otolaryngology, orthopedics, and plastic surgery. The rapid growth of ambulatory surgery has been due to a demand by insurance companies and government to provide surgery at lower costs. Hospitals perform close to 70 percent of all outpatient surgery and freestanding surgical centers perform about 30 percent.

These freestanding surgery centers are able to compete effectively with hospitals, because Medicare now covers many more kinds of procedures on an outpatient basis. Importantly, these centers typically have lower overhead costs than do similar services provided through the hospital outpatient department. Also, they frequently affiliate with HMOs and preferred provider organizations (PPOs), thereby ensuring a certain flow of patients to them.

Hospitals have responded to the growth of ambulatory surgery centers by establishing their own freestanding centers, by affiliating or going into partnership with some of the freestanding centers, and by aggressively marketing and expanding their own hospital-based outpatient surgical services.

Close to 75 percent of freestanding surgical centers are independently owned, mostly by surgeons who are competing with the very hospitals in which they perform their more complicated surgical procedures. Many of the independently owned facilities are small, single-specialty surgical

centers with fewer physicians than those owned by hospitals and corporate chains.

The development of ambulatory surgical centers in an area depends on such factors as state regulations, certificate-of-need requirements, competition, and reimbursement policies (3).

Freestanding Emergency and Ambulatory Centers

Freestanding emergency centers that provide episodic emergency care 24 hours a day are increasing, and it is estimated that there are over 5,000 in the nation. They provide primary care on a "walk-in" or appointment basis. They are sometimes store-front operations located in large shopping malls. Like the ambulatory surgical centers, they provide the opportunity for physicians and for-profit organizations to compete with hospitals and office-based physicians for patients. They are having an adverse effect on the use of hospital emergency departments and on other practitioners whose location or appointment systems are inconvenient for patients.

Family Planning Centers

Family planning centers were first established in 1970 when Congress passed Title X of the Public Health Service Act, which provided federal funding for establishing family planning services on the local level. These services are provided by local health departments, hospital agencies, and voluntary agencies, depending on the state and geographic area. Typically, the centers provide gynecologic examinations, breast or cervical cancer screening, contraceptive information and supplies, and other services related to reproductive health care. Many centers have expanded their services to include genetic screening; routine child health screening; and sexually transmitted disease diagnosis, treatment, and followup. Funding usually comes from the federal government, state government, private donations, fund raising, and sliding scale client fees. During the early 1980s, federal funding became less available as the administration cut back on many health and social services.

Clinical Laboratories

The physician may require a variety of laboratory analyses to facilitate diagnosis and treatment. Some physicians do their own tests or have their own technicians to carry out whatever tests are desired. However, some tests are very complicated and require rather costly equipment. For these tests, as well as some of the simpler tests, the physician may have an arrangement with the nearby hospital or may use a freestanding clinical laboratory run by a pathologist or by a registered medical technologist. Sometimes the physician sends the patient to the lab; sometimes the physician sends the specimen to the lab. In rural settings, the doctors may have to mail the specimen to a lab, or the lab may arrange for periodic pickup of specimens.

Although there is state licensing of clinical laboratories and federal monitoring of those labs that work across state lines, there has been concern over the years about the quality of laboratory analyses. Periodically, studies are completed that call into question the accuracy of clinical lab results. This is, of course, a serious matter, because a physician treats a patient on the basis of lab reports.

Ambulance Services

Ambulance services are provided by a variety of agencies. Funeral homes are frequently the source of this service, but it is also available, depending on the community, from the police and fire departments, hospitals, volunteer groups, and private ambulance companies. Considerable effort has been made in recent years to train ambulance crews in dealing with the kinds of emergencies they are likely to encounter.

Health and Welfare Councils

Health and welfare councils are voluntary agencies usually representative of the smaller health and welfare agencies in a community, though the larger agencies may sometimes belong. The councils serve a very useful service not only in terms of representing the small agencies but also in providing a research and planning capability that the agencies individually, because of their size, could not afford.

Voluntary Health Agencies

There are a large number of national health agencies that operate state and sometimes local chapters. These agencies are typically oriented toward special disease and are financed largely by charitable contributions. Some of the more prominent agencies include the American Heart Association, American Cancer Society, National Society for the Prevention of Blindness, National Tuberculosis and Respiratory Disease Association, American Association on Mental Deficiency, American Red Cross, and the National Association for Mental Health. Some of these agencies provide some direct service (e.g., diagnostic services, clinic consultation), some support research, some help finance needed services, and most conduct some health education activities to educate the population about the health problem of their concern.

Renal Dialysis Centers

Many renal dialysis centers are freestanding and are owned by physicians or for-profit organizations. Also, many hospitals have established dialysis centers. The number of these centers increased greatly after 1972, when Congress extended Medicare coverage for all persons, regardless of age, who had chronic kidney disease and who required periodic dialysis treatment. Some units also operate home dialysis programs.

Mental Health Services

The shortcomings of mental health services in the United States are brought forcefully to the attention of Americans by the large number of mentally ill homeless people who are seen in the streets, subways, and parks of our larger cities. It is estimated that about one third of the homeless are seriously mentally ill (4). This situation has come about because of the fragmented system of financing and responsibility as well as an inadequate amount of care that is not geared to the needs of many of these people. As a result, sufficient medical care, social support, and help with basic living needs for a prolonged period of time are not available. How this came about and what is being done to remedy the situation is the focus of this section.

Before 1800 the mentally ill usually were cared for by their families. They became a public concern only if they had no family support, were violent, or were unable to care for themselves. If that were the case, local officials assumed responsibility for their welfare by boarding them with families or placing them in public almshouses along with the very poor, or housing them in public jails.

As the population grew and urbanization increased, there was a growing awareness of social and medical problems. Some psychiatric hospitals were established. (In that era these institutions were often referred to as "mental hospitals" or as "asylums.") About this time Dorothea Dix became very interested in the condition of almshouses and jails in her native state of Massachusetts and found, among other problems, that insane persons were held in unheated jails. She convinced the state legislature to assume direct responsibility for the care of the mentally ill. Dix campaigned for improved conditions for the mentally ill in many other states. Dix's reforms led to the establishment of large state institutions in almost every state; thus an era of "moral treatment" began, in which patients were nourished and cared for until they became well again. The prevailing view at that time was that mental illness was the result of improper behavioral patterns that were associated with an unsatisfactory environment. It was thought that psychiatric institutions could provide a more appropriate environment, where patients could be improved physically, be treated with narcotics to calm violent behavior, and be provided with kind, individual care. Most patients were institutionalized for brief periods of time.

There were relatively few long-term or chronic cases in institutions during the nineteenth century, partly because a large proportion of the mentally ill were still kept at home or in municipal almshouses and partly because the funding of these institutions was divided between state and local governments. States provided funding to build and renovate psychiatric institutions, but local communities paid for the care and treatment of the patients admitted if their family or friends did not assume the cost. Sometimes local officials kept indigent mentally ill in almshouses, where the costs were less. Other times local officials pressured psychiatric hospitals to discharge patients prematurely if localities were paying for their care (5).

As the number of chronic patients increased, the conflicts that occurred because of the divided responsibility resulted in states assuming full responsibility for the mentally ill. Local officials then redefined senility as mental illness and transferred poor senile and elderly patients from almshouses to state mental institutions to save even more money. As a result, state psychiatric institutions that had good turnover rates saw those rates decline with the rapid increase of long-term patients. They became institutions largely for custodial care for the aged and those with conditions such as senility, cerebral arteriosclerosis, and brain tumors (5).

After 1945 psychiatrists who were associated with institutional care began to leave psychiatric hospitals and move into community and private practice. They were frequently replaced by international medical graduates with little or no training in psychiatry, and psychiatric hospitals deteriorated. Most psychiatrists in the community treated large numbers of patients with psychological problems and had little contact with the institutionalized mentally ill. As the links between psychiatric hospitals and psychiatrists weakened, there was a movement to strengthen outpatient care and community clinics. By the middle 1950s there were over 1,000 outpatient psychiatric clinics, most of which were state supported or state aided (5).

The support for community-based care and treatment grew steadily based on the assumption the outpatient psychiatric clinics could identify and treat early cases of mental disorders and serve as alternatives to psychiatric hospitals. At the same time a growing number of private psychiatric hospitals and psychiatric beds in community hospitals became available for short-term treatment and emergencies. Mental health treatment in the community was based on the assumption that patients had a home and a sympathetic family or others who would assume responsibility for their care—an assumption that turned out to be unrealistic. Even so, the concept of community care and treatment prevailed, supported by those who did not believe in the concept of mental illness, civil rights advocates who identified the mentally ill as a group deprived of their civil liberties, and social advocates who emphasized that psychiatric hospitals are inherently repressive and dehumanizing (5). The Community Mental Health Act of 1963 strengthened community facilities and weakened the central role psychiatric hospitals played in the treatment of the mentally ill.

After 1965 there was a rapid decline in the number of patients in psychiatric hospitals because of the introduction of psychotropic drugs; a belief that community care was an acceptable alternative to institutionalization; and the introduction of Medicaid, which paid the cost of nursing home care for the poor elderly and enabled them to transfer from psychiatric hospitals to nursing homes. The transfer of the elderly to nursing homes was encouraged because Medicaid was funded partly by the federal government and this reduced the cost of their care for state and local government. "Prior to 1940, public policy had been focused almost exclusively on the severely and chronically mentally ill. This policy was based on the assumption that

society had an obligation to provide such unfortunate persons with both care and treatment in public mental hospitals. The policies adopted during and after the 1960s rested on quite different assumptions" (5). They created a decentralized system of services that separated care and treatment, and often focused on mild mental illness to the detriment of the severely mentally ill who were more difficult to treat. The separation of care and treatment often resulted in a lack of social services to ensure that patients had their basic living needs covered while they underwent treatment.

Mental illness is difficult enough to define and identifying a large segment of that population, the chronically mentally ill, is even more difficult. There is disagreement about who to include in this category, but the following definition is generally accepted: "The chronically mentally ill population encompasses persons who suffer from certain mental or emotional disorders (organic brain syndrome, schizophrenia, recurrent depressive and manic-depressive disorders, and paranoid and other psychoses, plus other disorders that may become chronic) that erode or prevent the development of their functional capacities in relation to three or more primary aspects of daily life—personal hygiene and self-care, self direction, interpersonal relationships, social transactions, learning and recreation—and that erode or prevent the development of their economic self-sufficiency" (6).

It is estimated that nearly 1 percent of the U.S. adult population suffers from chronic mental illness that makes self-care impossible (7). The mean annual cost of care and treatment for an individual with chronic mental illness is about $32,000, of which treatment and residential and rehabilitation costs are more than half; the other costs are income support and the time burden borne by families (7). A study conducted for the federal government estimated the total cost of chronic and acute mental illness, including diagnostic and treatment costs as well as indirect costs such as lost productivity and premature death, was close to $130 billion in 1988—the latest figures available (8). Accurate figures are difficult to come by, but the above estimates show that mental illness is a major, costly problem.

Although ways to cure or prevent chronic mental illness are not known, much has been learned in the past 20 years about how to improve its management. Persons with chronic mental illness need in addition to treatment a range of services to provide a stable adjustment to community life such as housing, meaningful daily activities, and socialization. Absence of these leads to patient stress and may cause a relapse. Relapses are common in the chronically mentally ill (9).

Few communities have an integrated system of treatment and social support for the mentally ill. Hospitals and community programs often compete for funds and often do not coordinate nor collaborate in the provision of services, leaving many patients without care (9). A recent study reports that there are more seriously mentally ill persons in street shelters and prisons than in hospitals, largely because of the failure of deinstitutionalization, which resulted in the vast majority of those discharged from mental hospitals not being cared for in the community and drifting into homelessness and destitution (10).

Inpatient Services

Community hospitals with separate psychiatric services, private psychiatric hospitals, state and county psychiatric hospitals, and Veterans Administration (VA) medical centers provide inpatient treatment services today. The large majority of mentally ill inpatients are treated at community hospitals or in private, for-profit psychiatric hospitals. They are treated mostly for affective disorders such as anxiety, depression, and manic-depressive conditions, and their stay is relatively short. Only about 10 percent of mentally ill inpatients are treated at state and county psychiatric hospitals. The majority of these patients are schizophrenics or have organic brain disorders. VA medical centers treat a small percent of institutionalized patients, a large number of whom suffer from schizophrenia. As is evident, the case mix of institutions for the mentally ill

differs, with the state, county, and VA centers serving about 90 percent of the schizophrenics, who are difficult to treat, and the other institutions serving those with less difficult affective disorders (11).

Nursing and related care homes have become a major resource for residential care of the mentally ill. Nearly half of the total nursing home population was diagnosed with organic brain disorders, including Alzheimer's disease. Schizophrenia, other psychoses, and depressive disorders account for about one quarter of nursing home residents (11).

Outpatient Psychiatric Services

The majority of outpatient mentally ill are cared for by community mental health centers. About 15 percent are cared for by services provided by community hospitals and a much smaller percentage are treated through the outpatient services of state and county psychiatric hospitals and private psychiatric hospitals. However, all of these resources combined do not meet the needs of the mentally ill who live in the community.

In 1964, federal legislation provided construction money for community mental health centers to serve deinstitutionalized persons and others who could be treated on an outpatient basis. It was hoped that 2,000 centers would be established to meet the need throughout the nation, but the maximum number never exceeded 700. Very little money was obtained from other sources to staff and operate the centers. The federal government provided matching funds for operational costs for eight years and after that the funds decreased and the community was to assume the financial responsibility for operational costs. That didn't happen. States were forced to provide funds, but it was not enough. Services were reduced and some centers closed.

Funding and Expenditures for Mental Illness

Government pays for nearly 60 percent of the care of the mentally ill. State and local governments pay about 33 percent, while the federal govern-

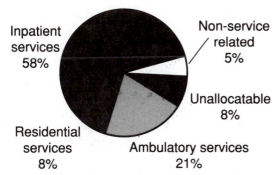

Figure 7–1. Percent distribution of state mental health agency expenditures: United States, 1990. Note: Residential services include treatment centers for emotionally disturbed children. (*Source:* National Association of State Mental Health Directors.)

ment pays 23 percent via Medicare and Medicaid. Insurance and patient fees pay the remainder. About 80 percent of inpatient care (mostly in state psychiatric hospitals and nursing homes) is funded by Medicaid. Medicare pays for psychiatric care in community hospitals, just as it does for other medical conditions. However, Medicare has a lifetime limit of 190 days and severely restricts outpatient care. The pattern of funding for mental health is summarized in Figure 7–1.

Although the number of patients in state psychiatric hospitals has declined dramatically since the 1960s, states still allocate most of their funds to inpatient care and only about 25 percent for outpatient services. State psychiatric hospitals continue to be overfunded, while community programs remain underfunded.

The difficulties of shifting funds to where they are most needed and maintaining adequate budgets is illustrated in New York State.

New York spends more per capita than any other state on mental health services. Part of the explanation is that about 75 percent of the state mental health budget is allocated to underused state psychiatric hospital facilities (12). There were more than 90,000 patients in these hospitals in the 1960s, but by the early 1990s that number had dropped

to less than 14,000. Nevertheless, the state continues to maintain 22 psychiatric hospitals that are part hospital and part nursing home for the mentally disabled elderly. Efforts to close four psychiatric hospitals stirred a heated debate. Although the psychiatric hospitals are underused and community services are inadequate because their funds have been cut, there has been great resistance to closing any psychiatric hospitals and using the released funds for community services. The biggest obstacle to closing state psychiatric hospitals is a political one. These hospitals typically are located in rural areas, where they are often the area's largest employer. For years the state legislature has been pressured by constituents who want to preserve their jobs and the economy of the area. There is additional pressure from the public employees' union to keep the institutions open to preserve hospital workers' jobs. A plan to convert psychiatric hospitals to prison space did not appeal to workers because the pay is much less. However, the severe financial problems of the state creates the opportunity for overcoming the opposition of local officials and labor unions and makes the transfer of some funds to community programs possible. Other states, facing similar obstacles to shifting funds from underused psychiatric hospitals to community programs, are finding their financial crises are forcing changes in mental health funding.

Many health insurance policies include some mental health benefits. There has been no incentive for the for-profit chains of psychiatric hospitals, which grew rapidly in the 1980s, and community hospitals to contain psychiatric costs nor to treat patients on a lower-cost outpatient basis, which has made limitations on the amount insurance companies will pay inevitable.

Mental health services need major changes in terms of organization, financing, and services to cope with current realities. The large number of untreated and homeless mentally ill will continue to remind us of the serious shortcomings of mental health services for a long time to come. A major problem in gaining support for the care and treatment of the mentally ill is that the diagnosis, treatment, and cure are not as precise, certain, and assured as other types of illness—the broken hip, heart disease, or cancer—which can be precisely diagnosed and definitively treated to yield a cure or an alleviation of symptoms or pain. Management of mental illness still has as a large element simply helping patients live with their condition.

SUMMARY

Although most ambulatory care is provided by physicians in their offices, the number and kinds of other types of ambulatory care services have sharply increased in recent years. Many of the procedures formerly performed in hospitals are now able to be done on an outpatient basis for less cost. In addition to the usual ambulatory care services such as hospital outpatient departments and community health centers, new types such as surgery centers, diagnostic imaging centers, and even cardiac catheterization laboratories are increasing rapidly. Many of these new ambulatory care facilities are for-profit and operated by chains.

The demand for mental health services far exceeds their availability. Until the 1960s seriously mentally ill persons were housed mostly in state psychiatric hospitals. The advent of psychotropic drugs and the dismal conditions in state institutions facilitated the deinstitutionalization of many of the mentally ill, who were to be treated in community-based facilities. Unfortunately little money was transferred from the state institutions and other funds were not available, so the community mental health centers were not funded adequately. As a result, too few centers have been built and services are limited. Social support services for those receiving treatment and to prevent relapses are also inadequate. Therefore, many of the chronically mentally ill in the community receive little or no treatment. It is estimated that up to one third of homeless people are seriously mentally ill.

Most of the mentally ill who need to be institutionalized are admitted to community hospitals with psychiatric units or to private, for-profit psychiatric hospitals for relatively short periods of time. The more difficult and long-term patients are in the state and local government hospitals or at VA centers.

Government funds most of the cost for the care and treatment of the mentally ill. Private insurance and patient fees account for the rest. The mental health services need major changes if they are to cope with the current problems of the mentally ill.

DISCUSSION QUESTIONS

1. What impact do you think the rapid growth of for-profit ambulatory care chains will have on the quality and cost of those services?
2. In general, many community health services are experiencing financial difficulty because of a reduction in federal funds. What should and can be done about it?
3. What roles should local, state, and federal governments play in assuring adequate mental health services?
4. Should seriously mentally ill persons be removed from the streets and treated against their will? Give reasons for your answer.

REFERENCES

1. U.S. Department of Health and Human Services, National Center for Health Statistics: *Advance Data,* No. 213, April 30, 1992.
2. Pear, R.: Community Health Clinics Cut Back as Malpractice Insurance Soar. *New York Times,* August 21, 1991.
3. Henderson, J.: Surgicenters Cut Further Into Market. *Modern Healthcare,* May 18, 1992. 108–110.
4. Pardes, H.: Problems in Providing Future Services to the Mentally Ill, in Fransen, V., ed: *Mental Health Services in the United States and England: Struggling for Change.* Princeton, NJ, The Robert Wood Johnson Foundation, 1991.
5. Grob, G.: The Chronic Mentally Ill in America, in Fransen, V., ed: *Mental Health Services in the United States and England: Struggling for Change.* Princeton, NJ, The Robert Wood Johnson Foundation, 1991.
6. Goldman, H., Gattozzi, A., Taube, C.: Defining and

Counting the Chronically Mentally Ill. *Hospital and Community Psychiatry,* Vol. 32, No. 1, January 1981, pp. 21–27.

7. Shore, M., Dickey, B.: The Dimensions of the Challenge, in Fransen, V., ed: *Mental Health Services in the United States and England: Struggling for Change.* Princeton, NJ, The Robert Wood Johnson Foundation, 1991.

8. Rice, D. Kelman, S., Miller, L., Dunmeyer, S.: *The Economic Cost of Alcohol and Drug Abuse and Mental Illness: 1985.* Washington, D.C., Alcohol, Drug Abuse and Mental Health Administration, U.S. Department of Health and Human Services, 1990.

9. Stein, L.: Filling in the Gaps: Service Gaps and Exemplary Programs in the Treatment of Chronically Mentally Ill Persons, in Fransen, V., ed: *Mental Health Services in the United States and England: Struggling for Change.* Princeton, NJ, The Robert Wood Johnson Foundation, 1991.

10. Hilts, P.: U.S. Returns to the 1820s in Care of Mentally Ill, Story Asserts. *New York Times,* September 12, 1990.

11. Manderscheid, R., Sonnenschein, M., eds: *Mental Health, United States, 1990.* DHHS Pub. No. (ADM) 90-1708, Washington, D.C.: National Institute of Mental Health, 1990.

12. *New York Times:* Collapsing the Mental Health Featherbed. February 5, 1991.

Chapter 8

Long-Term Care

Long-Term Care

Long-term care refers to a range of health and social services that are needed to compensate for the functional disabilities of people. They may be persons under 65 years of age with conditions such as birth defects, spinal cord injuries, mental impairment, or other chronic debilitating conditions, but most often they are the very old whose ability to function independently is deteriorating. To assist these people numerous services are provided that are based both in communities and in institutions. These services are very expensive and future costs are difficult to estimate. The government has no coherent policy, believing that the foundation of long-term care is the family and that services should not replace family efforts, but complement them. The basic policy questions for government are who should be eligible for services and who should pay for them. The kinds of long-term care—how it is delivered, evaluated, and financed—are among the most critical health issues facing the nation.

People of any age who are unable to cope with the tasks of daily living for extended periods of time because of physical or mental impairment need social and health care services. The risks of functional disability increase with age, however, and in the United States the number of people age 65 and older has increased from 8 percent in 1950 to almost 13 percent in 1990 and is expected to grow to 14 percent by 2010. Those 85 years and older are increasing faster than any other age group and they are expected to make up almost 15 percent of those over 65 by the year 2000. It is the 85 and older group who consumes the majority of long-term care services.

Most people who are unable to cope with the tasks of daily living are helped by families, friends, and neighbors, not by an organized service or agency. For a growing number of others, home care and other community-based services are relied on and are significant alternatives to institutional care. However, an increasing number of people, namely, the chronically and mentally ill, impaired children, and especially the frail elderly, need some level of institutional care. This is typically available through long-term care facilities that provide inpatient care for those who need care over a longer period of time than would be provided by an acute-care general hospital. Long-term care facilities include nursing homes, psychiatric and mental retardation facilities, chronic disease hospitals, and rehabilitation hospitals. The large majority of long-term care facilities are nursing homes that care primarily for the elderly. It is estimated that almost half of those Americans who survive to age 65 will spend some time in a nursing home before they die (1).

Nursing Homes

The nursing home, which is one type of long-term care facility, represents one of the more difficult problems. With fair regularity scandals erupt in homes that cheat patients, physically abuse and neglect patients, provide inadequate medical and nursing care, and are fire traps. To make matters worse, there is an insufficient number of good nursing home beds to deal with the growing number of aged people who need such care.

The roots of this problem lie in history. Nursing homes have their origins in the county poorhouses (or almshouses) of the eighteenth and nineteenth centuries. Local governments established these institutions to care for the poor, to provide them with shelter, food, clothing, and with work to help pay the costs of their care. As might be expected, many, if not most, of these people were older folks who had no families to care for them; being older, many were also invalids. Over time, these almshouses became the community dumps for all society's cast-offs, not only the poor and the physically ill but also the mentally ill, the mentally retarded, and the alcoholics, because there were often no places for them to go except the local poorhouses. Generally, conditions in these homes were not good, for they had to get along on meager public appropriations and on charity. The appropriations were meager because the public had little sense

of identity with these institutions or with the people in them; the inmates were poor and noncontributing to the general welfare, and many were transients without a previous history of community contributions. Why reward them with ideal facilities? Why tax the hard-working, thrifty citizenry to support those who were not that way? The politicians gave the almhouses the level of support the electorate wanted: bare minimum.

But a society gets what it pays for; periodically scandals erupted, as they do today, and public consciences were pricked. Over time, the mentally ill and retarded were pulled out and sent to more appropriate institutions that were mostly state rather than locally administered. In Maryland, the conditions in some county almshouses were so bad that the state set up a state-run chronic disease hospital to care for the infirm in return for closing of the county almshouses. In other states, improvements were made from time to time, and these county homes, as patients were reassigned, were left mainly with the aged poor and the physically disabled who did not need hospital care but who were unable to subsist without some form of health service support.

In recent decades, the state governments began to regulate these homes along with church, fraternal, and proprietary nursing homes, inspecting them and setting standards for performance. But the hands of state regulation were generally lightly applied. Few states were prepared to close many of the county, voluntary, and proprietary homes, because that would force the state to assume full responsibility.

As noted above, nursing homes developed under other sponsorships. Church groups and fraternal organizations started homes for care of their members. These were mainly homes for the aged, but over time they had to develop supporting health services to meet the needs of their residents. These homes received strong support from their sponsoring bodies, not only direct financial aid but also much "in kind" support in terms of gifts of equipment, volunteer maintenance, and, where there were farms, harvesting services, as well as a variety of volunteer, direct-patient care services such as help in feeding patients, occupational and play therapy, and social visiting. It is widely acknowledged that the quality of service in church- and fraternal-sponsored homes is high, and one rarely finds in them the shortcomings often found today in local government nursing homes and in some of the proprietary nursing homes.

The private (for-profit or proprietary) nursing homes emerged during the 1930s as a result of the Social Security Act of 1935, which provided welfare benefits for patients in nongovernmental institutions. The original exclusion of benefits for patients in public institutions (since repealed) apparently stemmed from congressional concern about conditions in county poorhouses and a desire to get them closed.

Many health professionals and civic leaders were concerned about the resulting rapid growth in the private nursing home sector, believing that high-quality care could not be developed and maintained if the homes depended on income derived primarily from welfare recipients, because these homes not only had to provide the needed care but also had to leave enough profit to make the owner's investment of money worthwhile. Resulting scandals in the proprietary sector have borne out the fears of these people. Not only were the payments insufficient both to maintain quality care and to ensure a reasonable return on the owner's investment, but also the very availability of large sums of money to pay for care in facilities that were in short supply proved to be an open invitation to the unscrupulous to enter the business. As it turned out, the poor who were chronically ill and needed nursing home care were also often at the bottom of the list for admission to the proprietary homes. Even after the advent of Medicare and Medicaid, many of these homes gave preference to private applicants for admission regardless of the need for care, because the low payments by government programs did not permit a reasonable return on the owner's investment and still permit quality of care. Many proprietary nursing homes also restricted the number of patients they would

admit who required a great amount of care, so as to avoid the greater costs of such care. There developed in many states, as a consequence, long waiting lists for admission of Medicare and Medicaid patients, particularly of those who needed the most care.

Foreseeing the development of these circumstances, health professionals and civic leaders encouraged the development of nonprofit nursing homes. Congress responded by amending the Hill-Burton Act in 1948 to make construction grants available for public and nonprofit nursing homes, and some states also developed grant programs. The resistance of the proprietary sector to such grant programs was vigorous and highly political. One of the successful efforts of the proprietary sector was to get Congress to approve its eligibility for FHA (Federal Housing Authority) guaranteed construction loans. The distribution of nursing homes and beds among the public, proprietary, church and fraternal, and other nonprofit sponsorships shifts constantly, but the proprietary sector is clearly dominant, with more than 72 percent of the beds and 75 percent of the homes. Growth in the public and nonprofit sectors is slow, and many factors affect this slow growth. Local governments, for one, are financially hard pressed and may be reluctant to extend their commitments in the nursing home area, because the population is aging, costs are rising, and insurance and government programs do not pay all of the costs. The length of benefit periods is also limited, and sometimes there are retroactive denials of payment. The fear is that local government will be saddled not only with the initial investment, but also with the unmet costs and the costs forced by changing federal requirements for Medicare and Medicaid and changing state requirements for state licensure. Add to this the bureaucratic hassles and paperwork that a nursing home has to put up with, and the motivation to launch an expanded effort often dissipates. Similar considerations affect the nonprofit sector. This, then, leaves the field open to the proprietary sector, in which one finds some very good homes as well as many that are very bad.

The unmet need for nursing home beds has persisted for some years and is, in fact, becoming more critical. Our population is aging, and with it comes an increased amount of chronic disease. As family units become smaller and all able persons are working, no one is at home to care for the older folks, thus further increasing the demand for facilities for care of the aged. The demand accelerated enormously with the implementation of Medicare and Medicaid, which paid for some of this care, and also with the rapid growth of catastrophic (major medical) health insurance coverage, which also paid for some of this care. The demand also increased as government and health insurance companies sought to reduce the lengths of stay in acute hospitals by moving patients to a lesser level of care.

With the advent of Medicare and Medicaid and the accompanying large sums of money that would become available for nursing home care, the federal government had to establish definitions for the types of institutions that would fall within the framework of those eligible for reimbursement, as well as standards to govern and ensure quality of care in those homes eligible to participate. No longer could a "home for the aged" be synonymous with "nursing home." If a home for the aged wanted to be paid under Medicare or Medicaid for care to eligible patients, the home had to meet certain standards. The federal government now recognizes two types of homes as being eligible. The first is a *skilled nursing facility* (SNF) and the second is an *intermediate care facility* (ICF). The U.S. Department of Health and Human Services (HSS) provided these definitions:

A *skilled nursing facility* (SNF) is a nursing home that has been certified as meeting Federal standards within the meaning of the Social Security Act. It provides the level of care that comes closest to hospital care with 24-hour nursing services. Regular medical supervision and rehabilitation therapy are also provided. Generally, a skilled nursing facility cares for convalescent patients and those with long-term illnesses.

An *intermediate care facility* (ICF) is also certified and meets Federal standards and provides less extensive health-related care and services. It has regular nursing service, but not around the clock. Most intermediate care facilities carry on rehabilitation programs, but the emphasis is on personal care and social services. Mainly, these homes serve people who are not fully capable of living by themselves, yet are not necessarily ill enough to need 24-hour nursing care.

Most nursing homes now provide a combination of skilled and intermediate care.

There were 15,324 nursing homes and 1,609,677 nursing home beds (53 per 1,000 persons over age 65) in the United States in 1991. More than one half (54 percent) of all nursing home beds were for skilled nursing care and the remaining beds were for unskilled (intermediate) care. The nursing home occupancy rate has remained steady at 95 percent. Seventy-five percent of all nursing homes are operated by for-profit groups (Table 8–1). Nine large chains operate more than 100 homes each, with the largest chain, Beverly Enterprises, operating more than 800 nursing homes.

The average length of stay in nursing homes is about two years, but varies greatly according to the type of patient. The average length of stay for Medicare patients (those recovering from an illness or disability) was 57 days, but Medicaid patients (mostly those who receive unskilled care) had an average length of stay almost 20 times longer than Medicare patients (Table 8–1). Most nursing home patients need unskilled care. Over 90 percent of nursing home patients are 65 years or older. The remaining are younger people who cannot care for themselves because of chronic diseases or accidents.

Many general hospitals have SNFs under their management, developed in part to provide a more efficient use of their acute beds. Some hospitals are experimenting with "swing beds," which can handle acute cases one day and SNF cases the next. This allows a hospital some flexibility. It is a particularly inviting approach to a hospital that has low occupancy, and, it is doubly inviting if there is a shortage of SNF beds in the area. Rather than close beds or keep them unoccupied, they can

TABLE 8–1. Nursing Home Data by Type of Owner, 1991

	Gov't	Church-Related	Secular Nonprofit	Profit	Average
			Owner		
Nursing home facilities (%)	5.0	5.5	14.9	74.5	
Nursing home beds (%)	14.4	8.0	22.1	74.2	
Occupancy rate (%)	95	97	95.8	94.9	95.4
Patient mix (%)					
Medicare	6.2	2.4	4.9	6.1	4.9
Medicaid	70.1	44.9	53.0	64.7	58.2
Private pay	25.0	52.9	45.5	29.5	38.2
Average length of stay (days)					
Medicare	67.9	40.2	58.1	56.9	57.2
Medicaid	1,162.9	1,120.3	1,379.2	941.6	1,151
Private pay	1,192.1	1,045.9	962	964.6	993
Semiprivate room rate ($)					
Skilled	77	74	83	80	
Unskilled	65	62	60	72	

SOURCE: Marion Merrell Dow, Inc.: *Managed Care Digest–Long Term Care Edition,* Kansas City, Mo., 1992.

use them and produce income with them, providing a level of care less than acute general hospital care. If the hospital is pressed for acute beds at any time, it then has the option of converting the long-term care beds back to acute beds.

Though federal standards were meant to raise the quality of nursing homes, at the time of Medicare and Medicaid implementation, the standards were applied liberally, that is to say, homes were approved even though they did not fully meet the standards. The decision by the government to do this was, of course, political: the homes were already in business, and not to certify them and thus deny benefits to the population who thought they were getting benefits would be a political liability for the president and for the legislators who passed the legislation. However, another consideration undoubtedly operated: getting marginal homes in would, over time, provide an opportunity to force them to raise the quality of their services, which would be easier to bring about the more dependent the homes were on Medicare and Medicaid payments.

The process for elevating the quality of nursing homes and of the care they provide continues.

Apart from upgrading the notorious homes that provide substandard care and that abuse both the patients and the agencies that pay the bills, the process of reform and improvement is still uphill because of the rising number of people needing care, the increased recognition of new types of care needed, and the rising costs of care in an economy that is experiencing difficulty.

The typical person in a nursing home is older (43 percent are 85 years or older), female (76 percent are women), alone (86 percent have no spouse, many have no living relatives), and mentally ill (60 percent have a major psychiatric diagnosis) (2). The costs of providing nursing home care have exploded; costs rose from $2.1 billion in 1965 (5.8 percent of all *personal* health expenditures) to $7.1 billion in 1973 (8 percent of all personal health expenditures) to $27.3 billion in 1982 (9.5 percent of all personal expenditures).

In 1990 spending for nursing home care reached $53 billion with an average cost of $86 per day for each resident, an increase of 11.4 percent from 1989. Public programs, mainly Medicaid, financed 55 percent, while residents paid directly for 45 percent (Fig. 8–1). Medicaid finances long-term

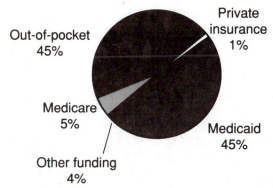

Out-of-pocket
45%

Private
insurance
1%

Medicare
5%

Medicaid
45%

Other funding
4%

Figure 8–1. Who paid for nursing home care, 1990? (*Source:* National health expenditures, 1990. Health Care Financing Review, Vol. 13 No. 1, Fall 1991.)

care for the poor elderly and those who have exhausted their savings as private paying resident. Two out of three private paying residents deplete their financial resources within one year after entering a nursing home and apply for Medicaid benefits.

Private insurance paid for about 1 percent of nursing home costs in 1990. About 135 insurance companies are selling long-term care policies. A typical policy pays a specific amount for each day in a nursing home and each home visit by a nurse or home health aide up to a certain limit. The policies may not cover the entire cost of care and typically do not take inflation into account. Many do not insure persons above a certain age unless they have purchased a policy at an earlier age. Annual premiums for long-term health care vary enormously, from $200 to $8,200, depending on age, medical condition, the amount of the daily benefit, and the number of days not covered when first admitted (3). Because most long-term care patients require intermediate or custodial care, it is important to include those provisions as well as home health care in policies; it is also important that persons with mental disorders (for example, Alzheimer's disease) not be excluded. Unfortunately, few people can afford or have the foresight to obtain private insurance. A few employers are beginning to offer long-term care insurance plans

to employees so they can get group rates, but the entire premium is usually paid by the employee.

Most people dread the prospect of entering a nursing home largely because of the lack of privacy, loss of autonomy, and regimentation. Nursing homes' operations are largely determined by regulations governing them and the payment system, chiefly Medicaid, on which they depend. Faced with the increasing numbers needing care, some believe it is time to rethink the concept of nursing homes and to experiment with new forms and combinations of care, and new residential programs and types of personnel. One innovative proposal to change the concept of nursing homes and improve the quality of life for its residents is to separate the cost of the nursing component (i.e., rehabilitation and help with bathing and feeding), which averages about 3 hours a day, and the housing component (room and food). Nursing needs would be provided for all residents by universal insurance coverage, but the housing component would be financed primarily on the resident's ability to pay. Under this model, housing for the poor would be subsidized by government, but those with higher incomes could pay for more comfortable living arrangements and amenities. This would be an incentive for people to save for the time when they might need long-term care and avoid transferring their assets to become eligible for Medicaid (4). This could reduce Medicaid costs and improve the quality of life in nursing homes.

Community-Based Care

It is generally felt that many of the elderly (who represent about 90 percent of the nursing home population) would neither need nor prefer nursing home care if the necessary long-term care services were available in the community. In fact, studies have shown that 20 to 40 percent of the nursing home population could be cared for at less intensive levels if adequate community-based care were available (2). However, even when community services are available, many people are still tempted to stay in nursing homes. Medicaid pays for nursing home care but not for community-based services, unless the state receives a waiver from the federal government. Beginning in 1981 waivers were granted to some states to offer certain kinds of social services (for example, help with bathing, cooking, or cleaning) to people living at home, in the hope that nursing home care could be delayed or avoided and the high government expenditures for nursing home care could be reduced.

The most extensive study on community-based care was financed by the federal government from 1982 to 1984. It involved 6,300 elderly people, whose average age was 80, in 10 states (5). The states were granted Medicaid waivers and funds to provide a broad base of community services to help impaired elderly to remain in their own homes rather than enter nursing homes. Comprehensive case management called "channeling" was used, whereby a person, called a case manager, identified the participating elderly's specific problems and services needed, and developed a plan of care. The case managers helped their clients get access to needed services, and they coordinated community services and informal help given by family and friends. They monitored the services to be sure that they were delivered and that they met the needs of the client. The results of the study showed that the community-based programs did not reduce nursing home costs and, in fact, increased the cost to the government. The community services had little effect on the number of nursing home admissions. Most of the elderly studied would have remained in their own homes whether or not the community services were provided.

Mechanic points out that the reason for admission to a nursing home may be factors other than need, because many living in the community may have as great a need level. Rather, admission may be the result of the loss of a spouse or other significant support person(s), or a major illness or accident that makes a person lacking support unable to care for himself or herself (6).

The services provided in the "channeling" project did not replace the care family and friends gave, but it complemented that care and enabled the informal caregivers to maintain their efforts rather than become overwhelmed. The channeling long-term care study "indicates that the expansion of case management and community services beyond what already exists does not lead to overall cost savings. But it does yield benefits in the form of in-home care, reduced unmet needs, and improved satisfaction with life for clients and informal caregivers who bear most of the burden. Whether these benefits are commensurate with its costs is a decision for society to make" (7). The National Long-Term Care Demonstration results agree with other community-care demonstrations. Kemper suggests that policy makers should move beyond asking whether expanding community care saves money and should address the issues of how much community care society is willing to finance, who should receive it, and how it can be delivered efficiently (8). A recent synthesis of 27 studies of home and community care for the chronically ill elderly, including the 10 state multi-million-dollar National Channeling Demonstration Project, concluded that the health benefits were small. Longevity and mental functioning were unaffected. Physical functioning either remained the same or decreased, apparently because the client became dependent on the home care aid. Only life satisfaction or "contentment" was favorably affected, but even this improvement was small and dissipated after several months despite continuing care. Most of those using home care services were not at risk of entering a nursing home, and although nursing home use was reduced in some studies, the cost of home care offset any savings from the reduced use of nursing homes. These results make it hard to justify home care on the basis of health benefits or cost savings. However, expanding home care is still popular because it is "the right thing to do" (9).

Home Health Care

Home health care agencies typically provide care for the disabled in the community. They supply a combination of medical and social services such as changing dressings, monitoring medications, helping clients bathe and dress, changing bed linen, and cooking. They provide some or all of the following: part-time skilled nursing care, physical therapy, speech therapy, occupational therapy, medical social services, and some medical supplies and equipment (e.g., crutches, walkers, wheelchairs) for people confined to their homes. Some agencies provide homemaker services under certain conditions. In most cases the services supplement the care the clients receive from family and friends. Although most of the agencies' clients are elderly, there are also younger clients who are recovering from an illness or accident or who have chronic medical conditions and need prolonged care. These agencies operate under various names, have varying organizational ties, and offer differing services. There are independent, hospital-operated, or health department-managed agencies. Forty-eight percent of home health agencies are for-profit agencies. They are usually financed by Medicare, Medicaid, government grants, insurance company payments, patients' fees, and charitable contributions.

A visiting nurse association (VNA) is one type of home health service in which a nurse, usually a nurse with public health training, visits a patient's home to provide some type of nursing service, for example to change a dressing or give an injection. Many of these VNAs also provide physical therapy and speech therapy services by qualified personnel.

Home health care expenditures reached almost $7 billion in 1990, with public programs financing 75 percent. Medicare, which provides home services for persons recuperating from a hospital illness, paid for more than half, while most of the rest was financed by Medicaid. Out-of-pocket expenditures accounted for about 12 percent and the rest from other private sources (10).

Meals-on-Wheels, an agency that supplies usually one hot meal a day to those confined to their homes, are common in many cities and towns today. They typically provide the noon meal, the assumption being that someone is at home in the

morning and evening to provide the other meals. Many of these agencies use volunteers to deliver the meals. The meals are secured from various agencies, the hospital or the school kitchen being two common suppliers.

Unfortunately, the government has been cutting back on home care benefits by increasing restrictions on coverage for Medicare patients at a time when the need for these services is increasing.

Adult Day Care

Another long-term care program that enables some elderly to remain in the community is adult day care. These programs can maintain or improve overall functioning, increase social interactions, offer respite care for family caregivers or even allow caregivers to remain employed. They differ from senior centers in that participants are evaluated and activities prescribed. Adult day care programs are operated by hospitals, nursing homes, social agencies, and freestanding centers established by both nonprofit and for-profit groups.

Adult day care centers in the United States have been influenced by programs in Great Britain, where a "day hospital" is part of an integrated program of geriatric services. The "day hospital" evaluates conditions and provides therapy and is sometimes an intermediate step between the hospital and the community. They provide more medical services than the United States. Adult day care is less developed and transportation is sometimes a problem in the United States. According to Kane and Kane adult day care is a much less promising investment than home care (11).

Hospice Care

In medieval times, hospices cared for the sick, wounded, and dying; the modern hospices care only for the dying. Modern hospices began in England in 1967 and operate on the principle that the dying have special needs and wants that busy hospitals, preoccupied with treating the curable, cannot provide. The first hospice service in the

United States, the Connecticut Hospice in New Haven, Connecticut, began offering home care services in 1974. In 1980, it opened a bed care facility to back up its home care program. Hospice care emphasizes the management of pain and other symptoms associated with dying when conventional treatment is no longer of value. It provides an opportunity for dying people to express their feelings about dying to people sensitive to their needs, and to spend their last days in an optimum environment. In other words, the hospice tries to improve the quality of a person's last days. About 90 percent of hospice users are cancer patients and their families. Many hospices offer only home services, but increasingly they are adding bed care facilities.

Funding is a major problem. Blue Cross and Blue Shield and other commercial carriers often do not cover hospice services. Before 1983, Medicare did not have a category for hospice care but it was paying for home care and physician services, and reimbursing as hospitals some freestanding hospice units that provided bed care. In 1983, Congress passed a bill providing limited hospice coverage under Medicare in order to reduce the rising cost of hospital inpatient care for the terminally ill. The major question concerning hospice care is not the humanity issue, but whether it is cost effective. Although there is no definite answer yet, a research firm that "studied the studies" concluded that there would be significant cost savings by adding comprehensive hospice services to Medicare (12).

Continuing Care Communities

Continuing care communities became popular about 20 years ago as an arrangement that provides for the needs of the elderly, including nursing care. These communities require a large entrance fee of $50,000 to $100,000 or more (often obtained through the sale of a home) and a monthly payment to contribute to operating costs (often financed by pension or assets). For this, housing and nursing care is ensured, along with housekeeping and some meals. Persons with high-risk health problems are either excluded or required to pay more. Medicare pays for acute medical care. People are encouraged to enter after retirement while still in good health. Accommodations are usually apartments and, when residents can no longer cope in apartments, single rooms. Until recently most communities were run by nonprofit groups, but now for-profit communities are being developed, some of which do not require a large entrance fee, but charge a monthly fee according to the amount of care needed. Continuing care communities are only available to those with adequate financial resources who want the security they provide. However, there are some government-subsidized housing complexes with facilities and services for the poor elderly who cannot manage housekeeping and personal tasks.

Financing Long-Term Care

Total public and private spending for long-term care (nursing and home care) was about $60 billion in 1990. Government paid for approximately 55 percent of the total cost. Out-of-pocket payments accounted for more than 40 percent (9). The elderly pay a much higher percentage out-of-pocket for long-term care costs than they do for acute care.

Persons receiving government-financed services generally fall into two categories. One is Medicare enrollees who are recovering from an acute illness. Because Medicare provides the elderly protection from the high costs of an acute illness, its coverage of nursing home and home care is narrowly targeted to those persons requiring skilled care during recovery from an acute illness; it does not cover custodial care.

Unlike Medicare, most Medicaid programs pay for both skilled and custodial care for persons with long-term disabilities, but only if they are poor enough to qualify for coverage. Medicaid is run by the states and eligibility for coverage and the services provided vary greatly among the states. Generally Medicaid coverage is only available to persons having less than $2,000 in financial assets. This has resulted in the practice of "spending down" among some elderly, which is the transferring of assets such as real estate and securities to trusts and relatives in order to become poor enough to qualify for Medicaid. Most persons who pay out-of-pocket for nursing home care deplete their resources and qualify within a year. Legislation has recently been enacted to protect the spouses of nursing home residents from financial devastation. Assets are now divided, with half used to pay nursing home expenses incurred before the resident becomes eligible for Medicaid, and half remains with the spouse living in the community. Medicaid now pays for about 42 percent of the total cost of long-term care and about 46 percent of nursing home costs.

Home care services account for about 12 percent of the total cost of long-term care. The government pays for about three fourths of it through numerous federal, state, and local programs. These programs vary greatly among the states and regions. In addition to Medicaid and Medicare, federal matching grants are allocated to states under Title III of the Older Americans Act of 1965 to develop comprehensive and coordinated community-based systems of services for the elderly. These include homemakers, home health aids, and nutritional services such as Meals-on-Wheels. The Title XX Social Services Block Grant to states, although not specifically intended to finance home care services, is used by many states to augment home care programs financed by other sources. The Department of Veterans Affairs operates a range of programs for disabled veterans living in the community and many states support home care programs with general revenue funds.

There have been a number of strategies to slow the rate of growth in government expenditures for long-term care. Medicare has controlled costs by maintaining a clear distinction between skilled care needed for rehabilitation following an acute illness and unskilled or custodial care. It also requires a very high copayment after 21 days of skilled nursing home care.

Medicaid also employs a number of cost-containment strategies. One of the most effective is limiting the number of nursing home beds by Certificate of Need programs and moratoria on the addition of new nursing home beds. This is based on the belief that if a nursing home bed is available, it will be filled. Other measures include tightening the criteria for Medicaid eligibility and preadmission evaluations to determine whether applicants meet the level of care criteria to be eligible for Medicaid. Because of escalating costs and access problems, new approaches to financing long-term care are being explored.

There are two basic views regarding public and private roles in financing long-term care. One view is that the government should take the leading role in solving the problem, leaving the private sector to offer supplementary policies. The other view is that the government should step in only if the private sector is unable to meet the social and financing goals.

A major study by the Brookings Institution entitled "Caring for the Disabled Elderly: Who Will Pay?" advocates a leading government role. It contends that long-term care should not be treated as a form of public charity that requires people to impoverish themselves before government helps with costs—which is now the case. The report recommends that Medicare be extended to provide nursing home care and community-based services, but only for those with rather severe disabilities regardless of their income level and that additional benefits for community-based care be provided to enable the elderly to remain in the community as long as possible, even though the costs of nursing homes and hospitals would not be reduced. Money for the increased coverage could come from taxing Social Security on the entire amount of a person's earnings rather than up to a certain level, as is now the case, higher real estate taxes, higher Medicare premiums, and an income tax surcharge (13). Another advocate of government taking the lead role is Glaser, who proposes that there be obligatory public insurance to cover basic long-term care for all and that private insurance be voluntary for amenities and services to maintain one's standard of living (14).

Another approach, based on the belief that neither public nor private sectors alone can provide affordable and comprehensive coverage for long-term care, is to limit the amount of private insurance needed to make it more attractive and affordable. Several states are involved in demonstration projects in which the elderly would buy insurance to cover the initial costs, and after a specific time, government programs would pay for home care or nursing home services (15). Because the amount of insurance needed is limited, the insurance would be affordable for many middle-income elderly. The elderly who purchase the insurance would not have to "spend down" to become eligible for Medicaid, thus preserving their assets while being assured comprehensive long-term care coverage. The government would also benefit because the elderly with insurance would not begin to use government resources as soon as they would under the present system, which would reduce the strain on Medicaid.

New York State has begun a program whereby the elderly can buy insurance from private companies that will pay for the first three years of nursing home care or six years of home care. If they need additional care, they automatically will be entitled to Medicaid without having to "spend down" their assets. The insurance is expected to appeal to people 65 years and over and they would need an annual income of at least $20,000 to afford them. State officials hope the program will help slow the steep growth of New York's $6 billion a year Medicaid budget for long-term care (16). Critics say the program is not fair to the less affluent elderly, who cannot afford the insurance and will still have to "spend down" to qualify for Medicaid. They argue that the national government

should develop a national program for long-term care. Given the realities of the federal government's financial condition, it appears unlikely it will assume any more responsibility for long-term care and that any changes will have to come from state initiatives.

SUMMARY

Long-term care refers to a range of health and social services that are needed to compensate for the functional disabilities of people of any age. Although many are under 65 years old with chronic conditions that prevent them from functioning independently, most are the very old who are no longer able to cope with the activities of daily living without help. Nursing home care is for those persons who are no longer able to live in the community and its cost is financed almost entirely by Medicaid and by out-of-pocket payments of residents. Private insurance pays for only about 1 percent of nursing home costs.

Community-based services provide home care to enable the functionally disabled to remain in the community. Unfortunately, home and community services have not been shown to improve physical functioning or significantly reduce nursing home admissions, but do appear to improve the quality of life. Other community-based services include adult day care, hospice care, and nutritional services like Meals-on-Wheels. Most long-term care is financed by the state and federal government via Medicaid. The costs have risen sharply and the demand for services continues to increase, making the question of who should pay for long-term care a prime policy issue. Many policymakers believe that neither government nor the private sector alone can provide long-term care and are seeking new ways of financing it. The states (which pay part of Medicaid) have initiated a number of reforms. One approach being tested is to encourage middle-income elderly to purchase limited long-term care insurance. If they do, they will be eligible for Medicaid when their insurance runs out regardless of their assets. Financing is only one major problem; others are determining the appropriateness and quality of services.

DISCUSSION QUESTIONS

1. How desirable is it to have such a large number of for-profit nursing homes? What are the alternatives?
2. What do you think will be the financial and humanitarian effects of the trend away from institutional care of the disabled elderly?
3. Is it ethical for the elderly to pass their wealth on to their children while passing their long-term care expenses to taxpayers via Medicaid?
4. What responsibility do children have for meeting the long-term care needs of their parents?

REFERENCES

1. Kane, R.A., Kane, R.L.: Time to Rethink the Nursing Home. *New York Times,* August 21, 1991.
2. National Conference on Social Welfare: *Long Term Care, In Search of Solutions.* Washington, D.C., 1981.
3. Maryland Office on Aging and Maryland Insurance Division: *Medicare and Medigap: A Senior Citizen's Guide to Medicare and Medigap Health Insurance in Maryland.* Baltimore, 1987.
4. Kane, R.L., Kane, R.A.: A Nursing Home in Your Future? *N Eng J Med,* Vol. 324, No. 9, 1991.
5. Department of Health and Human Services: *National Long-Term Care Demonstration.* Washington, D.C., 1987.
6. Mechanic, D.: Challenges in Long-Term Care Policy. *Health Affairs,* Vol. 6, No. 2, Summer 1987, pp. 22–34.
7. Department of Health and Human Services. The Evaluation of the National Long-Term Care Demonstration: *Final Report Executive Summary.* Washington, D.C., 1987.
8. Kemper, P.: Community Care Demonstrations: What Have We Learned? *Health Care Financ Rev,* Vol. 8, No. 4, Summer 1987, pp. 87–100.
9. Weissert, W.G.: A New Policy Agenda for Home Care. *Health Affairs,* Vol. 10, No. 2, Summer 1991, pp. 67–77.
10. Levit, K., Lazenby, H., Cowan, C., Letsch, S.: National Health Expenditures, 1990. *Health Care Financ Rev,* Vol. 13, No. 1, Fall 1991, p. 36.
11. Kane, R.A., Kane R.L.: *Long-Term Care: Principles, Programs, and Policies.* New York, Springer, 1987.
12. Ohio Blue Cross and Blue Shield: *Hospice Perspective.* Cincinnati, 1982.
13. Rivlin, A.M., Weiner, J.H.: *Caring for the Disabled Elderly—Who Will Pay?* Washington, D.C., The Brookings Institution, 1988.
14. Glaser, W.A.: *Health Insurance in Practice: International Variations in Financing, Benefits, and Problems.* San Francisco, Josey-Bass, 1991.
15. McCall, N., Knickman, J., Bauer, E.: A New Approach to Long-Term Care. *Health Affairs,* Vol. 10, No. 1, Spring 1991, pp. 164–176.
16. Freudenheim, M.: Medicaid Plan Promotes Nursing Home Insurance. *New York Times,* May 3, 1992.

9

Health Costs

If one were to place a current dollar value on all goods and services produced by a country during any one year, the resulting sum would constitute what is known as the *gross national product* (GNP) or gross domestic product.* Economists have been able to use such figures as a rough index of a nation's economy, as a measure from one year to the next of the increasing or decreasing wealth in a society as measured by its productive capacity, and as a comparative measure of the economic vitality and productive capacity of one country against another. The U.S. has historically used the GNP figure but in late 1991 began to switch to using the GDP. In the transition from GNP to GDP one will find both figures used at different times for a number of years. The health sector has long accounted for one of the largest shares of the GNP in the United States as measured by the percentage of the GNP credited to it: the physicians, nurses, optometrists, dentists, physiotherapists, and other health workers; and the hospitals, nursing homes, health insurance companies, community health agencies, public health departments, and support for medical research. The health sector has, over the years, captured a growing share of the GNP. In 1960, for example, national health expenditures constituted only 5.3 percent of the GNP. Since that time they have risen steadily to 7.3 percent in 1970 and to 12.2 percent in 1990 (Table 9–1). All indicators point to a continued rise.

Another important point to note is that the public (government) sector has, over the years, paid for an increasing share of all national health costs. In 1929, for example, only 13.6 percent of the total health expenditures was from tax sources. The 13.6 percent was for the health services provided by the armed services, the Veterans Administration and other federal government hospitals; health ser-

---

*The technical difference between the GNP and the GDP: the GNP measures what United States' residents and corporations produced regardless of their location in the world and excluded the productivity of foreign owned businesses in the United States; the GDP measures only the value of goods and services produced in the United States whether by US or foreign owned businesses. The figures are roughly comparable.

TABLE 9–1. National Health Expenditures Aggregate and per Capita Amounts, Percent Distribution, and Average Annual Percent Growth, by Source of Funds: Selected Years 1960–1990

Item	1960	1970	1980	1985	1990	1991 †
			Amount in billions			
National health expenditures	$27.1	$74.4	$250.1	$422.6	$666.2	$738.2
Private	20.5	46.7	145.0	247.9	383.6	—
Public	6.7	27.7	105.2	174.8	282.6	—
Federal	2.9	17.7	72.0	123.6	195.4	—
State and local	3.7	9.9	33.2	51.2	87.3	—
			Number in millions			
U.S. population*	190.1	214.9	235.3	247.2	248.7	—
			Amount in billions			
Gross national product	$515	$1,015	$2,732	$4,015	$5,465	—
			Per capita amount			
National health expenditures	$143	$346	$1,063	$1,710	$2,566	—
Private	108	217	616	1,003	1,478	—
Public	35	129	447	707	1,089	—
Federal	15	83	306	500	753	—
State and local	20	46	141	207	336	—
			Percent distribution			
National health expenditures	100.0	100.0	100.0	100.0	100.0	100.0
Private	75.5	62.8	58.0	58.6	57.6	57.0
Public	24.5	37.2	42.0	41.4	42.4	43.0
Federal	10.7	23.9	28.8	29.2	29.3	29.2
State and local	13.8	13.3	13.3	12.1	13.1	13.7
			Percent of gross national product			
National health expenditures	5.3	7.3	9.2	10.5	12.2	13.1
			Average annual percent growth from previous year shown			
National health expenditures	—	10.6	12.9	11.1	10.5	—
Private	—	8.6	12.0	11.3	9.5	—
Public	—	15.3	14.3	10.7	11.9	—
Federal	—	19.8	15.0	11.4	11.7	—
State and local	—	10.2	12.8	9.0	12.5	—
U.S. population	—	1.2	0.9	1.0	1.0	—
Gross national product	—	7.0	10.4	8.0	5.1	—

SOURCE: Health Care Financing Administration, Office of the Actuary: Data from the Office of National Health Statistics.
*July 1 Social Security area population estimates.
†Projected.
Note: Numbers and percents may not add to totals because of rounding.

vices provided by state and local health departments; care in state and local government general, psychiatric and mental retardation hospitals; and comparatively limited monies provided by the federal government for medical research and to the states for public health services for mothers and children. Since that time, there has been a growth in government expenditures, to the point where in 1990 government at all levels was responsible for 42.4 percent of all health expenditures. This percentage has been relatively constant since 1980.

The rise in terms of government's share of the GNP for health can be attributed to new or expanded government activities such as medical research, the Hill-Burton Construction Act, which for many years provided construction grant monies for hospitals and other health facilities, and such health services programs as crippled children's services, mental health, Medicare, Medicaid, as well as a vast number of other programs that, in their own way, added to the total public share. By 1970 we note a sharp rise in federal government expenditures. This was largely due to the implementation of Medicare and Medicaid. The growth in the public sector in subsequent years can, for the most part, be attributed to growth in the expenditures for these two programs.

By 1990, of all monies spent for health, 88 percent was for personal health care, which consists of the cost for hospital care, physician services, dental and other professional services, drugs, eyeglasses, nursing home care, and related personal care items (Table 9–5). The remaining 12 percent is accounted for by government public health activities, research and construction of medical facilities, costs related to program administration, and the net cost of private health insurance (the difference between the premiums collected and the benefits paid).

Factors accounting for the health sector's increasing share of the nation's GDP can best be seen if we focus on personal health care expenditures, for this is where the big growth occurs. The principle factor in the rise in the health sector's share of the GNP is inflation—inflation that affects all sectors of the economy and as well as that which is specific to the health sector. Economy-wide inflation during the 1980s accounted for nearly half of the rise in personal health care costs. The cost of everything—food, electricity, telephones, gasoline, automobiles, and labor—rose. Health sector inflation, commonly referred to as excess medical inflation, accounted for 22 percent of the growth—the introduction of new technology and the costs associated with its operation, the costs of equipment and drugs, and the rising cost of highly skilled professional personnel. For some of these items, the health sector must simply pay the going rate. It cannot do much about the cost of fuel, electricity, telephones, or food. It cannot do much about the prevailing wage rates: as a labor-

intensive sector and as a traditionally heavy employer of unskilled labor (as well as skilled labor), it is acutely sensitive to congressionally mandated rises in Social Security payroll deductions, to rises in the minimum wage, and to state or federal legislation mandating new employee benefits. In the hospital sector alone, labor costs in 1990 represented nearly 54 percent of total costs. Not to be forgotten is the fact that when the value of the dollar falls on the international money market, as it has in recent years, the cost of imported medical equipment rises accordingly.

Economies can sometimes be achieved in hospitals and in the health sector generally through group purchasing, consolidation of facilities and services, the establishment of medical society and hospital association liability (malpractice) insurance companies, and other steps. Critics of the health field often focus on the inefficiencies that allegedly drive up costs unnecessarily. However, most of the critics who cry "inefficiency" have few data to support their assertions. Their citations typically refer to equipment and services that are not life-threatening but that may improve patient quality of life, contribute to the quality of care, and serve to protect the physician and hospital against possible malpractice claims. Although true inefficiencies do exist in medicine, as in every enterprise, it is questionable whether all of the inefficiencies in the health sector amount to a significant component. The economic pressures on the health sector in recent years have driven out the bulk of the inefficiencies that allegedly existed.

Ways of getting an effective handle on the critical components for effective cost control still elude the critics. They do not want to spend more money on the health sector so they cry "fat" and "inefficiency," and they advocate ceilings on expenditures by cutting many of the poor off Medicaid, by forcing the elderly under Medicare to pay more for their care, by underfunding public health department immunization programs and other preventive services, and through such mechanisms as diagnosis-related groups (DRGs), fixed fees, and capitation payments, as well as other regulatory devices such as requiring a certificate of need from many of the state governments before a hospital or nursing home development or major service expansion is permitted. Some of these efforts tend to suppress demand and decrease services. Others assert that these mechanisms limit access for many who need care and that they contribute to a lesser quality of care, and higher costs later on. The remaining factors that account for the health sector's increasing share of the GNP are population increases and increases in the use and intensity of services. There has been a continuing increase in our population owing to a greater number of births than deaths, and to more immigration than emigration. These increased numbers of people make basic demands on the health care system. The aging of our population also accounts for a significant share of these increased costs. People are living longer, and along with that comes a variety of acute and chronic debilitating diseases, the diagnosis and treatments for which are very costly.

As we look at the health sector and its rising costs we note immediately that technological advances have been enormous: new drugs, which permit the more effective treatment of disease; organ transplants; new anesthetics that are safer and often more effective; new instrumentation, permitting the electronic monitoring of patients requiring intensive care and high-risk surgery; a variety of sophisticated diagnostic and therapeutic radiologic devices [such as the positron-emission tomography (PET) and computed tomography (CT) scanners, magnetic resonance imaging (MRI) and cobalt therapy units, as well as diagnostic units that do exactly what other units do except with much less radiation exposure to the patient]; renal dialysis equipment; autoanalyzers and an array of other laboratory equipment that allow faster and more accurate and more sophisticated analyses; heart-lung machines that aid in open heart surgery; new metals and materials that permit the replacement of hip and knee joints; lithotripters; and so on.

The developmental costs of new equipment are typically high; many require highly trained techni-

cians to operate them, and they cost money. The very development of this new technology increases utilization and accompanying expenditures. New drugs and new anesthetics likewise frequently lead to expanded services and increased utilization and costs. It has been estimated that 40 percent of the annual increase in health insurance premiums can be attributed to expensive technologies (1).

Increased concern over quality of care, accompanied by an increase in malpractice suits, has caused both hospitals and physicians to accelerate their technological capabilities and to utilize various tests and procedures more frequently. The substitution of tests for professional judgment may or may not always improve the overall quality of care; it certainly increases costs.

There are some technological advances that cost money but could be considered by some as unnecessary. For example, therapeutically, we could probably provide as effective care in hospitals by using the hand-cranked iron posted beds of old. Instead, we have shifted mostly to more expensive, electronically controlled beds in which the patient is able, by the push of a button, to raise and lower the head, the foot, and the knees.

Another change in the health system, but not a technological advance, is the availability of semi-private and private rooms rather than the use of the open wards, though the construction of open wards would be less expensive. The questions here are really ones of social choice: what a society wants in respect to the setting in which care is to be provided. Does it want a stripped-down, bare essentials model, or does it want some of the comforts and conveniences that are possible? We have opted for the latter, and believe that they contribute to patient recovery.

Along with technological advances have come a number of other changes in the organization and utilization of health services that have affected the overall cost picture. The number of patient visits to physician offices has increased. At the same time the number of hospital days decreased, as did the average length of stay.

It is true, of course, that the way we have paid

for hospital care until recently—reimbursement at cost or close to cost, or, frequently, payment of hospital charges that are above costs—encouraged expansion and did not encourage either provider or consumer economies. But this in itself should not be construed as inefficiency, though critics of the health sector are inclined to do so. In fact, the goals of health insurance and of many pieces of legislation—Medicare, Medicaid, community and mental health center, and others—were to facilitate access to care by removing the cost barriers, by assuring the hospitals through proper reimbursement that they would be able to provide all of the services necessary and of the highest quality. The enormous expansion of the National Institutes of Health (NIH) further encouraged the development of new technology. Furthermore, it was, after all, the Congress that passed Public Law 89–749 in 1966, which declared that "fulfillment of our National purpose depends on promoting and assuring the highest level of health attainable for every person, in an environment which contributes positively to healthful individual and family living. . . ."

Although mechanisms to pay the hospital are changing to systems of negotiated rates and to DRG systems, many insurance companies still pay costs, and others still pay charges, on a retrospective basis.

Our population is an aging one (Table 9–2) and the impact of this has been particularly significant on the overall cost picture: the elderly do not have the resiliency of younger people; it takes longer for them to recover from illnesses. In addition, they are afflicted more than other age groups with a number of debilitating and degenerative conditions, such as heart disease and cancer, which make a heavy demand on health resources. Their conditions are more life threatening and complicated, and are often multiple. The results are longer lengths of stay in the hospital, use of more specialized hospital services, and attention of more personnel. In 1990, for example, while the average length of stay in short-stay hospitals for all surgical patients was 6.4 days, for those 65 and older it was 8.7 days (Table 9–3).

In addition, the number of surgical operations for the aged was nearly twice more per 1,000 population than for those in the 45-to-64 age group (Table (9–3). Because of advances in knowledge, surgical and anesthesia techniques, and monitoring devices, more and more elderly people can be successfully treated surgically than in years past. Combine the fact of an aging population that has more days of hospitalization with longer than average lengths of stay than other age groups, higher surgical rates, and costs per hospital stay that average much more than the overall U.S. average, and one can appreciate not only the continuing concern for the solvency of the Medicare health insurance trust fund but also the more fundamental policy question of whether we will be able to afford the continued allocation of resources at current growth rates. Table 9–4 shows the growth of room charges and costs of inpatient stays for selected years.

Table 9–5 provides a detailed breakdown of the nation's health expenditures for 1990. The $585

TABLE 9–2. Age Distribution of Population: Under 65, 65–84, 85 and Over; Selected Years 1950–1985

Year	Total All Ages	Under 65	(%)	65–85	(%)	85+	(%)
1950	150,697	138,502	91.9	11,618	7.7	577	0.4
1960	179,323	162,764	90.8	15,630	8.7	929	0.5
1970	203,212	183,147	90.1	18,554	9.1	1,511	0.7
1980	226,546	200,996	88.7	23,310	10.3	2,240	1.0
1990	248,710	217,468	87.4	28,161	11.3	3,080	1.2

SOURCE: U.S. Department of Health and Human Services: *Health United States, 1987*. Washington, D.C., 1988 and later editions.

TABLE 9–3. Operative Procedures for Patients Discharged from Short-Stay Hospitals by Patient Age, 1979–1990

Patient Age (Years)	Number of Operations (in Thousands)	Rate/1,000 Population	Average Length of Stay (in Days)
1979			
Under 15	1,864	37.2	4.3
15–44	12,434	125.7	5.2
45–64	5,274	121.3	8.2
65 and older	4,286	183.4	10.8
All ages	23,858	110.5	7.2
1983			
Under 15	1,786	34.6	4.6
15–44	12,556	115.4	5.0
45–64	5,686	127.7	7.6
65 and older	6,192	226.1	9.7
All ages	26,220	112.9	6.9
1990			
Under 15	1,011	18.4	4.8
15–44	10,385	89.6	4.6
45–64	5,085	108.3	6.8
65 and older	6,569	207.9	8.7
All ages	23,051	92.4	6.4

SOURCE: National Center for Health Statistics: *Utilization of Short-Stay Hospitals, United States, annual summaries, 1979–86, and unpublished data 1979–86.* U.S. Dept. HHS, Government Printing Office; American College of Surgeons: Socio-Economic Factbook for Surgery 1988, and later editions.
Note: Sum of operative procedures by age may not equal total of ages because of rounding. Average length of stay is for all patients discharged, not only for patients undergoing operations. Excludes newborn infants and federal hospitals.

TABLE 9–4. Average Cost to Community Hospitals per Patient Day and per Patient Admission; Average Length of Stay in Community Hospitals in the United States

Calendar Year	Average Cost to Hospital per Adjusted Inpatient Day*			Average Length of Hospital Stay (in Days)	Average Cost to Hospital per Adjusted Admission*
	Total	Payroll	Other		
1946	$ 9.39	$ 4.98	$ 4.41	9.1	$ 85.45
1950	15.62	8.86	6.76	8.1	126.52
1960	32.23	20.08	12.15	7.6	244.95
1970	81.01	47.30	33.71	8.2	664.28
1980	245.12	119.13	125.99	7.6	1,850.96
1985	460.19	213.07	247.12	7.1	3,244.74
1990	686.83	368.14	318.69	7.2	4,946.68

SOURCE: American Hospital Association: *Hospital Statistics* (various annual editions) and Health Insurance Association of America.
*Adjusted expenses per admission is the average expense to the hospital in providing care for *one inpatient stay.* These expenses are derived by subtracting outpatient expenses from total expenses, and dividing the resulting amount by total admissions. Adjusted *expenses per inpatient day* covers expense of inpatient care only and is derived by dividing expenses by inpatient days.

TABLE 9–5. National Health Expenditures, by Source of Funds and Type of Expenditure: 1990 (in $ billions)

Year and Type of Expenditure	Total	Private All Private Funds	Private Consumer Total	Out-of-Pocket	Private Insurance	Other	Government Total	Federal	State and Local
National health expenditures	$666.2	$383.6	$352.9	$136.1	$216.8	$30.6	$282.6	$195.4	$87.3
Health services and supplies	643.4	374.8	352.9	136.1	216.8	21.8	268.6	184.3	84.3
Personal health care	585.3	343.5	322.2	136.1	186.1	21.3	241.8	177.2	64.6
Hospital care	256.0	116.0	102.2	12.8	89.4	13.8	140.0	104.6	35.3
Physician services	125.7	81.7	81.7	23.5	58.2	0.0	43.9	35.1	8.8
Dental services	34.0	33.1	33.1	18.0	15.1	—	0.9	0.5	0.4
Other professional services	31.6	25.2	21.5	8.8	12.8	3.6	6.4	4.9	1.6
Home health care	6.9	1.8	1.3	0.8	0.5	0.5	5.1	4.1	1.0
Drugs and other medical non-durables	54.6	48.5	48.5	40.2	8.3	—	6.1	3.0	3.1
Vision products and other medical durables	12.1	9.4	9.4	8.2	1.3	1.0	2.7	2.4	0.3
Nursing home care	53.1	25.5	24.4	23.9	0.6	1.0	27.7	17.2	10.5
Other personal health care	11.3	2.2	—	—	—	2.2	9.1	5.5	3.5
Program administration and net cost of private health insurance	38.7	31.2	30.7	—	30.7	0.6	7.5	4.8	2.7
Government public health activities	19.3	—	—	—	—	—	19.3	2.3	17.0
Research and construction	22.8	8.8	—	—	—	8.8	14.0	11.0	3.0
Research	12.4	0.8	—	—	—	0.8	11.5	10.0	1.5
Construction	10.4	8.0	—	—	—	8.0	2.5	1.0	1.5

SOURCE: Health Care Financing Administration. Office of the Actuary: Data from the Office of National Health Statistics. *Health Care Financ Rev*, Vol. 13, No. 1, Fall 1991.
Notes: 0.0 denotes amounts less than $50 million. Research and development expenditures of drug companies and other manufacturers and providers of medical equipment and supplies are excluded from "research expenditures," but are included in the expenditure class in which the product falls. Numbers may not add to totals because of rounding.

billion for personal health care represents 88 percent of all monies spent that year on health. Personal health care, it should be noted, is the treatment and caring function of the health sector; it excludes public health activities, research, and construction of health facilities. Although planners are seeking to slow construction and to cut in other areas, the principal focus for cost containment is in the personal care sector. The reason is clear once we examine Table 9–6.

Hospital care accounts for $256 billion, or 43.8 percent of all personal health care expenditures. Physician services come next, accounting for $125.7 billion, or 21.5 percent. Nursing home care accounts for $34.6 billion, or 9.3 percent. These three components account for 74.7 percent of all personal health care expenditures, and it is these three elements that government is seeking most urgently to address. The other two components that are significant consumers of resources—dental services and drug and medical sundries—do not make a heavy demand on government resources. Drug and medical sundries consist of over-the-counter purchases; drugs that are provided in hospitals, nursing homes, and directly by physicians are charged to those categories. One should also note that the monies paid for salaries to hospital-based physicians appear as hospital costs, not physician services. Because these dental and outpatient drug costs do not make a heavy demand on government funds, government has not paid much attention to these items. This suggests to some that government today is more concerned with public finance than it is with public policy.

The first column of figures in Table 9–5 shows the total amount spent in a number of health categories. Who pays for each (the public or private sector) and how (patient payments, health insurance, federal government, state/local government, or other groups) is shown for each category by reading across the table on each line. We might note that of the $256 billion spent on hospital care (Table 9–6), about 5 percent, or $12.8 billion, was paid out-of-pocket because the patients had no

health insurance or because their benefits had been used up; or because they incurred extra charges for private rooms, telephone calls, and television rental; or because they used the outpatient departments or emergency department, where the insurance did not cover all of the charges. For the remaining $243.2 billion (95 percent of the expenditures for hospital care), third parties made the payments. (*Third parties* are principally the insurance companies and government.) Medicare accounted for 26.7 percent of all hospital expenditures, or $68.3 billion; Medicaid accounted for 11.1 percent or $28.5 billion. Private health insurance was responsible for 34.9 percent, or $89.4 billion. These figures represent expenditures for hospital care, not hospital costs or hospital charges. Why the federal government focuses on hospital costs should be evident from these figures.

When we examine the physician service figures in Table 9–6 we find that the patient paid $23.5 billion, or 18.7 percent, of the total 125.7 billion spent in that category. At first glance this would suggest how woefully inadequate health insurance is in this area. It is true that there are shortcomings, particularly with regard to the elderly and the poor who are not eligible for Medicaid but who are able to pay the physician for routine care, although not for more costly care in hospital. However, this figure needs interpretation: most of this money is for routine care in physicians' offices, a type of care not usually covered by health insurance. Many would argue that such *first dollar coverage* (i.e., insurance coverage for all visits to a physician's office) should not be part of any insurance package because it does not encourage judicious patient behavior in deciding whether or not to visit a physician. Indeed, first dollar coverage encourages frivolous visits to the physician, and it encourages the billing for extra visits by the physician. Of a more serious nature is the fact that a significant portion of this patient payment figure represents out-of-pocket payments by Medicare patients. Some of this is to pay the upfront required deductible

TABLE 9–6. Hospital, Physician, and Nursing Home Expenditures by Source of Funds, 1990

| | | | | | | Third Parties | | | | |
| | | | | | | | | Government | | |
Year	Total	Direct Patient Payments	All Third Parties	Private Health Insurance	Other Private Funds	Total	Federal	State and Local	Medicare*	Medicaid†
Hospital Care Expenditures										
1990 *(Amounts in Billions)*	256.0	12.8	243.2	89.4	13.8	140.0	104.6	35.3	68.3	28.5
1990 *(Percent Distribution)*	100.0	5.0	95.0	34.9	5.4	54.7	40.9	13.8	26.7	11.1
Physician Care Expenditures										
1990 *(Amounts in Billions)*	125.7	23.5	102.1	58.2	0.0	43.9	35.1	8.8	30.0	5.2
1990 *(Percent Distribution)*	100.0	18.7	81.2	46.3	0.0	34.9	27.9	7.0	23.9	4.1
Nursing Home Care Expenditures										
1990 *(Amounts in Billions)*	53.1	23.9	29.2	0.6	1.0	27.7	17.2	10.5	2.5	24.1
1990 *(Percent Distribution)*	100.0	45.0	49.0	1.1	1.4	52.2	32.4	19.8	4.7	45.4

SOURCE: Health Care Financing Administration, Office of the Actuary: Data from the Division of National Cost Estimates.

*Subset of federal funds. Percentages are of the total expenditures for that category.

†Subset of federal and state/local funds. Percentages are of the total expenditures for that category.

under Part B of Medicare. Much of it, however, represents payments to the physician after the deductible has been met.

Under Medicare, after the deductible has been met, a physician who accepts "assignment" agrees to accept from Medicare 80 percent of what Medicare determines to be a reasonable fee, and the physician agrees to bill the patient only for the balance—that is, only 20 percent of the fee set by Medicare. In a growing number of states, state laws require physicians to accept assignment in all cases as a condition for retention of their license to practice medicine in that state. Federal legislation is lowering the amount physicians may charge in nonassigned cases, and will likely require assignment in all cases throughout the country within a few years. Nearly half of the Medicare population has taken out additional health insurance, which pays the deductible and the co-insurance (the 20 percent) portion of the allowed charges. These supplementary insurance policies also cover the deductible and co-insurance charges under Part A—the hospital portion—of Medicare.

Another significant component of the sum paid directly by patients to physicians represents monies paid by non-Medicare patients for surgical and in-hospital medical care to cover charges over and above what the insurance company pays. Also in this category are payments by people who do not have health insurance.

As one looks at nursing home care in Table 9–6, one finds that in 1990 patients paid some 45 percent of the total amount spent ($23.9 billion out of a total of $53.1 billion). Though the cost per day in a nursing home is substantially less than in a hospital, the length of stay is typically much longer, and the population in nursing homes is virtually all over 65 years of age. Medicare pays for skilled nursing facility (SNF) care up to only 100 days, provided the patient had first spent three days in a hospital. After the twentieth day the patient has to pay a significant part of the cost. Many elderly people do not meet the initial hospitalization requirement. Other Medicare patients do

TABLE 9–7. Estimated Distribution of Expenditures Among the Private Sector, Federal Government, and State and Local Government

Expenditure	1990	
Private expenditures	383.6	57.5%
Federal expenditures	195.4	29.3%
State/local expenditures	87.3	13.1%
Total	666.2	99.9%

not need the level of care a skilled nursing facility provided, but instead a lesser level of care for which Medicare does not pay.

Though federal expenditures for nursing home care under Medicare have been slight, under Medicaid they are substantial; the federal and state governments under the Medicaid program paid 45.4 percent of all nursing home expenditures. The economic pressures on government under Medicaid beginning in 1983 led some states to adopt a policy of reclassifying SNF patients to the lower cost intermediate care facility (ICF) category, for which Medicaid also pays. On being reclassified, a patient's condition may not have changed, but the intensity and quality of services certainly did, illustrating government's obsession with the cost of everything.

Finally, of all national health expenditures in 1990 ($666.2 billion) the estimated distribution among the private sector, federal government, and state/local government was as shown in Table 9–7.

Resources for Health: Are There Limits?

The rise in health costs, and the likelihood of a continued rise owing to the aging of our population and the development of new technologies, raise the question of how much of the nation's resources should be allocated to the health sector. In 1990, 12.2 percent of the nation's GNP was spent in the health sector, a growing portion over the years. Latest figures for 1992 indicate a rise to 14.6 percent of the GDP. The increased spending has brought high-quality health services to the population, contributing to its health and quality of life. But the use of money for health services does not permit it to be used for something else.

To the extent that the consumer pays out-of-pocket for health care, the money cannot be spent for travel, clothes, restaurants, automobiles, stereo and video equipment, or a number of other things. Fortunately, the consumer only has to pay for 20 percent of this directly by out-of-pocket payments (Fig. 9–1). The remainder, *all* citizens pay indirectly through taxes and in the price paid for purchases, which usually include a component to cover the employers' contributions for employee health insurance. As the costs of health care go up and as the health sector commands a growing percentage of the GNP, the citizens pay one way or another. Although the population may feel that costs are getting out of hand, it is very likely that it is getting good value for its direct personal

expenditures, as well as for its combined direct and indirect expenditures. The population is nonetheless displeased when it has to spend more for insurance or out-of-pocket, because it means that other wants cannot be met. Part of the difficulty may be due to the fact that the population is not sufficiently aware of the benefits it derives from increased health spending.

There is a certain public ambivalence about this issue. Although most Americans express concern over the rising cost of care and believe that the trend "has made the costs of their own medical care unreasonable," most (54 percent) still "believe that federal spending for health care should be *increased,* [and] 71 percent still favor some form of national health insurance . . ." (2, p. 52).

The principal worriers over rising costs are business and industrial leaders, health insurance companies, governments, those who cannot afford health insurance, and those who have to purchase health

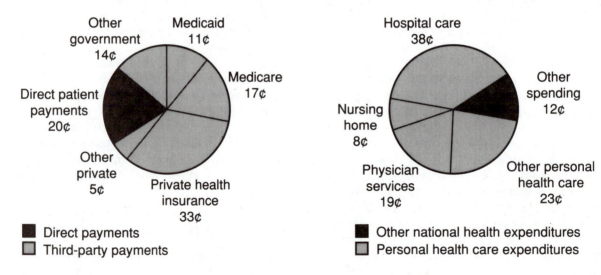

Where it came from

Where it went

Figure 9–1. The nation's health dollar: 1990. Eighty percent of national health expenditures was channeled through third parties. Forty two percent was channeled through government. The bulk of that expenditure was for patient care, and the remaining 12 percent was spent for research, construction, administration, and government public health activity. (*Source:* Health Care Financing Administration, Office of the Actuary: Data from the Division of National Cost Estimates.)

insurance entirely on their own. Most companies today pay all or part of the health insurance premiums for their employees. Company contributions are tax-deductible as a bona fide business expense. In a very real sense, the company's contributions can also be viewed as nontaxable employee income. In order to increase its tax revenues, the federal government is increasingly seeking to limit the amount that business can deduct and also to tax some of these contributions as employee income. In any event, the cost of these employer contributions must be recovered if the business or industry is to make a profit. The costs are therefore built into the price of the product or service. The concern that employers have is that if costs continue to rise, or if the insurance benefits they pay for are expanded and cost more, the passed-on costs could jeopardize their competitive position in the marketplace.

The auto industry is a case in point. In recent years it has been hard pressed by Japanese competition. Several years ago, as part of the strategy to be more competitive and to cut costs, the Ford Motor Company asked its 56,000 salaried workers to pay up to $750 a year for health benefits, thus eliminating the existing first dollar comprehensive benefits the employees had (3). The significance of that shift of costs is more evident if one recognizes that the savings to the Ford Motor Company would have amounted to $42 million in 1984. General Motors announced in 1992 that its health benefits cost the company $3.4 billion, or about $929 for every car it produced (4).

For government, and for all who are concerned with public policy, there is concern that, to the extent the health sector commands a greater share of the GNP, there will be less money in the economy for development in other sectors—improvements in public education, space research, and defense, to cite just a few examples—which affects the profitability and employment in these sectors. Profitability is, as suggested earlier, also affected if consumers cannot afford new products because of expenditures they make in the health area. Small wonder then that business and industrial executives are among the leaders in the drive to contain health costs. The rise in health costs is threatening to them.

The commercial insurance companies are also unhappy about the rise in costs. As their payments rise, they have to recover the costs through increased premiums from the insurance purchasers. When this occurs, they run the risk of losing business to competitors, and they also get pressure from the employers to do something about rising costs. The loss of business might entail not only health insurance but life and retirement policies as well. Blue Cross and Blue Shield meet some of these same problems, but also, because they are regulated by state insurance commissioners, they frequently have limits placed on the amounts they can pay in benefits and on how much they can charge for their policies; if the constraints make them less competitive, their insured may shift to the competition.

The other group most concerned about rising health costs is government—federal, state, and local. Government paid 42.4 percent of all monies spent for health in 1990—29.3 federal, 13.7 percent state/local. In recent years these levels of government have sought to contain the rise in costs in several ways, such as by regulation (e.g., certificate of need and rate control); by reducing their efforts in some areas (e.g., eliminating support for a variety of health education and health service programs); by shifting costs to the providers or to the consumers (e.g., paying hospitals less than cost or by paying some physicians less than their usual charges, and by releasing patients from state psychiatric hospitals without providing the necessary money for noninstitutional and community services). At the state level, the increases in Medicaid costs have outpaced increases in revenue in most states. The ability of a state, under these circumstances, to expand health services, improve education, or strengthen any of its other services is severely constrained. About all it can do is trim costs, cut back on Medicaid eligibility and services, cut back in other areas, and ask the federal government to help it do the job through new federal mandates or federal monies. Alternatively, it can raise taxes. But whatever a state does, except for securing federal action, it runs the risk of alienating voters. Legislators and governors can and have been voted out of office because of tax increases. Small wonder that federal solutions are sought; besides it all started largely because of new federal initiatives.

At the federal level, the largesse began when the economy was booming and the population was expanding. In recent years, however, the economic boom has subsided, and the population is aging. The resulting drain on the Medicare trust fund has already been noted. Apart from a conservative ideology that in the Reagan-Bush years deemphasized federal initiatives and actions in the health sector, the growing demands of other sectors precluded much action in the health area. As one White House spokesman put it, "The clash over resources comes down to a choice between the armed services and the old folks, or between free school lunches and troops in Korea" (5). The author of the article in which that quote appeared went on to say, "Social security retirement benefits and Medicare together consume today as much of the budget as the armed services. These are the programs that old people have come to depend on; they feel they have a contract with the Government and it must be honored."

Uwe Reinhardt believes that the perceived cost crisis is actually a moral crisis (6, p. 8). He points out that German and French firms pay a "larger share of the nation's health bill than do American firms." There are, he says, "more compelling reasons why American business firms find it hard to compete abroad." He goes on to note, "In 1983 we spent $22 billion on farm support programs—expenditures designed to pay farmers not to grow food or to grow surplus food the government must store in its warehouses. A nation that can do this year after year has no case arguing that it cannot afford additional public health care expenditures." He also says that "the dimension of the crisis before us: an apparent unwillingness of society's well-to-do to pay for the economic and medical

maintenance of the poor. It is not an externally imposed economic or cost crisis; it is a moral crisis." Rather than face the real, troublesome issue directly, we try to "finesse" it by focusing on a symptom of the problem. The symptom is costs, and to deal with this is easier.

To increase the share of spending by the health sector denies the opportunity to fill other needs and wants. To find the resources to permit health sector expansion is difficult because it requires the other sectors to give up the resources. Very unpopular! A political dilemma!

The easy way out is to restrain the sector that is making the claim for additional resources. This is being done with defense, but here restraining growth can affect employment and profitability in many sectors (construction, automobile, aerospace, and other weapons areas) that fuel the nation's economy by stimulating production in those areas that supply them with materials. In other words, defense spending has an enormous ripple effect in terms of stimulating the nation's economy. Another approach, the one we are trying to take, is to restrain the growth in the health sector: as a labor intensive sector its spending does not *seem* to have a positive ripple effect; it does not appear to spawn as much economic activity in as many other sectors as defense spending despite the fact that in many cities the hospital is the largest employer. How then do we restrain health spending in light of an aging population and major technological advances?

The fight, and it is a fight, is over resources, over which sector of the economy gets a bigger piece of the pie. Ideology plays a role, as does propaganda. The health sector, we are told, is expanding too rapidly and commanding too great a share of the GNP, but on what basis is such an assertion made? Is there a right percentage? That the health sector commands more than most other nations means very little. Though the ripple effect of defense spending is significant, the ripple effect from health sector spending, while not as dramatic or as visible, is also significant. As a major employer of both skilled and unskilled labor, health workers pay taxes and spend money, thus fueling the nation's economy. As a heavy purchaser of supplies, drugs, and equipment, this sector generates employment in these firms, as well as in the construction industry because of the need for new buildings and for modernization of existing plants. One cannot help but observe the relative ease by which a new weapons system is sold, a weapons system that may never be used, whereas the health system still has difficulty in selling the need for new scanners, additional renal dialysis equipment, more long-term care beds, and the needed community health and social services that would demonstratively be used to improve health and the quality of life in general, as well as contribute to the nation's economy.

There are inefficiencies and excesses in the health sector, but these exist in all sectors. They are not to be condoned, but should be dealt with as they are identified and as effective solutions are devised. In the battle for resources between sectors, however, it may be that the health sector has allowed itself to be judged by rules that deemphasize societal values to too great an extent. It is fashionable, for example, for health sector people to use the language of business and economics: cost effectiveness, marketing of services, vendor payments, multi-institutional management, corporate structure, risk management, and the health *industry* (as though it were comparable to the automobile, banking, or airplane industries). It is businesslike language, and it even speaks of health sector competition, though what this typically means is price competition and not quality competition.

Cunningham addressed this when he asked, "What has become of the underlying, care-before-cost philosophy—the system of motivating beliefs and concepts that created our hospitals and guided their activities for so many years? Given all the pressures of inflation, regulation, competition, and now the determination of government, insurers, and employers to cut down the amounts they are spending for health care, how could the direction of our ideas and convictions have shifted so far so fast?" (7). He was concerned that the hospital has

overreacted to the pressures and that "the danger now is that there could be a confusion of means and ends; acceptance of the methods of commerce could lead to acceptance of the values of commerce." He concluded that "there is time still to moderate the march on the market. . . ."

The health sector certainly is not an island; it must coordinate with other sectors in society. However, in doing so, there is evidence to suggest that the health sector may be failing to maintain and emphasize adequately the value component of its claim for resources, because it is the value element that can assist society in making a more balanced choice in the allocation of resources.

SUMMARY

In 1990, 12.2 percent of our GNP was spent on health. This is the highest percentage ever recorded and the percentage is continuing to rise. The enormous growth in health expenditures can be attributed to inflation, population increases, technological advances and other changes in the health system.

Economy-wide inflation and population increases are factors that largely reflect occurrences outside of the health sector; they affect the health sector but cannot be significantly controlled by it. Technological advances and other health system changes, however, are health specific, and are often referred to as medical-specific inflation. The cost increases relate to new drugs such as for AIDS and other diseases; technological developments (such as lithotripters, MRI scanners, and organ transplants), which permit the treatment of people in more effective ways; increased utilization of services because they are physically more accessible and more easily paid for by insurance, government programs, or the patients who have more disposable income; and the aging of our population, which has greater morbidity, slower recovery, and longer hospital and nursing home stays.

It is the aging of the population that most threatens the other claims for the use of resources. The extent to which additional monies are consumed in the health sector owing to the aging of our population and new technological advances suggests that there will continue to be significant increases in health consumption, with the result that other sectors of the economy will not have access to these monetary resources. The other sectors that lose access to these resources include the defense industry, highway development, education, and so on. The political dilemmas that flow from these conflicting claims for use of the available monies are considerable. Though most consumers express concern over rising costs, they are insulated to a considerable extent because of their private health insurance, Medicare, Medicaid, and other government program protection. The principle groups that are most concerned in the clash over access to resources are business and industrial leaders, the insurance companies, government, and those who would like to buy health insurance but cannot afford it. The biggest contest in government over access to resources is between the defense and health sectors.

The easiest way to deal with the problem in the eyes of nonhealth sector people is to restrain health sector development. This is the course that the nation has chosen for the moment. By controlling hospital and nursing home construction, by slowing down the acquisition of expensive technology, and by shifting the burden of costs to the consumer, the hope is that the health sector growth will be slowed and the other sectors can continue to receive resources and "do their thing."

In the debate to slow health sector growth, assertions are made about the nation's being unable to provide such a high percentage of its productivity to the health sector. The implication seems to be that the health sector is a consumer of resources and is itself unproductive. However, the fact is that the health sector as a labor intensive sector is highly productive: it not only purchases large amounts of drugs, supplies, and medical equipment, but it also is a boon to the construction industry. It fuels the economy of those who supply it with its needs. As a labor intensive sector it employs people who pay taxes and buy goods, both of which encourage the nation's economy. In many communities, the hospital is by far the largest employer, and the local economy depends on it.

As important as the health sector's productivity is, there is another element that the health sector has allowed to slip from its grasp. That element is *values*. As one author expressed it: "What has become of the underlying care-before-cost philosophy—the system of motivating beliefs and concepts that created our hospitals and guided their activities for so many years? Given all the pressures of inflation, regulation, competition, and now the determination of government, insurers, and employers to cut down the amounts they are spending for health care, how could the direction of our ideas and convictions have shifted so far so fast?"(7) He goes on to express the concern that in the health sector's reaction to these pressures, it has overreacted and that "The danger now is that there could be a confusion of means and ends; acceptance of the methods of commerce could lead to a acceptance of the values of commerce" (7). Another author noted, after pointing to the billions appropriated each year to pay farmers not to produce food or to produce surplus food so that the government can warehouse it: "A nation that can do this year after year, has no cause arguing that it cannot afford additional public health care expenditures" (6). The cost crisis, he went on to say, is a moral crisis.

DISCUSSION QUESTIONS

1. Are health costs commanding too great a share of the nation's gross national product? Why?
2. What are some of the consequences for patients of cost-containment efforts?
3. To what extent do you believe that societal values should influence the allocation of the available resources?
4. How can the health sector effectively introduce value considerations into its claim for an increased share

of the nation's resources? What would be the effect if education, social welfare, and defense also introduced value factors in their claims for resources? How could dilemmas created by conflicting claims be resolved?
5. What kind of restrictions should there be on the acquisition of new technology by hospitals? What would be the implications for the patient? For the physician? For overall hospital quality of care?
6. If a community with only one hospital raised the money by public donations or by a local bank loan for a very expensive piece of equipment, such as a CT scanner or MRI unit, and a large teaching hospital 50 miles away had a unit with unused capacity, and if the state authorities said that the community could not justify its need for such equipment, should the community be allowed to purchase it regardless?

REFERENCES

1. *The New York Times,* August 16, 1992.
2. Blendon, R.J., Altman, D.E., in Schramm, C.J., ed. *Health Care and Its Costs,* New York, Norton, 1987.
3. *The New York Times,* August 5, 1983.
4. *The Wall Street Journal,* August 31, 1992.
5. White, T.H.: Weinberger on the Ramparts. *The New York Times Magazine,* February 6, 1983.
6. Relman, A.S., Reinhardt, U.E.: Debating For-Profit Health Care. *Health Affairs,* Vol. 5, No. 2, Summer 1986.
7. Cunningham, R.M., Jr.: More than a Business: Are Hospitals Forgetting Their Basic Mission? *Hospitals,* January 16, 1983.

10

Health Insurance

Most people in the United States have some protection against the costs of medical care. For most, all or nearly all of the major costs are covered by health insurance or some government program, but for others the protection leaves much to be desired. Estimates vary concerning how many people are protected. Some say that insurance and government programs cover about 85 percent of the U.S. resident population, leaving some 35 million Americans without any protection at all. Whatever figure one chooses to accept, the fact remains that many people are still unprotected from health care costs and must rely on charity to pay for care or on whatever out-of-pocket funds they might have available to them. For some of the unprotected, securing access to care can be difficult. It is also recognized that many in our population, even those who are insured or enrolled in a government program, do not have adequate protection against hospital, physician, nursing home, dental, and drug charges. There are shortcomings in both private insurance and government programs, and these should be a cause for social concern.

Most people have health insurance policies taken out through the place of employment (hence, *group policies* or *group enrollment*), but some policies are taken out on a *nongroup* or *direct payment* basis by the self-employed and by others who are not eligible for group enrollment. The principal differences between group and nongroup coverage are that the former generally costs less and has a broader range of benefits.

Most insured people (an estimated 153 million in 1991) have policies with Blue Cross and Blue Shield or with one of the large commercial insurance companies such as Prudential, Cigna, and Metropolitan. Many, some 32.5 million people, were protected against health care costs in 1991 under the Medicare program, a government entitlement program principally for those over the age of 65, which also protects a small number of younger people (approximately 3 million) who fall into certain disability categories. Some 21.7 million people received benefits in 1991 under Medicaid, a federal-state government program designed to pay for health care of the poor. Many of these people (some 2.6 million) were Medicare enrollees who became eligible for Medicaid because of their low income (Table 10–1).

Protection against health care costs is also available through various other government programs: for military personnel; for their dependents in the military system and through a program known as the Civilian Health and Medical Program of the Uniformed Services (CHAMPUS); for Native Americans and Alaska Natives through the Indian Health Service; for veterans who are totally dependent on the Veterans Administration system for care; and for long-term residents of federal, state, and local psychiatric hospitals and prisons.

We must emphasize that the figures cited about the number insured and otherwise protected are estimates, and the estimates vary depending on the rate of unemployment in the country, business conditions, and the changing eligibility standards for Medicaid and other government programs. Those not protected by health insurance or by government programs are the unemployed (including many high school and college graduates who enter the workforce and because of age—typically over 19—or graduation automatically go off their parents' policies), those between jobs, those too well off to be eligible for Medicaid but not well off enough to afford health insurance, those working in some small businesses that do not offer

health insurance, some part-time workers, and some who choose not to have health insurance. It is worth noting that most of those without insurance in 1990 are in paid employment (Table 10–2).

The extent to which people have protection is a source of satisfaction, but when one considers the adequacy of that coverage against the costs that people must bear, there is cause for great social concern.

Some policies exclude coverage for conditions that existed at the time of enrollment. Other policies insist that the insured must wait a certain period of time (typically 11 or 12 months) before a preexisting condition is covered. Most policies place a limit on how much is paid for hospital care, physician care, nursing home care, and the like. Many policies have deductibles, money the patient must pay first, before the insurance policy provides benefits. The shortcomings with existing policies become particularly pronounced when one notes (Table 10–3) that, whereas 95 percent of hospital costs in 1990 were covered by insurance, government programs, or other third-party payers, the percentages for other categories are depressingly low, and the patients have to pay a much greater share of the overall costs.

Why do we have such a variety of policies with so many limitations that ultimately force the patient or patient's family to meet a significant portion of the costs of care? Why can't we have a compre-

TABLE 10–1. Number of Persons With Health Insurance or Government Program Protection Against Health Care Costs, 1990

	Population (Millions)	% U.S. Population
Medicare enrollments	32.5	13.6
Medicaid recipients under 65	21.7	8.7
Health insurance, under 65*	153.2	61.6
Military and military dependents	3.7	1.5
Indian Health Service	1.000	.004
Total U.S. population (estimated)	246,191	

SOURCE: *Health Care Financing Review*, Vol. 14, No. 1, Fall 1992.
*Unduplicated count of recipients.

TABLE 10–2. Persons Without Health Insurance Coverage, by Attachment to the Workforce, 1990 [Thousands]

	Workers	Dependents	Total	Percent of Uninsured
Nonworker	0	4,958*	4,958	14.3
Full year/full time worker	8,976	8,083	17,059	49.3
Full year/part time worker	1,511	716	2,227	6.4
Part year/full time worker	5,387	2,414	7,801	22.5
Part year/part time worker	2,047	538	2,584	7.5
Total	17,921	16,708	34,629	100.0

SOURCE: CRS analysis of data from the March 1991 Current Population Survey.
*Includes both heads of household and dependents with no workforce attachment.
Note: Items may not sum to total because of rounding. Full-year workers were employed 50 or more weeks during the year. Full-time workers worked an average of 35 or more hours per week during the weeks they were employed.

hensive benefit structure for all people? What good is all the insurance if it does not *protect?*

There are two general answers to these questions. The first is by Victor Fuchs from his book *Who Shall Live?* (1, pp. 17–19):

The most basic level of choice is between health and other goals. While social reformers tell us that "health is a right," the realization of that "right" is always less than complete because some of the resources that could be used for health are allocated to other purposes. This is true in all countries regardless of economic system,

regardless of the way medical care is organized, and regardless of the level of affluence. It is true in the communist Soviet Union and in welfare-state Sweden, as well as in our own capitalist society. No country is as healthy as it could be; no country does as much for the sick as it is technically capable of doing.

The constraints imposed by resource limitations are manifest not only in the absence of amenities, delays in receipt of care, and minor inconveniences; they also result in loss of life. The grim fact is that no nation is wealthy enough to avoid all avoidable deaths. . . .

Within limits set by genetic factors, climate, and other

TABLE 10–3. Personal Health Care Expenditures, Percent Covered by Third Parties, and Patients in Selected Categories—1990

Category of Expenditure	Total Expenditures ($ Billion)	% Covered By			
		Health Insurance	Government Programs	Patients	Other*
All expenditures for personal health care	585.3	31.8	41.3	23.3	3.6
Hospital care	256.0	34.9	54.7	5.0	5.4
Physician services	125.7	46.3	34.9	18.7	—
Dentist services	34.0	44.4	2.6	52.9	—
Other professional services	31.6	40.5	20.3	27.8	11.4
Drugs and medical sundries†	54.6	15.2	11.2	73.6	—
Eyeglasses and appliances†	12.1	10.7	22.3	67.8	—
Nursing home care	53.1	1.1	52.2	45.0	1.9
Home health care	6.9	7.2	73.9	11.6	7.2
Other health services	11.3	—	80.5	—	19.5

SOURCE: Gibson, R.M., Waldo, D.R., Levit, K.R.: *Health Care Financ Rev,* Summer 1987; Levit, A. L., et al., *Health Care Financ Rev,* Fall 1991.
*Spending by philanthropic organizations, industrial in-plant health services, and privately financed construction.
†Outpatient expenditures only purchased by consumers from retail trade outlets. Excluded are expenditures for patients in hospitals and nursing homes and items dispensed through physician offices.

natural forces, every nation chooses its own death rate by its evaluation of health compared with other goals. . . .

If better health is our goal, we can achieve it, but only at some cost.

Although Americans are very lightly taxed compared with people in almost every other industrialized nation, we have been unwilling to provide comprehensive coverage even for a limited population group—the elderly. As each year passes, benefits are cut, and the elderly are forced to pay more.

A second answer to the questions posed earlier lies in the history of health insurance in America, and in the principles of health insurance rate structuring.

Historical Developments: Blue Cross and Blue Shield

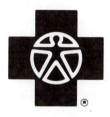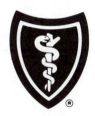

The year 1929 is generally credited as marking the birth of modern health insurance. It was in that year that Justin Ford Kimball established a hospital insurance plan at the Baylor University Hospital for the schoolteachers of Dallas, Texas. As a one-time superintendent of the Dallas public schools, he was sensitive to the plight of schoolteachers, particularly so when he found many of them had unpaid bills at the hospital. Working from hospital records, he calculated that the schoolteachers as a group "incurred an average of 15 cents a month in hospital bills. To assure a safe margin, he established a rate of 50 cents a month" (2, p. 19). In return, the school teachers were assured of 21 days of hospitalization in a semiprivate room.

Kimball's success spread, and over the years his approach was the model for what became the Blue

Cross plans around the country—the concept of assuring the benefit not of cash but of *service,* the emphasis on semiprivate accommodations, and even the time frame of 21 days of benefits.

Though 1929 is cited as the beginning, there were antecedents. Anderson notes, for example (2, p. 17):

Between 1916 and 1918, attempts were made by 16 state legislatures from New York to California to establish some form of compulsory health insurance, essentially a mechanism to help families pay for health services, which were already being felt as costly and unpredictable episodes. The necessary mass political support in the states was not present, however, and the solid opposition of the American Medical Association, insurance companies, and the pharmaceutical industry, not to mention business and industry opposed to unaccustomed payroll taxes, stopped the movement.

The Health Insurance Institute also cites antecedents (3, p. 7):

When health insurance began some 130 years ago, it met a far simpler need—coverage against rail and steamboat accidents.

The nation's first health insurance company came into being in 1847. Three years later another company was organized specifically to write accident insurance. By 1864, coverages were available for virtually every type of accident. At the turn of the century, 47 companies were issuing accident insurance.

In addition, the mutual aid society concept, which originated in Europe, was adopted in the United States in the latter half of the 1800s. Small contributions were collected from members of workers' groups in return for the promise to pay a cash benefit for disability through accident or sickness. Fraternal benefit societies also were important early providers of health insurance in the U.S.

Mutual benefit associations, or "establishment funds," began in 1875 in the United States. These funds—sometimes financed partially by employers—provided small payments for death or disability of workers in a single organization.

Both accident insurance companies and life insurance companies entered the health insurance field in the early 1900s. At the beginning, the insurance largely covered the policyholders' loss of earned income due to a limited number of diseases, among them typhus, typhoid, scarlet fever, smallpox, diphtheria and diabetes. . . . .

This was the birth of modern health insurance. The demand for the new product grew as the Depression of the 1930s deepened. Out of this emerged the Blue Cross service concept, which foreshadowed insurance company reimbursement policies for hospital and surgical care. Also during the 1930s, insurance companies began to emphasize the availability of cash benefit plans for hospital, surgical, and medical expenses. The first Blue Shield type of plan for surgical and medical expenses was formed in 1939.

In addition, there was the single hospital benefit plan organized in 1912 at Rockford, Illinois; the Grinnell, Iowa, hospital plan in 1921; the Brattleboro, Vermont, plan in 1927. Each offered payment for limited hospital services. But the idea as developed at Baylor by Kimball was the model that spread. The American Hospital Association (AHA) requested Kimball to describe the Baylor plan at its annual meeting in 1931. Other hospital people also developed interest, and by 1935 there were 15 hospital insurance plans in 11 states, and six additional plans developed during 1936. "Concurrently, there was a move to create a coordinating agency of some sort to give the now rapidly growing movement a national focus and a broad base" (2, p. 36). This was done within the framework of the AHA, evolving over the years to a semiautonomous body and eventually to a completely independent Blue Cross Commission and, later, Blue Cross Association.

Anderson notes that the early leadership came not from hospitals but from early pioneers, farsighted individuals, some of whom were hospital accountants. The hospitals, says Anderson, were "timid in their backing of prepayment" (2, p. 42). It was, after all, a new idea, an experiment. "Originally, the plans covered only employees and not their dependents; the dependents were an unknown and feared quantity actuarially. But common sense and equity would shortly have it that dependents should be covered too, and so they were" (2, p. 43).

Anderson goes on to note that the Blue Cross movement surged ahead in the 1940s, with a nationwide enrollment of 6 million subscribers in 1940 spread through 56 independent Blue Cross plans. "By 1945, the enrollment was up to 19 million in 80 plans, and by the early 1950s, it was 40 million. By that time, private insurance companies were also coming up from behind after an early lack of interest in insuring against hospital costs" (2, p. 45).

The Health Insurance Institute states (3, p. 8):

During World War II, as a result of the freezing of wages, group health insurance became an important component of collective bargaining.

Even greater impetus came in the postwar era when the U.S. Supreme Court ruled that employee benefits, including health insurance, were a legitimate part of the labor-management bargaining process.

After that, health insurance protection expanded rapidly. For instance, in 1950 some 77 million people had hospital expense insurance. By 1976, some 177 million Americans were protected, or more than eight out of ten of the civilian noninstitutional population.

Traditionally, the greatest emphasis has been on hospital coverage because health services revolve around the hospital as the center of medical technology.

The dramatic progress of surgery and its increasing cost also spurred the demand for insurance for these expenses. In 1950, 54 million people had surgical expense insurance. By 1976, this coverage had tripled, with 167 million having such protection.

In 1950, more than 21 million people had coverage for physicians' fees other than surgery. In 1976, 163 million persons were covered.

In general, coverage for the cost of hospital care, surgery, and physicians' services is called "Basic Protection."

As Blue Cross began to demonstrate the feasibility of covering hospital expenses through the insurance mechanism, pressures to do likewise for physician services also developed. The pressures accelerated following the report of the Committee on Costs of Medical Care, with its challenge to organized medicine. In 1939, the California Medical Association established the California Physicians

Service, which was the first of what became known as the Blue Shield plans for payment of doctors' bills. Like Blue Cross, Blue Shield operated on a *service benefits* principle: the California plan provided complete physician's service at a rate of $1.70 per month (4, p. 36):

Enrollment was limited to employed persons earning less than $3,000 per year. Physicians were reimbursed on a "unit" basis, the unit having a par value of $2.50 (the fee for an office visit), with other services being valued at multiples of this unit. Experience in the early years, however, was unfavorable, as demand of services far exceeded expectations, and the effect was to devalue the unit. So, beginning in 1941, all contracts were modified. This resulted in much more favorable experience, and the unit value now approximates par.

We might digress for a moment to note two things. First, California developed the unit-value scale, more recently known as the relative-value scale. Most Blue Shield plans did not, however, use this method for establishing their schedules of payments. Second, the need to devalue the unit was acceptable to the medical profession because the plan was medical society sponsored: the physicians were obligated to deliver the service regardless of what the plan could pay. This is acceptable if one has a say in the management, as the physicians did. Throughout the Blue Shield movement, physicians had dominated the boards of directors not only because they underwrote the plan but also because the plans were truly *their* response to the challenge for national health insurance and they met the AMA principles of keeping medical matters in the hands of physicians. A similar situation existed with Blue Cross. The participating hospitals agreed to accept the Blue Cross payment as full payment for care in a semiprivate room. If the Blue Cross plan could not pay the agreed-upon cost, then the hospital would accept whatever Blue Cross could pay and *not* bill the patient for any additional monies. Thus, Blue Cross offered its subscribers *service benefits* rather than lump-sum or *indemnity benefits.* In the early days of Blue Cross, quite a

few plans had to pay hospitals less than 100 cents on the dollar, and hospitals tended to dominate Blue Cross boards. More recently, both Blue Cross and Blue Shield have changed or are in the process of changing their board structures, since the underwriting of the plan by the providers of service is now less a fact of life. We might note here that even when Blue Cross paid a hospital full cost, it was frequently discounted and was acceptable to the hospital because it was assured payment.

Medical society sponsorship of the Blue Shield plans had its origins as early as 1917 in the state of Washington, in which county medical societies established "county medical service bureaus" that contracted with employers to provide medical care for employees. According to Hawley, these bureaus developed as a result of competitive abuses that arose among some of the medical care plans in the state (4, pp. 35–36).

Both Blue Cross and Blue Shield were service-benefit plans, the former relying mainly on type of accommodation (semiprivate room) as the determinant of service-benefit eligibility. Blue Shield relied on income of the patient or patient's family. Both Blue Cross and Blue Shield provided benefits for subscribers who used private rooms (Blue Cross) or were above income (Blue Shield), and the patient paid the additional charges, if any.

Blue Cross worked quite well. The Blue Shield service-benefit principle did not work well. The reasons for this failure were historical and developmental. When Blue Shield first began, physicians commonly charged patients on a sliding-fee scale: soak the wealthy to pay for care of the poor, and so on. The early Blue Shield payments for various services were pitched to the going rate in the service-benefit income category. As the economy developed, and along with it inflation, the Blue Shield schedule of payments provided service-benefit payments for fewer and fewer subscribers because they were increasingly above income. Blue Shield made the same dollar payment for services rendered, but because the patient was above the service-benefit income level, the patient frequently had to pay an additional amount to the physician.

This led some Blue Shield plans to develop different types of contracts with different service-benefit income levels, allowance schedules geared to each level, and, of course, premiums geared to the allowances. In time, many Blue Shield plans developed contracts with *usual, customary,* and *reasonable* (UCR) allowances. But still the Blue Shield service benefits, when geared to subscriber income, did not work well because of inflation and the difficulties in determining subscriber income. It was left to the patient to discuss his or her income level with the physician, and both parties were reluctant to talk about money when the patient was sick. Resulting misunderstandings were common.

More than half of Blue Shield enrollees are now covered under UCR payment schedules, but the patient must, of course, use a physician who has agreed to accept the Blue Shield UCR payments as full payment. If the physician is not a Blue Shield participating physician, then the Blue Shield payment is an indemnity payment, and the physician may charge whatever he or she thinks is appropriate.

Another problem faced by Blue Shield with regard to service benefits developed as a result of the changing health system. Initially, radiology, pathology, and anesthesiology were hospital services covered by Blue Cross. During the 1950s and 1960s, many of the hospital-based physicians in those specialities moved out from under the hospital umbrella to do their own billing while still housed in the hospital, and many also established their own offices. Blue Cross generally was not allowed by law to pay for physician services as such, only for hospital services. Blue Shield rate structures were not geared to pay these professional services because they had never been calculated or anticipated in structuring the rates. For a while, the subscribers were caught in a bind and had to pay the bills until such time as Blue Shield was able to adjust its rates to incorporate these benefits. But then Blue Shield had to get the groups, mainly the employers, to go along with the increased rates. As one can imagine, not all were

willing to do so unless they had to, and others would not do so until the next round of collective barganing sessions began, when these new benefits could become a management concession.

Both Blue Cross and Blue Shield also faced similar situations in later years as new, often expensive, technology developed. If they paid for equipment under existing rates because payments were close to or at cost, it would encourage hospitals to expand and to write off the increased costs on Blue Cross: the new equipment would be averaged with all other costs and be built into what all admissions would cost. If Blue Cross covered such items, it would eventually force a rate increase, and if there was a rate increase, then competitors would gain an advantage. The pressures on both Blue Cross and Blue Shield became even more acute as they acted as fiscal intermediaries (the agency handling the payments) for Medicare. The federal government, bitten by rising costs, sought to pressure the Blues (a frequently used word for the Blue Cross/Blue Shield movement) and others to stem rising costs; pressure also came from state governments, which were bitten by the rising costs of Medicaid—if the Blues held the line, the federal/state Medicaid program would benefit.

Generally, the Blue Cross plans provided great support and assistance to the developing Blue Shield plans. Typically, they used the same salaried sales forces, the same personnel systems, the same offices, and sometimes the same executive staffs, although the governing boards were generally different and the corporations generally separate from a legal standpoint. In nearly all states, there was special enabling legislation for both plans that made them legally different from ordinary insurance companies. In some states, there were bitter conflicts between the Blue Cross plan and local medical societies that sponsored Blue Shield. These conflicts even reached the national level in 1948, for example, when the AMA opposed a proposed merger of Blue Cross and Blue Shield at the national level for purposes of enrolling national accounts. Why the conflict? The AMA's position was based on fear that it would again be accused of restraint of trade, and well it might have been. It also feared that Blue Cross, representing the hospitals, would dominate the national joint venture and the views of medicine would not be adequately represented (2, pp. 53–67). This, like the conflicts within the states, reflected an age-old fear on the part of physicians that nonmedical people would tell doctors how to practice medicine. Hospitals, by the same token, were wary of physicians telling them how to run the hospital. These conflicts became more pronounced as one moves up the hierarchies. In small towns, the physicians and hospital people may get along fine (but not always) in their small hospital, but as organizations became larger, the need for a bureaucracy develops and, with it, the insensitivities and misunderstandings and resulting fears that pervade all large social institutions and organizational arrangements. Though a mechanism for enrolling national accounts was eventually successful, it was not until 1978 that there was a successful merger of the national Blue Shield and Blue Cross organizations. Part of the reason for the successful merger was that by 1978, under pressures from state insurance departments and the federal government, the Blue Cross and Blue Shield plans had become less than surrogates for the providers; they were becoming true third parties.

Some Elements of Health Insurance Rate Structuring

Blue Cross was initially underwritten by the hospitals. They agreed to accept less than 100 cents on the dollar (apart from the discounts) if Blue Cross was in a financial bind. This reduction in payments to hospitals did occur in some areas, forced largely by errors in calculation and setting the premiums and in enrollment procedures. A look at these errors may help us understand health insurance cost and benefits in general.

Premium errors in the early days of Blue Cross came about because the plans did not have available a reliable statistical base for predicting what their utilization would be. No one else had the data,

either. Thus, for a given premium, should Blue Cross provide 14 days of in-hospital care or 21 days or 30 days; should it cover maternity; what about medical conditions that existed at the time a person joined Blue Cross; if a preexisting condition exists when a person joins Blue Cross, should that person have to wait a period of time before Blue Cross covers it, or can it be covered immediately? Blue Cross and Blue Shield also had to weigh such questions and to build the answers into the equation for calculating what the premium should be.

To illustrate this in simple form, let us suppose that a community of 100 people is debating whether or not to join Blue Cross and be covered for only one kind of hospitalization: removal of gallbladder. Let us further assume that the cost of care in the hospital is $200 a day and that, on the average, a gallbladder removal case stays in the hospital for five days. Let us further assume that, on the average, one can predict five cases a year for every 100 people.

Given these assumptions, Blue Cross could anticipate for that community a cost of $200/day × 5 days × 5 cases, or $5,000. But the laws governing Blue Cross as a nonprofit company generally require Blue Cross to set aside an additional sum of money for the unforeseen. This would be a *contingency fund,* or *reserves.* In this instance, the law might require Blue Cross to provide for a possible sixth case, thus another $1,000 needed by Blue Cross. But the people at Blue Cross have to live; they need income and, therefore, must be paid for their services, which include selling the policy, negotiating with the hospital, and administering the claims. They also need an office in which to work, and that means rent, electricity, fuel bills, and so on. Typically, this will come, for Blue Cross, to about 6 percent of its income. Thus we must add about $360 for administration. The total cost to Blue Cross would thus come to $6,360.

Blue Cross can thus say to the community: We calculated a rate; it is a *community rate* to cover all of you for gallbladder removal. Since there are 100 people, it will cost each of you $63.60 a year for coverage, about 17 cents a day. That will cover you only for hospital care relating to gallbladder removal. It will not cover the doctor's bill or other conditions or admissions for gallbladder when surgery is not performed. You get what you pay for, and all you are paying for is gallbladder surgery. If all of you join *now,* you will be covered immediately—no waiting periods—and all of you are covered even if you have gallbladder problems before joining. We can do this because you represent the average, and we have calculated our premium rate on that basis.

It is this kind of exercise that Blue Cross went through originally in deciding what to charge and for what. In real life, however, it was much more complicated because Blue Cross covered most acute conditions. Moreover, since Blue Cross worked with the community rate idea, in the beginning it enrolled not communities but representative bodies or groups of the community, typically, groups of employees.

Let us carry our hypothetical model a step further. Let us suppose that not everyone in the community or group of 100 wants to join. Let us suppose that only 20 choose to do so. Blue Cross would probably refuse to let only 20 join, because the group of 20 is not a community average and, thus, does not meet requirements of a community rate. In all probability, more than one gallbladder case would occur in the 20. Blue Cross would probably not allow a group such as this to be organized even at a higher rate. But let us suppose that instead of only 20, 60 want to join. Now Blue Cross has a problem. Is 60 average enough? Probably not. But can't the rate be tinkered with to make the group financially acceptable? Though each Blue Cross plan has its own enrollment requirements, in this hypothetical case, Blue Cross might well say that it could enroll the 60 but that the rate would have to be adapted. It would change it not by setting a different rate but by imposing an 11-month waiting period for preexisting conditions, in this case, for any gallbladder surgery, if the subscriber had any reason to believe he or she had abdominal problems.

Let us assume now that in the next isolated community or employee group there are four people. They hear about the Blue Cross coverage and seek to join. But here Blue Cross would probably say that a community or group of four is not typical for its rate. However, Blue Cross might say that if any member of that group of four wants to join, it would write an individual contract or policy, but it would not cover any gallbladder operation if the subscriber had reason to believe something was amiss. Moreover, Blue Cross would charge more for the policy because of higher risks and higher administrative costs. Thus, Blue Cross and Blue Shield typically offer *nongroup* enrollment for those who are not eligible for *group* enrollment. But what about that group of 20? They cannot get nongroup enrollment because Blue Cross must rely on group enrollment if it is to succeed in its mission of covering everyone at a community rate. By denying the 20, they will encourage them to become a pressure group within the larger group, agitating for more to seek Blue Cross enrollment.

We can appreciate the need for minimum enrollment if we make another assumption. Let us suppose that two more groups of 100 each want to join, and let us assume that all 100 join in each group. The two groups contribute $2,000 to the contingency fund. The first group (60 subscribers) also probably contributes to that fund; we do not know for sure, but the waiting period (the Blue Cross equalizer) has probably assured us that instead of five cases, there will only be three. Proportionally, $600 from the 60-person group would go into the contingency fund. Thus, there is $2,600 in the fund.

Let us further suppose that a fourth group of 100 joins. As the year progresses, Blue Cross may find that this group has many more than five gallbladder operations. Let us say it has eight. The group's premiums cover five of those operations; the group's contingency fund contribution covers a sixth. That would leave Blue Cross $2,000 short if it did not have the contributions from the other groups to cover the high-utilization group. If there were no other groups, only this group with eight operations,

Blue Cross would have to seek a rate increase, and it might have to ask the hospital this year to underwrite the Blue Cross policy by accepting $6,000 as though $8,000 were paid. If Blue Cross had not adhered to its enrollment minimum, it would have fewer reserves and would have less money to pay the hospital. One can say, in fact, that enrollment minimums not only protect the hospital but also protect the subscribers against rate increases.

This is how Blue Cross and Blue Shield developed. They gambled, they made mistakes, but they won more than they lost.

Enter now another complication. Let us suppose that one of our groups of 100 is a community of young people in their twenties, working for the same company. The employer provides them with Blue Cross coverage as well as a life insurance policy and a good retirement plan. The complication is that some other large insurance company would love to get the insurance policy and the retirement plan away from a competitor. It has a handle on this business by way of health insurance. It could offer a health insurance policy with about the same benefits as Blue Cross at a lower cost because the group is low risk. It would base its rate on the group's experience (or performance). Alternatively, the insurance company would charge the same as Blue Cross but provide greater benefits. The commercial company does not need the unused premium money from the low-risk group to carry the losses incurred with a high-risk group, as does Blue Cross. If the commercial company enrolls a high-risk group, its rate would bear a relationship to its experience or anticipated claims performance. With an experience-rated policy, the commercial insurance company is thus not likely to lose even if it does not get the life policy and retirement plan business. At worst, it takes a loss for one year only and then adjusts its premiums accordingly the next year. But what is the effect on Blue Cross? Blue Cross would not have as much money in the contingency fund. If, moreover, the competition takes away too many low-risk groups, Blue Cross would be forced to seek a rate increase that, in turn might make it noncompetitive.

Blue Cross has thus had to engage in experience rating also, simply to remain competitive and to keep a few pennies of contribution in the contingency fund. But the process has undermined the concept of the community rate and has had the effect of driving up health insurance costs and of charging higher premiums for those who are more sick.

In practice, the group commercial insurance companies do not provide quite as high a ratio of benefits on the income dollar as Blue Cross and Blue Shield does (Table 10–4). Their indemnity benefit packages are, however, typically very good. In many cases, the competition has stimulated Blue Cross and Blue Shield to do better, but it has also had adverse cost effects on some groups because of the undermining of the community rate concept.

In recent years, the underwriting by hospitals and physicians has been inconsequential, because the economic pressures that exist today militate against any subsidization. Hospitals and doctors do not subsidize the inability of Blue Cross or Blue Shield to pay 100 cents on the dollar. Instead, rates rise, and subsidization by hospitals can be considered a luxury. As noted earlier, even in the best of times, in many areas, the Blue Cross plan never paid hospitals 100 cents on the dollar but negotiated a discounted rate because Blue Cross was assuring payment. In today's environment, hospitals have been rebelling against this cost squeeze practice, and a growing number are withdrawing from Blue Cross participation.

Nongroup commercial policies are available, and many are sold by mail and magazine and newspaper advertising. But while the Blue Cross and Blue Shield policies pay out generally in excess of 90 cents on the income dollar and the group commercial policies pay about 80 cents, the nongroup commercial policies tend to be highly selective and generally pay out less than 67 cents on the income dollar. These policies are almost all indemnity policies.

The percentages shown in Table 10–4, if totaled across each line, add up to more than 100 percent

TABLE 10–4. Financial Experience of Private Health Insurance Organizations, 1986 ($ Billions)— Provisional Estimates

Type of Plan	Total Premiums	Benefits Paid Out of Premium Income	Adminis- trative Expenses	% of Premium Income Paid in Benefits	% of Premium Income Absorbed by Administration	% Gain (Loss) for Year
Blue Cross and Blue Shield	44.6	41.1	4.4	92.0	9.8	(1.8)
Blue Cross	30.3	27.9	2.6	92.3	8.5	(0.8)
Blue Shield	14.4	13.1	1.8	91.3	12.5	(3.9)
Insurance companies	55.5	45	10.8	81.1	19.4	(0.5)
Group policies	28.2	22.3	6.6	79.2	23.4	(2.6)
Individual policies	6.3	4.2	3.4	66.7	53.9	(20.6)
Minimum premium policies	21.0	18.5	0.8	87.9	3.8	8.2
Self-Insured plans	30.3	27.7	1.5	91.4	4.9	3.5
Administrative services only	14.0	12.3	0.5	87.9	3.6	8.2
Self-administered	11.0	10.4	0.7	94.9	6.3	(1.3)
Third party administered	5.3	5.0	0.2	95.1	3.8	1.1
Other prepaid health plans	10.3	9.1	1.2	88.3	11.7	

SOURCE: Division of National Cost Estimates, Office of Actuary, HCFA: National Health Expenditures, 1986–2000. Health Care Financ Rev, Vol. 8, No. 4, Summer 1987.

of the subscription or premium income. This may indicate that a rate increase is imminent because of increased claims expenses (payment of benefits) or increased operating expenses. Operating expenses for Blue Cross and Blue Shield typically include state insurance department requirements and legislation mandating contingency and other reserves. For Blue Cross and Blue Shield, as well as for other insurance companies, the operating expenses include the costs of marketing, claims processing and associated activities, telephones, utilities, rent, and computer and other equipment purchases or rental. Personnel costs are, of course, a major element.

Health Insurance Today

Protection against the costs of health care services is provided by four basic groups: the commercial insurance companies, Blue Cross and Blue Shield plans, independent plans, and government. The first three groups constitute the category of *private health insurance.*

The commercial companies cover slightly more than half the people who have private health insurance. Some companies restrict their business

to group coverage, generally through place of employment; Prudential and Cigna are two such companies. Other companies focus primarily on individual policies, and, as Table 10–4 indicates, they constitute a relatively small part of the insurance scene and pay out the least amount in benefits, only 66.7 percent of their premium income in 1986, the latest year for which data are available. The benefits of these nongroup commercial companies tend to be most limited in terms of the amounts paid for care, what types of care are covered, and who can get coverage.

The group commercial companies, because they emphasize group enrollment, are able to be less restrictive: if a large group is enrolled, then all members of the group can be enrolled; no person will normally be excluded because of poor health. Some group commercial companies have in recent years selectively excluded some people from enrolling in small employee groups because of their health problems or have charged higher rates than for the rest of the small group members. This practice was designed to hold down the cost of the insurance for other employees. This practice of selective *medical underwriting* individuals out of small groups (i.e., excluding those with serious medical problems or are otherwise at high risk) undermines the very purpose of insurance as a way to spread the risk. Concern over this has led Pennsylvania and New York legislatures to prohibit the practice, and at least 26 other states have also followed suit. The benefits provided by the group insurance companies tend to be more liberal than those provided by nongroup companies, but what is covered and what is not varies depending on what the group wants and is willing to pay for. As with Blue Cross and Blue Shield, the benefits may vary in terms of the number of days covered in hospital, the dollar amounts paid for surgical and medical care, whether home and office medical care is included, and whether nursing home care, visiting nurse services, dental, vision, and major medical expenses are covered. For hospital coverage, some policies pay fixed amounts but some still pay hospital charges as differentiated from hospital costs, which may be lower than charges. As the federally mandated diagnosis related group (DRG) system of paying for Medicare admissions proves in the long haul to be an effective way to control costs, more commercial companies will likely adopt that mode of payment. The insurance companies are, moreover, becoming very active in sponsoring health maintenance organizations (HMOs) and preferred provider organizations (PPOs).

As Table 10–4 indicates, the group commercial companies now pay out in benefits less than the Blue Cross and Blue Shield plans, that is, 79.2 percent as against 92.0 percent. The commercial companies have higher operating expenses. The insurance companies showed a net underwriting loss for 1986 claim expenses (or payments) and operating expenses exceeded the premium income. Carroll and Arnett note that the insurance companies have a long history of underwriting losses in their health insurance business and offer the following explanation about how this situation has persisted (5, p. 71):

Two factors help explain how this situation has continued to exist for so long. First, due to competitive conditions, companies have to consider forces other than benefit and administrative costs when setting premiums. Pre-

mium rates that reflect costs may be too high to be competitive, with the subsequent loss of some large corporation or union contracts that include the insurance company's more profitable lines of business such as loss of income, dread disease, accidental death and dismemberment, and most important of all, the life and casualty lines. Probably a more significant factor is that companies are able to finance their losses in part by cash flow underwriting (that is, the investment income companies earn on premium dollars before they are paid out for benefits and administration), and in part by subsidizing health insurance through other lines of insurance. No information is available on the investment income earned by insurance companies from their hospital and medical expense business, as separate from their health insurance business, including loss of income line, but presumably this income has been large enough over time to help compensate for their net underwriting losses.

The commercial companies enroll more than 50 percent of the people covered by private health insurance; however, each of the companies is independent from the others. Each is in business for itself. This is in sharp contrast to Blue Cross and Blue Shield. Although there are 73 Blue Cross plans and Blue Shield plans in the 50 states and Puerto Rico, and though each has its own benefit packages, there are cooperating agreements. Perhaps one of the most important agreements is the ability of a person to transfer enrollment from one plan to another whenever one moves without having to meet any waiting periods or otherwise lose continuity of benefits.

Blue Cross and Blue Shield typically offer both group and nongroup coverage. About 85 percent of the Blue Cross and Blue Shield enrollees are covered by group policies. Many group commercial insurance companies still pay hospital *charges,* but Blue Cross plans typically pay costs only in *member* hospitals. However, the payment mechanisms are undergoing rapid change with the advent of negotiated rates under PPO and HMO arrangements that may or may not meet the hospital's costs or its charges, and as experiments with a DRG system of payment are explored by some Blue Cross plans. In nonmember hospitals, that is, hospitals that have not signed up with Blue Cross, payments for care are typically lower. However, some Blue Cross policies pay charges if the subscribing company is willing to pay a higher premium or subscription costs. It is the assurance of full coverage in a semiprivate room of a member Blue Cross hospital that made Blue Cross appealing to many people, and because of its nationwide connections, the same benefits were available no matter where one is traveling. The keys to these *service benefits* under Blue Cross were care in the semiprivate room and in a member hospital. However, while many Blue Cross policies still provide service benefits (full coverage) in hospital, a growing number of policies provide for deductibles and some patient copayments. In many parts of the country, hospitals are now reconsidering the benefits that accrue from membership in Blue Cross, and in some areas, hospitals are withdrawing from membership, preferring to have the lesser payments made for care as a nonmember hospital, collecting the balance from the patient, and preferring commercial policies that may still pay charges.

The independent health insurance plans represent a growing share of the market. The category includes many HMOs, such as the Health Insurance Plan of Greater New York (HIP) and Kaiser-Permanente, group cooperatives, and self-insured corporations. Many of these plans are nonprofit group plans.

Although studies have shown lower hospital utilization rates for HMOs, the results are not altogether persuasive on two accounts. First, some critics believe that many HMOs have enrolled groups that are not representative of the population, that they have sought younger groups of enrollees who would tend to be healthier, and that they have avoided those groups from which high utilization could be expected—principally the poor and the elderly. Second, many believe that some of the reduced utilization may stem from rationing—not doing some elective surgery, for example, which would serve only to improve the quality of life.

These, then, are the three private mechanisms

enabling people to meet the costs of health care—commercial insurance companies, the nonprofit Blue Cross and Blue Shield plans, and the nonprofit independent plans. Nearly all people enrolled in these insurance plans are covered for hospital and physician care; lesser numbers are covered for dental and eye care, though such coverage is growing. *Major medical expense insurance,* sometimes called *catastrophic insurance,* has experienced a very rapid growth since it was first introduced in 1951 by the commercial companies, and it is now also available through most Blue Cross and Blue Shield plans. Typically, major medical insurance covers 80 percent of all residual medical expenses (i.e., it covers 80 percent of all expenses not covered by the regular hospital, medical, and surgical policies) after the insured pays the deductible. The deductible may vary from $100 or $200 or more, depending on what the group wants and is willing to pay for. For the catastrophic illness, the bills can mount, so these policies tend to pay 80 percent up to a maximum of perhaps $250,000 or more.

Both deductibles and co-insurance are mechanisms designed to limit costs and to give greater assurance that the use of services is appropriate and that there is no unnecessary expense or use. To the extent that they are successful in this, we can appreciate them; but for the person who really needs the added services, the costs can be significant, and deterrence may not be in the best interest of the patient. In recognition of this problem, many policies now set a limit of $2,000 to $3,000, which the patient has to pay, after which the policies pay all costs. When the payment of costs is shared between an insurance company and the patient, or between two companies, it is said that the policy is *co-insured.*

The fourth basic group that protects people against the costs of health care is *government.* In this category are a number of programs that have already been cited such as those for military personnel and their dependents; for veterans for service-connected disabilities and for nonservice-connected disabilities if they are unable to afford private

TABLE 10–5. Medicare (Part A): Hospital Insurance-Covered Services for 1992

Services	Benefit	Medicare Pays	You Pay
Hospitalization: Semiprivate room and board, general nursing and miscellaneous hospital services and supplies.	First 60 days 61st to 90th day 91st to 150th day* Beyond 150 days	All but $652 All but $163 a day All but $326 a day Nothing	$652 $163 a day $326 a day All costs
Skilled Nursing Facility Care: You must have been in a hospital for at least three days and enter a Medicare-approved facility generally within 30 days after hospital discharge.†	First 20 days Additional 80 days Beyond 100 days	100% of approved amount All but $81.50 a day Nothing	Nothing $81.50 a day All costs
Home Health Care: Medically necessary skilled care.	Parttime or intermittent care for as long as you meet Medicare conditions.	100% of approved amount; 80% of approved amount for durable medical equipment.	Nothing for services; 20% of approved amount for durable medical equipment.
Hospice Care: Pain relief, symptom management and support services for the terminally ill.	If you elect the hospice option and as long as doctor certifies need.	All but limited costs for outpatient drugs and inpatient respite care.	Limited cost sharing for outpatient drugs and inpatient respite care.
Blood	Unlimited if medically necessary.	All but first three units per calendar year.	For first three units.‡

SOURCE: *1992 Guide to Health Insurance for People with Medicare.* Washington, D.C., Superintendent of Documents.

Note: 1992 Part A monthly premium: none for most beneficiaries; $192 if you must buy Part A (premium may be higher if you enroll late).

*This 60-reserve-days benefit may be used only once in a lifetime.

†Neither Medicare nor private Medigap insurance will pay for most nursing home care.

‡To the extent the blood deductible is met under one part of Medicare during the calendar year, it does not have to be met under the other part.

care; and for American Indians and Alaskan natives. But the principal programs with which we are concerned are *Medicare* and *Medicaid.* These programs were established when Congress amended the Social Security Act in 1965, adding to it Title XVIII and Title XIX. Title XVIII was Medicare; Title XIX was Medicaid.

Medicare

Medicare is a health insurance program for those age 65 and above, regardless of income or wealth, and it also covers people under 65 who have been entitled to Social Security or Railroad Retirement disability benefits for at least two consecutive years or who suffer from chronic renal (kidney) disease that requires a kidney transplant or routine dialysis treatment. The "under 65" provisions were added

to Medicare by the Social Security Amendments of 1972.

The program consists of Parts A and B. Part A (Table 10–5) is the hospital insurance portion of Medicare, providing coverage for in-hospital care, needed skilled nursing facility care and home health care. Financed by Social Security taxes, Part A benefits provided, in 1992:

1. Up to 90 days of inpatient care for each benefit period; a new benefit period begins after the patient has been out of hospital and/or skilled nursing facility for 60 consecutive days. But in 1992 this coverage did not cover all of the charges. The patient had to pay the first $652 of the hospital bill and, after 60 days, the patient paid $163 a day through the ninetieth day. If a patient stayed in hospital beyond 90 days, Medicare permitted the patient to draw upon a lifetime reserve of 60 extra days, with the patient paying $326 for each day used out of this reserve.

2. Up to 100 days in a skilled nursing facility, with Medicare paying the full cost for the first 20 days and the patient, in 1992, paying $81.50 a day for each day thereafter. To be eligible for this benefit, the patient must have been in the hospital for three consecutive days first. Intermediate or custodial nursing home care coverage under Medicare continues to be excluded.

3. Unlimited home health visits by a participating home health agency for part-time skilled nursing care, physical therapy, or speech therapy for patients confined to their home and, if certified, as needed by a physician. Some additional other home health agency services are available (if the preceding basic services are provided), such as occupational therapy, services by home health aides, equipment rental, and medical social services. The deductible does not apply to home health visits.

4. Hospice care in a home or homelike environment for the terminally ill. A wide range of medical and social services are available, including medical, nursing, and social work services, respite care, short-term inpatient care, as well as homemaker services. All services are available without charge to the patient except for some sharing of the cost for outpatient drugs and inpatient respite care.

As costs go up, Medicare payments to hospitals and to skilled nursing facilities go up, and they also do for home health care. At the same time, the amounts the patient must pay rise sharply. For prolonged illness, the patient's share for hospital and nursing facility charges, without additional insurance, can be substantial. Many of the elderly in 1992 had additional insurance to cover the Medicare deductible and co-payments.

There is a small number of people over 65 who are not automatically eligible for Medicare because they had insufficient work experience to accumulate the necessary Social Security credits; if these people want Medicare coverage they may secure it by paying a monthly premium.

There is one additional factor that patients must bear in mind. Hospital care must be needed and must be a type of care that can only be provided by a hospital. If the hospital's utilization review committee or some other peer review organization

(PRO) does not approve the hospital stay after being admitted as an inpatient because it was not needed, then there can be a retroactive denial of benefits, and the patient may have to pay all costs or the hospital bear the loss.

Part B of Medicare is Supplementary Medical Insurance (SMI); it is optional, and Part A-eligible people must pay for it if they agree to take it out; most people do subscribe to it. In fact, Part B enrollment is automatic unless the person informs Social Security that coverage is not desired and that deductions to pay for it should not therefore be made from their Social Security checks. Part B provides some important insurance benefits (Table 10–6):

1. Payment of *reasonable* physician charges (after the patient pays the initial $100 annual deductible). But the payment is not full payment, only 80 percent of what Medicare determines to be reasonable. If the physician accepts *assignment,* i.e., agrees to accept the Medicare fee, the physician bills Medicare, receives 80 percent of the fee, and is allowed to bill the patient for the remaining 20 percent. If the physician is unhappy with the amount Medicare determines as "reasonable," he or she may decline to accept *assignment* of the fee and may elect to have the 80 percent paid to the patient and thus be free to bill the patient for whatever amount the physician feels is appropriate. There are limits, however, on the amount a physician may charge for nonassigned cases: in 1992 the most a physician could charge for a Medicare service was 120 percent of the amount Medicare established as reasonable. In other words, the charge could not exceed 20 percent more than the fee schedule amount. In 1993, the most that could be charged was 115 percent. Congress is thus moving to the point where all cases will be on assignment. A number of states moved ahead of the Congress and had already made assignment mandatory for all Medicare cases in their states.

2. Hospital outpatient, ambulance, and emergency department services, subject to the same $100 deductible. Medicare pays 80 percent of the approved amount; the patient is responsible for the remaining 20 percent.

3. A number of other services and supplies such as

TABLE 10–6. Medicare (Part B): Medical Insurance-Covered Services for 1992

Services	Benefit	Medicare Pays	You Pay
Medical Expenses: Doctors' services, inpatient and outpatient medical and surgical services and supplies, physical and speech therapy, ambulance, diagnostic tests, and more.	Medicare pays for medical services in or out of the hospital.	80% of approved amount (after $100 deductible).	$100 deductible,* plus 20% of approved amount and limited charges above approved amount.
Clinical Laboratory Services: Blood tests, biopsies, urinalyses, and more.	Unlimited if medically necessary.	100% of approved amount.	Nothing for services.
Home Health Care: Medically necessary skilled care.	Parttime or intermittent skilled care for as long as you meet conditions for benefits.	100% of approved amount; 80% of approved amount for durable medical equipment.	Nothing for services; 20% of approved amount for durable medical equipment.
Outpatient Hospital Treatment: Services for the diagnosis or treatment of illness or injury.	Unlimited if medically necessary.	80% of approved amount (after $100 deductible)	$100 deductible, plus 20% of billed charges.
Blood	Unlimited if medically necessary.	80% of approved amount (after $100 deductible and starting with fourth unit).	First three units plus 20% of approved amount for additional pints (after $100 deductible).†

SOURCE: *1992 Guide to Health Insurance for People with Medicare.* Washington, D.C., Superintendent of Documents.
*Once you have had $100 of expenses for covered services in 1992, the Part B deductible does not apply to any further covered services you receive for the rest of the year.
†To the extent the blood deductible is met under one part of Medicare during the calendar year, it does not have to be met under the other part.

outpatient physical and speech therapy, diagnostic x-ray examinations, wheelchairs, artificial limbs, limited chiropractic services, and so on.

Part B (SMI) cost the insured person $31.80 per month in 1992. Additional costs come out of federal general revenue. As health care costs go up, so do the premium charges, but the law requires that the premium increase be limited to the percentage rise in the Social Security income.

HHS's Health Care Financing Administration (HCFA) oversees the Medicare program. It handles some payments directly, but most payments for care are made by *fiscal intermediaries* for Part A and *carriers* for Part B with whom HCFA contracts. The contractors are mainly Blue Cross, Blue Shield, and commercial insurance companies.

Medicare has clearly helped the aged and other

eligible pay for needed health services. Yet, these people are generally on fixed incomes and may still have to pay considerable sums when hospitalization and skilled nursing facility care are necessary, and there are some expensive items not covered that many elderly people require, specifically, most drugs, hearing aids, and eyeglasses. The medical insurance payments, though significant, still do not cover all of a physician's fee.

The physician's bills can be substantial, and it is the fortunate patient who can find a physician who accepts assignment. Although Medicare payments represent a sizable portion of most physicians' incomes, getting them to accept assignment has not been as successful as legislators and the elderly had hoped. Some accept assignment in all cases, but many more accept assignment on a selective or case-by-case basis, presumably basing their decision on whether the physician thinks the patient can afford to pay more than the fee Medicare has established as being reasonable. Some physicians never accept assignment. Massachusetts dealt with this issue by requiring that all physicians accept assignment in all cases if they wish to retain their license to practice there. A number of states have since adopted similar legislation. Congress began to deal with this problem first by instituting a Medicare Participating Physician (MPP) program, whereby physicians who agree to participate would accept all cases on assignment. Those who did not agree to accept all cases on assignment would have to bill all Medicare patients directly and not receive any payments directly from Medicare; there would be no case-by-case decision whether to accept assignment. Congress also directed that the names of all participating physicians be published so that Medicare patients could determine beforehand whether a physician was a MPP. The number of physicians accepting assignment has thus increased significantly due both to actions by various state governments and to the limitations Congress placed on the amount physicians can charge for nonassigned cases.

Although the direct costs of care borne by Medicare recipients are still considerable, the cost of benefits paid by the government has been frighteningly high, far exceeding the early calculations when the legislation was being considered. Expenditures by Medicare rose from 1967 fiscal year through 1986 an average of 15 percent a year. One can appreciate the political dilemma this poses if Medicare is to continue to meet its obligations: continuing to raise taxes to meet the rising demand and rising costs as we have in the past is not popular with wage earners, who have to pay the increased taxes, nor for business and government, which must also pay more. Capping payments to hospitals has been introduced through DRG payments. The hope was that the hospital will somehow manage by being more efficient, trimming corners, or finding the money somewhere else. But costs continue to rise. Some of the increased costs

are being shifted to the patient through higher deductibles and higher Part B premiums.

Denying access to care is tempting, and many countries do this, but it does violate our values, our sense of what is right. Many argue, however, that we will have to resort to rationing, but when the term is used we should be clear that it really means denying access to care, and this in turn may mean earlier death or lessened quality of life.

Medicaid

Medicaid, authorized by Title XIX of the Social Security Act, is a federal- and state-financed program to pay for health services for the *categorically needy* and the *medically needy*. The *categorically needy* are those receiving public assistance from the Aid to Families with Dependent Children (AFDC) program and those who receive Supplementary Security Income (SSI) because they are aged, blind, or disabled. All states must cover the categorically needy. (Some people are eligible for both Medicare and Medicaid.) The *medically needy* are those who have enough money to live on, but not enough to pay for medical care. They may be covered under Medicaid if their state has opted to provide coverage for the medically needy; well over half of the states have chosen to provide benefits for these low-income people. It is up to each state to define income eligibility for classification as medically needy, and this, as might be expected, varies from state to state. Lest one think that Medicaid is a generous government program, it should be noted that less than half of the nonelderly persons who are below the federal poverty standard qualify in their states for Medicaid.

The benefit structure under Medicaid also varies from state to state. If the state has a Medicaid program—and all but Arizona do—it must at least provide for inpatient and outpatient hospital services; skilled nursing facility services; physician services; home health care; family planning services; and early and periodic screening, diagnosis, and treatment (EPSDT) of children under 21 who are eligible. A state, at its option, may elect to pay for dental services, prescribed drugs, eyeglasses, intermediate care facility services, and other services.

Medicaid is financed from general tax revenues. The federal government share currently ranges from 50 percent in the most wealthy states to 80 percent in those states with the lowest per capita personal income. In some states, local governments share a portion of the state costs. The program is administered by each state under federal regulations and guidelines.

Like Medicare, Medicaid costs have risen rapidly. In 1992 Medicaid expenditures exceeded $75 billion, accounting for 14 percent of spending by all of the state governments, and 12 percent of all national health expenditures (6). These costs have been of growing concern to both state and federal governments. In most states, increases in Medicaid expenditures are outpacing increases in state revenues. Physicians who accept Medicaid patients must accept the full payment without charging the patient. Because payments have not grown with inflation, more and more physicians are limiting the number of Medicaid patients they treat.

Some years ago one congressional aide was reported to have said, "We can't sit by and watch the Medicaid program bankrupt our states." But the states are not sitting by idly. Many are reducing the number and scope of optional services and being more restrictive about eligibility of the medical needy. One common practice is not to change the income eligibility requirements. Thus, as inflation rises, and incomes rise to keep pace with inflation (or try to keep pace), some of the medical needy receive incomes above the eligibility scales. They are no better off in terms of paying for care, but the state and, in turn, the federal government, have thus washed their hands of many who were once eligible. Other states have imposed limits. Among the reductions are limitations on the number of days for in-hospital care, nuisance charges for certain services and supplies, and limitations on the amount paid physicians, hospitals and nursing homes.

State governments have tried many innovative approaches to secure additional funds. Early in the decade many latched onto the idea of levying taxes—sometimes referred to as *mandated donations*—on health care providers, "donations" dedicated to support the Medicaid program. This increased the amount of state government monies allocated for Medicaid and, in turn, made each of the states doing this eligible for additional federal matching monies. The new federal matching funds enabled the states to pay the providers more. The federal government viewed this as an open-ended raid on the federal treasury and eventually got Congress to agree to place a limit on the amount states could raise in this manner, the limit being 25 percent of the states' total Medicaid expenditures. It is expected that by 1993 these "donations" (provider taxes) will generate about $4 billion, which the federal government will have to match (6).

Another innovative approach was developed by the State of Oregon. The State proposed to extend Medicaid benefits to all residents who were below poverty level ($13,994 for a family of four people in 1992). This would add many more people to the Medicaid roles. To pay for the cost of care for these new Medicaid enrollees, the State proposed to mandate managed care for all Medicaid patients and it developed a list of medical services in priority order based on the effectiveness of the services, and proposed not to pay for those procedures which had little or no beneficial effect even though they were on the federal government's regular Medicaid list. The plan offered a basic benefit package that stressed prevention and would cover most, but not all, of the usual Medicaid treatments. It went beyond the customary Medicaid benefits by proposing to provide dental and hospice care, prescription drugs, routine physicals and most transplants (7). The list of medical treatments and their prioritization were developed by a broadly representative commission of health professionals and community leaders. The federal government, which had to approve the plan, rejected it in mid-1992 because the prioritized list might violate the federal Americans With Disabilities Act. The plan, according to Oregon's Governor, enjoyed the support of leading disability groups in Oregon because they believed it would help more than harm those who had disabilities. The Oregon commission reorganized the list and deleted references to "quality of life" and extended coverage to some controversial treatments such as treatment for newborns weighing 500 grams (1 pound, 2 ounces) or less, and transplants for alcoholics with cirrhosis. The Clinton Administration approved the revised plan in March 1993 for a 5-year demonstration period. This signals that the Administration recognizes the need for drastic action and will give the states flexibility in dealing with the problems associated with health care reform.

Abuses and Inefficiencies in Medicare and Medicaid

Inefficiencies in claims payments have plagued Medicare and Medicaid. Payments have been made for services not covered and for services previously paid. The former may reflect inadequate training for those who do the claims review. The latter may reflect the complexity of the system and the slowness of payments by the fiscal intermediaries. Abuses have also frequently been reported, including the "ping-ponging" of patients back and forth between physicians in a clinic to justify additional visits; ordering unnecessary lab tests and medications (with some kickbacks); and "gang" visits in which a physician visits all members of a family, or all patients in a nursing home, when visiting only one is necessary. We hear only of the cases discovered. Increasingly, the government is going after the cheaters; jail terms are more and more common on conviction. Computers are an invaluable aid in identifying fraud.

Hospitals, nursing facilities, pharmacies, physicians, ambulance services, and other health professions have yielded their share of cheaters. Although the number of cheaters among the total number of participants may be small, the sums involved have been considerable, newsworthy, and embarrassing to the groups from which the cheaters sprang. The abuses should also have been embarrassing to the governments, fiscal intermedi-aries, and insurance carriers who failed to set up more sound practices and controls at the outset. They failed to realize that whatever the enterprise or endeavor, when a large sum of money becomes available, it draws out the worst in some people, who do whatever they can to get more than they have earned.

National Health Insurance and Health Care Reform

Debates over the need for health care reform have accelerated because of the continued rise in health care costs and the fact that so many Americans do not have health insurance or government program coverage to pay for the costs of care. There is a widespread conviction that something has to be done to make the costs of the health system more acceptable to our society and that something also has to be done to make certain that everyone has easy access to needed services and the ability to pay for them.

While we tend to think of this as a new issue facing Americans, it bears remembering that in the 1930s and again in the 1940s there were major national proposals for reforming the health care system by instituting some form of national health insurance (NHI). In 1932 the Committee on the Costs of Medical Care issued its report calling for the provision of medical care by organized groups of physicians, dentists, nurses, pharmacists, and others, and that these services be financed by some form of a prepayment mechanism (8). Prominent among the unenacted bills in Congress was the Wagner-Murray-Dingell bill in 1943, which proposed "a national (i.e., federal) compulsory system of health insurance, financed from payroll taxes and providing comprehensive health and medical benefits through entitlement to specified medical service (service benefits) rather than through money payments (cash indemnity)" (9, p. 272). Subsequently, in the late 1940s, President Truman took a strong position in favor of NHI and sent proposed legislation to the Congress "which outlined a comprehensive prepaid medical insurance plan for all age groups, to be financed though a 4 percent raise in the Social Security tax . . ." (9, p. 273). Opposition from the AMA was largely responsible for the failure of Congress to adopt any of the legislative proposals.

Health insurance for those over the age of 65 captured the attention of national leaders during the 1950s and 1960s, culminating in the Medicare and Medicaid legislation, but these programs helped only a small segment of the population.

During the latter part of the 1970s NHI was once again a prime topic of conversation and concern. Congressmen, senators, presidents, union and business leaders, insurance companies, and professional and trade associations had their pet proposals. The "well informed" were certain that one of the proposals would be enacted.

Of the more than 19 bills considered by the Congress in 1976, no congressional consensus developed, and no formal action was taken. There was no agreement on the scope of benefits to be provided, nor on how the scheme would be financed. As appealing as some type of program was, the rising costs of health care, and in particular of Medicare and Medicaid, and the inability of anyone to control these costs, caused many political leaders to wonder if we could afford NHI at that point in time. By 1988 not a word was heard about NHI. But its time has come again and it is therefore important to consider it.

NHI is appealing because it would provide a uniform range of benefits for all citizens, enabling all to secure health care without being deterred by cost considerations, and it would assure all that they would not be bankrupted by the bills that come in following an illness.

Though an appealing concept, it is also misunderstood. NHI would not be free, nor would it pay for everything. NHI would cost money, through increased taxes and increased cost of manufactured goods (since employers are likely to be called upon to pay a major portion). Nearly all NHI proposals, moreover, have had limited benefit structures, particularly regarding care in skilled nursing home facilities.

NHI, moreover, is not the same as socialized medicine or a national health service. These latter concepts imply government ownership of facilities and government provision of services by salaried professionals and other personnel. NHI usually means the financing of health care by either of two approaches:

1. Government allocations of insurance monies collected from employers and others and then distributed directly or through intermediaries to pay for services provided.
2. Government-mandated universal health insurance coverage, whereby premiums are paid by employers and others directly to the insurance agencies or companies without passing through government hands. Where this approach is proposed, the proposals typically provide that those who are unemployed will have their premiums paid by government.

Some state governments, frustrated by national inaction, have initiated their own approaches. Most common is the "play or pay" approach, wherein the states mandate that all employers provide health insurance for their employees or pay a payroll tax to the state so the state could purchase the insurance for those employees and their families. Some of these proposals allow for the employer to require some employee co-payment of the premiums. Provision is also typically made for the state government to pay the premiums for those who are unemployed and in some cases for other groups of citizens. Implementation of such state "pay or play" approaches has been vigorously resisted by small businesses, and made difficult by the poor fiscal condition of the states.

Hawaii took a somewhat different approach. It simply mandated universal coverage: employers were required to provide health insurance coverage for all who worked more than 20 hours a week. Those not falling under that rule—the unemployed, seasonal workers, and others—were provided coverage by the state government from general revenues. Initiated in 1974, its approach has been very successful. Dr. John Lewin, Hawaii's director of health, commenting on the State's plan said, "One criticism I hear is that we are different, as if we're all sipping mai tais on the beach and dancing in coconut bras. We have a lot of poor people in Hawaii. We have all the health problems of the rest of the states. But what makes us different is that we decided to do something about it" (10).

Widely touted is the "managed competition" approach advocated by Alain Enthoven and Richard Kronick of California (11). Managed competition is a proposed mechanism for purchasing health care in a way that would obtain maximum value for both patients and employers by using the rules for competition derived from microeconomic principles. While the health sector is not a free market, the concept of managed competition proposes to use market forces within a framework of carefully drawn rules (12). It would have employers, government entities, and other large purchasers of health care forming health insurance purchasing cooperatives, or health insurance alliances, to negotiate with competing health insurance companies which would offer a comprehensive, standardized, federal government mandated range of benefits. The insurance plans would be required to accept all persons who apply—no exclusion of high risk employees who might be more costly—and they would have community based premiums. Starr and Zelman have proposed that managed competition alone does not control costs (13). The insurance companies would compete on the basis of price and quality of care. Since the benefits would be standardized—i.e., the same—meaningful competition would occur. Each insurance plan would have to be approved by the federal government.

In many respects this approach would resemble a nationwide system of competing HMOs or PPOs. It would appeal to many as less radical than other approaches in that it would retain the esteemed concept of "competition", and offer the hope of controlling costs. Interestingly, the Enthoven/Kronick proposal has influenced health system changes in The Netherlands and Great Britain, but it has its skeptics in the United States. Some feel that the

public will not accept limited choice of physicians and hospitals which characterize "managed competition". This has already been shown to be one of the shortcomings for some people with the HMO movement. Other critics believe that the savings envisioned will simply not materialize for the evidence is not yet clear that managed care will in fact control the costs of health care.

As in previous years, a large number of proposals for health care reform are pending in Congress. Most only seek to tinker with the existing system, trying to bring about an incremental change. Others seek fundamental reform. Whether an acceptable form of NHI will get through Congress and meet with presidential approval, remains to be seen. Large corporations want relief but whether they will agree to pay *community rates* is unclear. Small businesses, many of which have not provided any health insurance for their employees, are generally opposed to NHI which will require them to pay at least part of the premium costs for their employees. State governments are concerned that they might be forced to bear a heavy share of the costs of any reform, and want relief from the spiralling costs they already incur for Medicaid. Hospitals and physicians worry about regulations that would come with any NHI legislation, and worry even more about the possibility of a mandated cap on the level of health care expenditures. At the same time various consumer interest groups are pressing not only for a broad NHI program but one which will take care of all costs, even for services that the Oregon plan found unjustified.

Further controversy is likely if NHI proposals require patients to pass through a gatekeeper (i.e., primary care practitioner) before accessing specialist consultation and care. Medical equipment manufacturers, commercial insurance companies, as well as Blue Cross and Blue Shield, are concerned about the various proposals.

The pressures on Congress to pass some type of health reform legislation will be great, and because of the conflicting interests, development of a consensus may be difficult which is why states like Hawaii and Massachusetts have either moved ahead on their own or plan to do so just as soon as their state economies enable them to do so.

Advocates of health care reform are looking at various other national health systems to see if they provide any insights. The German and Canadian systems figure prominently in this regard, and we look briefly at those and some other systems in chapter 12.

SUMMARY

Most Americans are protected against major costs of health care by health insurance or some government program. Most of the insured secure their protection on a group basis through their place of employment. The insurers are generally Blue Cross for hospital coverage, Blue Shield for physician services, and some of the large commercial insurance companies such as Cigna and Prudential, which cover both hospital and physician services. The chief government programs are Medicare for those over 65 and Medicaid for low-income people.

The extent to which people have protection is a source of satisfaction, but when one considers the adequacy of that coverage, there is cause for concern. Many policies limit the benefits; some exclude coverage for certain conditions, require waiting periods before covering preexisting conditions, limit the number of days covered in hospital and nursing home, and limit the amount paid the physician and the circumstances under which payment is made.

Notwithstanding these limitations, there is a clear trend toward more comprehensive coverage, the principle deterrent being the willingness of the employee or employer to pay the premium costs. Nearly all hospital costs incurred by the insured are covered by their insurance. Though only two thirds of physician costs are covered by insurance, the bulk of the consumer payments are for routine office medical care that many feel should not be fully covered because of the need to ensure judicious use of such services, which is accomplished

when the patient pays at least part of the cost. One of the fastest growing types of health insurance is major medical, which protects against the cumulative costs of chronic conditions and against the very large costs that are fearsome but seldom encountered. A growing area of need in view of our aging population is improved coverage for nursing home care.

It was intended that the needs of the elderly would be met by Medicare, but the costs of Medicare have outstripped the predictions of almost everyone owing to new technology, inflation, and a rapidly aging population. The drain on the Medicare health insurance trust fund is so great that its resources eventually will be depleted unless corrective action is taken. DRGs are a step in this direction. Part of the corrective action is also to shift more and more costs to the patient.

Costs are also a factor in Medicaid, which is financed jointly by the federal and state governments. To control these costs, states are imposing a number of barriers that they hope will be successful: restricting the benefits available, reducing payments to hospitals or at least paying them less than cost, keeping physician payments low, and getting people off the Medicaid eligibility rolls.

The continued rise in health care costs and the fact that so many Americans are uninsured or underinsured gives rise to pressures for reform of the health care system. Mandating some form of national health insurance has once again risen to the top of the agenda for the nation.

DISCUSSION QUESTIONS

1. As we consider improvements in health insurance, should we try to secure first dollar coverage, that is, coverage for all health care costs without deductibles and co-insurance?
2. Instead of first dollar coverage, would it be more advisable to have limited health insurance benefits coupled with major medical insurance?
3. What are the advantages and the disadvantages of competition between Blue Cross and Blue Shield and group commercial insurance companies?

4. Under Medicare, are the benefit limitations and the co-payments that the elderly have to pay appropriate? Should the elderly have to pay more? Less? If changes are warranted, what might be the political and economic consequences?
5. What additional steps can and should be taken to increase the number and percentage of physicians who take Medicare assignment?
6. Are there lessons to be learned from our experience with Medicare and Medicaid? What are they?

REFERENCES

1. Fuchs, V.R.: *Who Shall Live?* New York, Basic Books, 1974
2. Anderson, O.W.: *Blue Cross Since 1929: Accountability and the Public Trust.* Cambridge, MA, Ballinger, 1975.
3. *Source Book of Health Insurance Data 1977–78.* Washington, D.C., Health Insurance Institute, 1978.
4. Hawley, P.R.: *Non-Profit Health Service Plans,* Chicago, Blue Cross Commission and Blue Shield Commission, 1949.
5. Carroll, M.S., Arnett, R.H.: Private Health Insurance Plans in 1978 and 1979: A Review of Coverage, Enrollment, and Financial Experience. *Health Care Financ Rev,* September 1981.
6. *American Medical News,* August 24/31, 1992.
7. *The New York Times,* August 11, 1992.
8. *Medical Care for the American People: Final Report of the Committee on the Costs of Medical Care.* Chicago, The University of Chicago Press, 1932.
9. Stevens, R.: *American Medicine and the Public Interest.* New Haven, Yale University Press, 1971.
10. *The New York Times,* July 23, 1991.
11. Enthoven, A., Kronick, R.: A Consumer-Choice Health Plan for the 1990s. *New Eng J Med,* Vol. 320, Nos. 1, 2, January 5, 1989, January 12, 1989.
12. Enthoven, A.; The History and Principles of Managed Competition. *Health Affairs,* Vol. 12, Supplement 1993, pp. 24–48.
13. Starr, P. and Zelman, W.: A Bridge to Compromise: Competition Under a Budget. *Health Affairs,* Vol. 12, Supplement 1993, pp. 7–23.

11

Public Health

Public health activities emphasize prevention of disease, disability, and premature death by the organized efforts of government. The first public health activities in the United States began in the early nineteenth century in the large cities and focused on sanitation. The major health threats at that time were epidemics of such infectious diseases as smallpox, typhoid fever, and diphtheria. Local boards of health were formed to combat these epidemics, and their main function initially was to improve sanitation. They developed ordinances regarding waste disposal, street drainage, removal of filth, drainage of swamps, and other measures that would improve the sanitary environment. Quarantine of homes and ships, and, much later, immunizations, were also important functions of local boards of health aimed at preventing the spread of infectious diseases.

In 1869 the first state board of health was formed in Massachusetts. By 1900 all states had boards of health. Their main functions remained the same as those of local units, but they focused on the statewide control of infectious or communicable diseases and the enforcement of sanitary regulations. They accomplished this mainly by encouraging the further development of local boards of health and then working through them, as well as by handling directly the issues that extended beyond the jurisdiction of a single local board or that required the organizational efforts and legal authority of the state government.

Departments of public health with fulltime professional staffs headed by a medically trained health officer evolved to support the work of the health boards. In the early 1900s, the work of health departments began to broaden. The New York City Health Department set up neighborhood health centers in slum areas to offer maternal and child health care services for the poor to deal with their high maternal and infant mortality rates; to detect (and in some cases treat) tuberculosis, the leading cause of death in 1900; and to control venereal (sexually transmitted) disease. The expansion of the public health departments into personal health care, particularly maternal and child health, initially drew opposition from the medical profession, which considered it an intrusion into its domain.

Local and state public health departments were strengthened in 1935 by the infusion of federal monies, which earmarked grants for maternal and child health and for general public health activities. By the 1970s the earlier threat of communicable diseases had largely been replaced by new concerns for chronic and degenerative diseases associated with modern life, such as heart and lung diseases, cancer, stroke, and mental illness. Public health officials have made smoking as well as alcohol and drug abuse important public health issues, with programs geared to prevention and with financing by local, state, and federal funds. Recently, communicable diseases have again become prominent with the rise and rapid spread of the acquired immunodeficiency syndrome (AIDS), which is now a major public health problem, and with the reemergence of tuberculosis.

Although physicians have always done some preventive work, including checkups and the education of their patients on matters relating to their health, the bulk of their activities has focused on crisis intervention, on dealing with the vast array of concerns and complaints registered by patients when they consult their physicians. This is not to suggest their lack of interest in, or concern for, prevention, but it does point out two fundamental facts.

First, the major preventive thrusts are beyond the organizational capacity of the individual physician. What is required is a communal effort organized under the police powers of the state. The individual physician can do little, for example, to ensure purity of water and air; the elimination from the environment of noxious substances, protection of people from a large number of communicable diseases and from the antisocial and self-destructive behavior of the mentally ill, protection from unsafe social and occupational environments, and safety of marketable products such as drugs, foods, and automobiles. The physician's authority is limited, but the physician can, as an expert in matters relating to health, advise those who have authority to order and to take all necessary steps to protect society, that is, state government along with its agencies and subunits that exercise delegated authority. Individual physicians and medical societies have given this kind of advice throughout our history; indeed, if one looks at the leadership of government health departments in terms of their salaried directors and the boards of health that provide legislatively delegated policy or administrative direction to the departments, one finds medical practitioners predominate. Health officers are mostly physicians, and boards of health that exercise policy or administrative authority tend to be controlled by physicians. In the extreme, Gossert and Miller report (1, p. 488):

In nine states professional societies or associations are mandated by law to provide a list of nominees from which the governor is obliged to make his selection. In two states, Alabama and South Carolina, the medical association is by statutory provision the state board of health; committees of the medical societies carry responsibility on behalf of the state for its public health functions. . . .

Boards with policy-making and administrative functions tend to have more professional representation than boards with only advisory functions. In every instance but one where physicians constitute a majority of the membership the board functions in policymaking and administrative capacities. . . . In no instance do physicians constitute a majority where the board functions only in an advisory capacity.

Medical domination of health departments stems largely from the fact that, in the early days, legislators and governors and mayors felt it necessary to delegate to "the doctors" all matters that related to health, for the doctors were recognized as the ones who were most knowledgeable in such matters. How deeply ingrained this notion is is perhaps illustrated by an experience one of the authors had in Maryland in the early 1960s. A medically dominated planning committee was considering a recommendation to the governor for a reorganized state board of health. Although the board was to be a policy board, the physicians on the committee all agreed that in the 1960s there was no need for a board of health to have physicians on it so long as the board had medical advisory groups. A layman on the committee, a prominent and able legislator, objected and said that it was inconceivable to him to have a state board of health without physicians on it, and that if the committee stuck to its thinking and did not specify some physician membership, he could predict legislative bewilderment and subsequent legislative action—not sponsored or led by him—to create a board of health consisting of mostly physicians.

We will return shortly to boards of health, but let us now note the second reason for physician concern for crisis intervention. Despite all that the theoreticians say about the primary importance of prevention, the fact remains that society will always demand that the crises of life that call for physician intervention—the injured child, the complicated pregnancy, a heart attack—be addressed and that prevention, if necessary, be deferred. Medical crises come first, and society demands physician intervention with whatever armamentarium is appropriate.

Having actively supported the creation of government health agencies, physicians in various states have nonetheless, from time to time, been in conflict with these health departments, sometimes in disagreement about how health department programs should develop professionally, sometimes in reaction to what the private physicians felt was government intrusion into their domain. The AMA, for example, though long supportive of many federal health initiatives, took issue with the Sheppard-Towner Act (1921) and unsuccessfully opposed that grant program for development of child health programs in the states. At the time, the AMA saw this as the opening wedge for the provision of all medical care by government. On the other hand, the AMA recognized and supported the need of government action to provide medical care for the poor but has vigorously opposed proposals for compulsory national health insurance.

Similar patterns appear at the state level. In some states, a happy and progressive relationship developed between the medical societies and the health departments. In Maryland for many years, leaders in the medical society and in private practice worked closely with the state health department to develop some of the most progressive public health programs in the nation. The qualities of leadership and political skill on the part of medical and government leaders often made the difference, along with some of the key issues of the time to which we all occasionally respond but over which we have little control. Miller and co-workers, in a 1974 survey of local health departments, found that in only one of 10 of the large city health departments and in only one in five of the small local health departments was the medical society viewed by the department as a constraint on the development of services (2, p. 935).

State Health Agencies

Administrative Organization

The traditional public health functions include *communicable disease control, maternal and child health services, environmental sanitation, health education, laboratory services,* and *vital statistics.* Until recently, these were placed administratively in state health or public health departments. In recent decades, there has been a tendency in some states to remove some of the environmental health activities and place them in new environmental protection agencies. But a state government's health responsibilities (and being government health activities, they are appropriately *public health* activities) go far beyond these basic six functions. Not only have the basic six functions spawned a large number of related program activities far beyond the original range of services, but the states have also been responsible for care of the mentally ill and mentally retarded, and for professional and institutional licensure. It is important to emphasize that the right to practice medicine, nursing, pharmacy, dentistry, and many other professional activities is a right granted by the issuance of a license from a state government, not from the federal government or a professional association, or by virtue of a university degree.

How a state government organizes its public health functions varies. History, personalities, federal grant programs, and chance all play a role. Some states place all activities in a single agency. Some states place them in separate agencies. In any one state, the organizational pattern may change from time to time as new problems arise and as new opportunities are seized. As might be expected, reorganizations within bureaucracies are resisted by some and favored by others.

There are three basic models. In the first, the health agency is headed by a board of health with policy or administrative functions over the agency. The board is typically appointed by the governor and approved by the state senate. Board members are usually nonsalaried and, as we have noted, when the boards have policy or administrative roles to play, physicians tend to be in the majority. In addition to overall direction of the agency, boards of health (including boards that have only advisory functions) very frequently have authority to enforce public health laws by holding hearings on violations, hearing appeals on health officer actions, and by issuance of *board orders* for compliance with the laws. Board orders must be enforced by law enforcement agencies, although the recipient of a board of health order can, of course, appeal it in the state courts. Many boards either appoint key agency personnel or have a strong influence in their appointment. As one might expect, there have been good and bad boards of health, progressive as well as nonprogressive boards. Some boards have been highly politicized by the types of people appointed to them; other boards have been highly professional with no partisan politics or political hacks. Advocates of policy boards argue that they provide not only good professional advice to the agency (which they could get, of course, equally as well from advisory boards) but also a buffer when the chief health officer must take unpopular stands on public health issues or when the political leaders want something done or not done for political reasons, such as when they close their eyes to a problem, withhold advice that might

prove costly and therefore politically difficult for the elected official to deal with, or support a budget cut. Critics of policy boards argue that they inhibit political accountability. How can a governor be held accountable if he or she must work through a board that is mostly inherited? This criticism has not always been persuasive, given the frequently held belief that politicians, if at all possible, avoid accountability when the going gets tough. Political escape acts have been common in the areas of mental health and mental retardation when poor conditions were publicized, and are common today when government leaders complain about high costs; supposedly everyone is at fault except them.

The second model of health agency governance has a governor-appointed secretary or commissioner of health. Like boards, this type of leadership can be good or bad, depending on the quality of the appointed official and the quality of the governor. If a governor avoids tough issues, if a governor tends to appoint incompetents or political hacks, then the board system might be preferred. If, on the other hand, there is an unprogressive board, then a strong governor with a competent secretary of health would be preferred. The political style of a state often dictates how well each of the systems works. There is a tendency in recent years to move away from policy boards to the cabinet system of government in which the health agency head is the secretary of health. In at least one state in which this occurred, there has been a marked deterioration in the quality of health programming. The cabinet approach allows greater political management and fiscal control, which has clear political advantages, but it can also be professionally disadvantageous.

In recent years, a number of states have sought to create a third model—umbrella organizations, bringing together under one secretary several human service agencies of state government. These super agencies (frequently called a *department of human resources,* or *department of human services*) do not include a set pattern of agencies, though health, mental health and retardation, education, and welfare are most common. Other agencies may also be included, such as corrections. The rationale for these superagencies stems from the fact that many of the clientele of one agency are clientele of one or more of the other agencies, and by placing these agencies under one authority, improved coordination would take place, resulting in more effective and more efficient services. Though success stories abound for this approach, the "successes" are usually reported by those who created these superagencies or whose jobs benefited by their creation. There are considerable anecdotal data to suggest that while the theory is true, the practice has, in fact, not been operationalized at the state levels because of jealous guarding of prerogatives by the various bureaucracies. A health professional, for example, may be very supportive of new initiatives in education or corrections as long as they are not at the expense of the health budget.

State Health Activities

Hanlon cites a 1961 unpublished survey of activities engaged in by 50 state health departments (3, pp. 299–300). There were 103 different activities, some (environmental health, health education, maternal and child health, nursing) engaged in by all 50 departments. Other activities reported by at least 40 departments included communicable diseases, dental health, engineering, hospital survey and planning and construction, licensure, laboratories, local health services, tuberculosis control, and vital statistics. Other frequently reported activities (more than 20 departments) included cancer control, chronic disease control, crippled children's services, food and drug control, heart disease control, industrial health, mental health, nutrition, sexually transmitted disease control, and water and sewage.

The categorization of activities was based on the organization charts for 50 state health departments. What the summary indicates, therefore, are those activities in the various states that have been given organizational chart identity. The activity may well exist in other departments, or in the health department, but be submerged under another organizational unit. For example, 19 states had general sanitation units on their charts. The other 31 states probably had that activity but it was not on the organizational chart. General sanitation in the other 31 states might have been subsumed, at least in part, under engineering, environmental health, industrial health, water and sewage, and like categories. The listing is useful, however, in its identification of some of the major programmatic areas for health department programming.

Miller and associates conducted years later a similar analysis but used state laws instead of the organization charts (4, pp. 940–945). They identified 44 public health areas specified in state laws:

Communicable disease control
Vital statistics
Promulgation of rules and regulations
Sexually transmitted disease control
Quarantines
Tuberculosis control
Water/stream pollution control
Facilities inspection
Facilities licensure
Laboratory services
Refuse disposal
Air pollution control
Abating of nuisances/filth
Health education
Radiological health
Food inspection
Mental health
Prevention of blindness
Maternal/child health
Immunizations
Occupational health
Care of indigent
Qualifications of local health officer
Chronic disease control
Crippled children
Milk inspection
Health planning
Housing inspection
Phenylketonuria/metabolic screening
Alcohol and addiction control
Dental health
Establishment of local hospitals
Rabies control
Ambulance service
School health
Health personnel registration
Home health
Needs and resource assessment
Nursing care
Family planning
Extermination services
Compulsory hospitalization
Nutrition program
Emergency medical service

Miller and associates discuss the problems that flow from the language of the statutes. For example, although only 60 percent of the states authorized immunizations by statutory language, 100 percent authorized communicable disease control activities. Miller and associates assumed, probably correctly, that immunizations in 40 percent of the remaining states are authorized under the broader mandate of communicable disease control.

Some public health programs are operated directly by a central department of state government (typically, state psychiatric and mental retardation hospitals; licensure of professional personnel, hospitals, nursing homes, and other health facilities). Some programs are decentralized to regional offices of the state agency if regional organization is employed. More frequently, programs have a shared responsibility between state and local government health agencies. When this shared responsibility occurs, the state agency typically sets performance standards under which local programs operate, in return for which some state monies are allocated to supplement local government resources. State standards often govern the operation of nongovernmental agencies; these standards must be met in order to be eligible for a license or for payment under some state-administered programs.

Some programs for which there is shared responsibility entail some state service along with complementary local services. Standards are typically minimal standards; if one proposes to provide a service, it must at least meet those standards. Standards are, in a sense, a floor below which a program is not considered acceptable. Standards have rarely been optimal standards because few, if any, could reach such levels without significant tax increases. Standards in public health, as in other areas, have been evolutionary in nature, initially the bare essentials which most could meet or which so clearly affected the public's health that no government could resist establishing them. As with medical education and hospital accreditation standards, after they are established public health standards become a mechanism for improving marginal programs. Often, the standards by themselves are not enough; an added inducement is the offer of a grant of money for development or operation of a program that meets the standards. Grant monies for local programs come from the state government and also from the federal government. Sometimes federal monies have paid all of the costs of the program; sometimes federal monies have paid only part of the cost. The federal strategy has been to offer to pay a sufficient proportion of the costs to stimulate the desired state or local action.

The mix of programs, the sophistication of programs, and the population served by programs vary considerably from state to state and from unit to unit within a state. Most states serve all the people through environmental health programs, ensuring the quality and safety of the environment through such program activities as were identified by Miller and associates and as reported by Hanlon. These activities involve health agency inspections, citations of deficiencies, and board of health or police action if deficiencies are not corrected. The variability from state to state in programs is illustrated by the rules and regulations governing restaurants in two large Eastern states. In one state the local health ordinances require all restaurants to have two separate doors leading to the street to inhibit the flow of flies and animals into the restaurant. Also prohibited is the use of chemically treated flycatching materials in the restaurant. In the nearby state, none of these requirements or prohibitions is present. The former state was practicing good public health, ensuring the quality and safety of the environment. Whether it in fact prevented disease is not known, but it represented an attitude toward health matters that, along with other attitudes and measures, contributed to a pattern that militated against opportunities for disease-causing agents to make inroads. An analogous situation occurs in surgical operating rooms. One break in sterile technique does not necessarily lead to infection, but a string of breaks may. If operating room people are finicky about technique, opportunities for infectious agents to make inroads are limited; when sterile technique is casual or sloppy, the chances of wound infection are greatly increased.

It is easy to demonstrate the value of immunizations as well as water quality control measures. It is more difficult to demonstrate and persuade people of the value of many other public health measures. To do so often requires able professional and political leadership and an informed public.

Sometimes public health laws and ordinances serve not the public's health but the public's aesthetic tastes. The prohibition against swimming in reservoirs is an example: because impounded water is almost always treated, there is really no reason why one cannot swim in the reservoir.

Although all states engage in environmental health activities, the degree and extent of activity varies. Similarly, all states have some personal preventive service programs, particularly in areas relating to maternal and child health, school health, and immunizations. Most, moreover, have program activities relating to crippled children's services, with a variety of diagnostic and treatment services available. In some states, however, access can be a problem, particularly when the state may require referral from a private physician or makes access to the service difficult through lack of public information about the service, infrequency of services, and remoteness of service. Some of these barriers are intentional, some accidental.

In a great many states, public health agency services have moved far beyond the traditional areas of environmental, personal preventive, mental health, and mental retardation services. These states, directly or through local public health agencies, offer many of the services that are provided by hospitals and private physicians in other states. Where this occurs, one often finds the public health agencies paying for care in general hospitals and hiring private physicians to provide special medical services, thus supplementing the more general services provided by the fulltime physician staff. Though most of the personal preventive and the medical care services are provided to the poorer people of the state, some programs are available to all citizens regardless of income status. This, again, varies considerably from state to state.

Mental Health and Mental Retardation Agencies in State Administrations

Mental health agencies were frequently spun off administratively. In the nineteenth century and for a great portion of this century, there was, in fact, little that could be done clinically for the mentally ill, and the mainstream of medical practice more or less washed its hands of the problem. The medical schools were not very helpful either during the first half of this century; few had psychiatric departments, and the psychiatric component of undergraduate medical education programs was thin at best. Professional interest lagged largely because of the absence of knowledge of how to treat these patients, so the state assumed responsibility for warehousing them in large, remote, custodial institutions. Typically, the facilities were understaffed and poorly maintained, for what useful purpose would be served by pouring tax monies into them?

Efforts at reform were spotty at best and usually only temporary. But as the appalling conditions in most state institutions became known; as professional interest grew in the 1950s because of new knowledge and new insights into how to deal with the mentally ill; as tranquilizers were developed that, by suppression of symptoms, made possible the treatment of many patients in out-of-hospital settings; and as the nation's economy improved and tax monies became more readily available, reformers began to be heard. Professionals argued that it was now time for psychiatry to reenter the mainstream of medical practice, to subject its theories and its treatment modalities to the scrutiny of other medical people. Professionals and lay people also called for new monies for improved staffing and for community programs. Moreover, in many states, inadequate and incompetent administration within the mental health units led to cries for administrative reform. Among the reforms suggested was the merger of the health and mental health agencies where they were separate. In some states, this was accomplished. In other states, it was successfully resisted by the mental health bureaucracies. Though the clinical justification for merger is clear-cut, merger may at times be inadvisable for other reasons, particularly when the absorbing agency has a greater level of incompetence or is so highly politicized that merger would run the grave risk of inappropriate interference in the clinical programs.

The placement of mental retardation agencies in state bureaucracies also varies. They are sometimes separate, sometimes in the health department, very often in with mental health, and sometimes in other state agencies. These institutions have also suffered along similar lines and for similar reasons as the mental health institutions. Periodic efforts to change the organizational placement of mental retardation agencies by merging them with other agencies or by making them independent agencies are usually controversial. For example, a controversy still exists between the psychiatrists and the pediatricians, the former having handled the mental retardation problem historically by default. These two medical specialties often debate with educators, who argue that since mental retardation cannot be cured, special education must play the most prominent role, educating the mental retardation patients to as high a functioning level as possible. The controversy around mental retardation, while sometimes a question of merger, is more often a question of professional responsibility for mental retardation program leadership.

Reformers have called for more modern residential facilities, improved staffing, and the development of a variety of nonresidential and community services such as day hospitals, community mental health centers, and emergency services. But state governments, faced with rising demands from many sectors of society along with rising costs, generally have given measured responses to the new demands. Major improvements have been made in many states, but in many states progress is slow. The work environment of many state institutions leaves much to be desired; physically remote, old, and without adequate support services, they have proved unattractive to many professionals. In addition, professional positions

have become vacant in many states because of low salaries; in others, they have been filled by international medical school graduates (IMGs), many of whom have language problems and only temporary medical licenses. On the whole, the record of state governments has not been good, even in the second half of the twentieth century.

The movement for community-based care loomed as a solution to the state governments. If community care was the most appropriate locale for the mentally ill and retarded, why make heavy investments in state hospitals? Why not get the patients out to the communities in which they belong? Not only did this encourage states not to allocate large sums of new monies for hospitals and staff upgrading, but it also encouraged some states to accelerate the discharge of patients to the community. In California and New York, the dumping of patients reached scandalous dimensions, because the communities did not have the money to develop an adequate range of services, and the states released the patients without services in place. In New York City, many patients ended up in what are aptly called flophouses. In California, the Santa Clara County sheriff's department reported in 1974 that the jail population there had more than tripled as a result of former psychiatric hospital patients who were arrested for loitering and mischievous conduct. This, of course, has prompted citizens to resist both the release of patients to the communities and the placement of community facilities near their homes. But the problem exists not only in California and New York. In a great many states, newspapers periodically report on community homes and nursing facilities that burn down or that drug, beat, or starve patients because the state governments have not enforced standards that, if upheld, would force the state to take back the patients. Becker and Schulberg concluded (5, pp. 255–261):

The majority of patients currently cared for in state hospitals could be adequately treated in the community if a comprehensive spectrum of psychiatric services and residential alternatives were established. The failure to establish this network of community services before the discharge of thousands of patients has discredited the deinstitutionalization programs in many states, including California and New York, and forced California to abandon its plan to phase out all its state hospitals. Thus, although phase out of state hospitals is clinically feasible, it is unlikely at present since the fiscal and ideological commitment to shift to community-based care is lacking.

It should be noted that two additional factors preventing the closure of state hospitals are the hospital employee unions and the communities around the hospitals. The unions fear unemployment and the communities fear an adverse effect on the local economy. Pressures brought by both on state legislatures have slowed the process of closing hospitals.

Local Health Activities

There are about 3,000 local health departments in the United States. Nearly two thirds of these departments serve populations of under 50,000 people. Seventy percent of the local health departments have a board of health. These boards may be governing or advisory boards. The governing boards are commonly the local county commissioners; advisory boards are typically representative of the area's professional interest groups and the general citizenry. The 1990 National Profile of Local Health Departments, a survey conducted by the National Association of County Health Officials, reported that more than half of the local health departments had some activity in the following areas (6):

- Data collection and analysis (vital records and statistics, reportable diseases)
- Epidemiology and surveillance (chronic disease and communicable disease)
- Health code development and enforcement
- Health planning
- Inspection activities (food and milk control, health and recreational facility safety/quality)
- Health education

- Water supply safety
- Sewage disposal systems
- Solid waste management
- Vector and animal control
- Water pollution
- AIDS testing and counselling
- Child health
- Chronic disease
- Family planning
- Home health care
- Immunizations
- Prenatal care
- Sexually transmitted diseases
- Tuberculosis
- Women, Infants, and Children (WIC) food supplement program

The larger the population served by the local health department, the greater range of services provided. A high percentage of the larger departments also provide services in the areas of air quality surveillance and control, hazardous waste management, occupational health and safety, dental health, handicapped children services, laboratory services, and primary care. Where appropriate public health services are not provided by the local health department, they are typically provided by the state health department, particularly laboratory, environmental, and mental health services.

The person in charge of a local health department is typically called the *local health officer* or *county health officer*. Slightly more than half of them are medically qualified but only one third of these have had advanced graduate training in public health or related areas. The larger departments tend to have physicians with advanced training in public health in charge.

Miller and associates conclude their 1974 survey of local health departments by noting that despite all of the recent federal efforts to influence health services in the United States, there has been "little acknowledgment that local health departments are part of that scene." They go on to note that "increasingly, when the nation's leaders speak of existing patterns of health service they refer to private professional practice, ignoring important resources and potentials in the public sector" (4, p. 937). This lament is well taken. Critics cite inadequacies of local health departments to justify the diminished recognition given these public agencies, but one cannot resist observing that some of the diminished recognition stems from ignorance about what health departments do, some stems from irritation or frustration over the fact that an entrenched lower-level bureaucracy exists that has its own expertise and its own honestly held views on needs and on ways to do things, and some stems from individuals who are from those relatively few states in which the state health department is weak and the local scene and potential goes unrecognized or undeveloped.

It is important for us to appreciate more fully what a health department does, for it should go without saying that were it not for organized public health efforts, our nation would not be as stable, as successful, or as livable as it is. It is the work of local health officers and their collaborators that makes our society one in which it is safe to live and that is conducive to the healthy development of the individual.

The pattern of local health department organization varies from state to state. A few states (Hawaii, Vermont, Rhode Island, and Delaware) have no local units; whatever services are provided are provided by the state. Most states do have local departments; typically, some of their monies come from state and federal coffers. In New England, local departments tend to be on a city or town basis, county government being weak or nonexistent. In the South, local departments tend to be organized on a county basis. And there are inbetween arrangements, as in Pennsylvania, in which there is a provision for county health departments (but very few in existence) and local government (subcounty, town, borough, etc.) units with largely environmental responsibilities, as well as regional state health department offices. In some parts of the country, we find metropolitan and other kinds of multijurisdictional departments, that is, multicounty or combined city-county departments. How much autonomy the local (county, town, city, or

multijurisdictional) department has from the state authority varies from state to state and even within the state, depending on the extent of state support, the dynamism of the local health officer, the relative political strength of the different local governments, as well as the administrative style of the state health agency leaders.

The state health department sets the minimum standards for local department operations. Typically, the local units submit their budgets and plans to the state authority for review and approval. With state approval, the local department is then approved to receive state funds. In many states, the local unit can, if it wishes, exceed the standards set by the state and use its own resources to accomplish that end. The level of state support varies but is usually based on a minimum program expected of the local unit and funds distributed accordingly to some kind of formula.

To illustrate what a local health department does, let us focus on the Baltimore County Health Department in Maryland.* The county has a land area of 610 square miles and surrounds the city of Baltimore (Fig. 11–1). The county seat is Towson. The county population in 1990 was 692,134, 85 percent of which was white. Twelve percent of the population lived below 185 percent of the poverty level. Nearly 3.9 percent of the population received medical assistance.

The county is well served by medical resources. There are four acute care hospitals in the county, 51 licensed nursing homes, and a wide range of public and private psychiatric services. There were in 1990 562 primary care physicians, backed by a full range of medical specialists. The proximity of the county to Baltimore, with the city's two medical schools and teaching hospitals, provides Baltimore County residents with ample access to both hospitals and physicians. The closeness to the city of Baltimore and its vast medical resources illustrates the fact that standard ratios as a means of deter-

---

*We are indebted to the health officers for Baltimore and Anne Arundel counties for their help in providing us with the data from which this account is drawn.

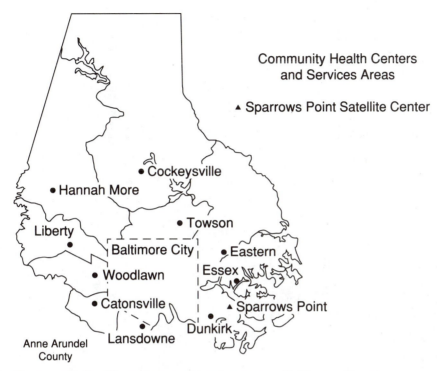

Figure 11–1. Community health centers and service areas—Baltimore County.

mining need (such as the standard of four beds per 1,000 population, or a desired ratio of physicians per population) should be assessed in a large context and may be of limited value in state and substate jurisdictions because of the ability of a population to be served by resources in the neighboring jurisdiction.

The county health officer also serves as deputy state health officer, and is thus accountable both to the elected county council and to the secretary of the State Department of Health and Mental Hygiene. The organizational structure for the Department is shown in Figure 11–2. Headquartered at the county seat in Towson, the Department carries out its activities throughout the county in 11 centers. The range of services provided by each center is shown in Figure 11–3. Services at the centers begin at 8:30 A.M., and some are available to as late as 7 P.M.

The work of the county health department is carried out by a professional staff of 296 people, including 8 fulltime salaried physicians, 67 public health nurses, 99 school nurses, 35 social workers, and 3 dentists (Table 11–1).

The formula used in Maryland to finance local health services until mid-1992 was known as the Case Formula, after the chairman of the committee that recommended its use. The formula provided for the state to pay 50 percent of all approved local health services, with the exact amount in any one county bearing a relationship to population and assessed value of property. Baltimore County was thus close to the economic average for the state: the state paid 50.85 percent of the approved budget and the county paid for 49.15 percent. But these percentages apply only to the approved budget of $13,783,663. The county, in addition, proposed to appropriate another $6,178,785, bringing the total budget for local health services to $19,962,448.

Baltimore County Department of Health
Organization Chart

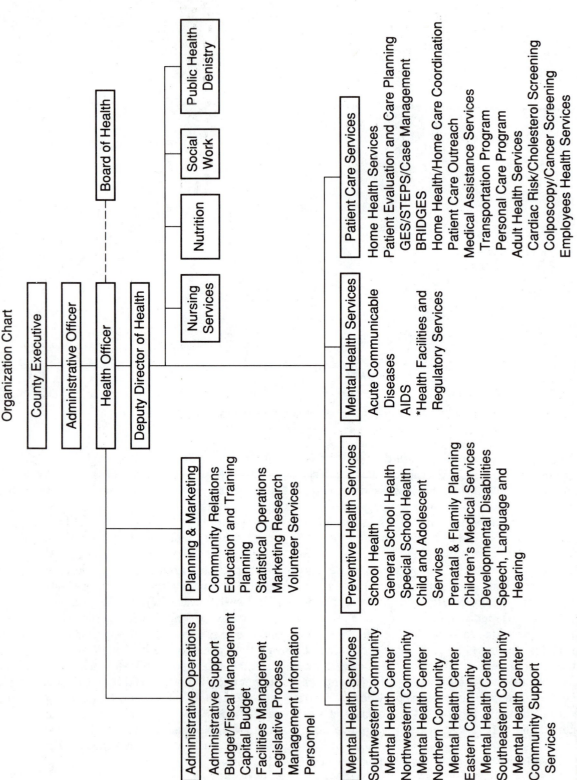

* This will function as a support unit

Figure 11–2. Baltimore County Department of Health, Organization Chart.

FIGURE 11–3. Health Center Locations and Services: Baltimore County

Baltimore-Highlands-Landsdowne
3902 Annapolis Road 21227

PPD screening/education
Child health
　Nurse assessment
　Well child
Family planning
　Teen family planning
　Nurse clinic
Pregnancy testing/counselling
Family centered home care
WIC
HIV risk assessment/counselling
Nutrition counselling
Pediatric nurse practitioner clinic
Adolescent prenatal clinic
Healthy start services
Cancer screening
Colposcopy

Catonsville
18 Eggs Lane 21228

Child health
　Nurse assessment
　Well child
Family planning
　Pregnancy testing/counselling
　Prenatal clinic
WIC
Tuberculosis screening/education
Hypertension screening/monitoring
Family centered home care
WIC voucher distribution
HIV risk assessment/counselling
Healthy start services

Cockeysville
10746 York Road 21030

Prenatal
Family planning
Child health
Attention deficit disorder
WIC
Colposcopy
Pregnancy testing/counselling
Hypertension screening/monitoring
Family centered home care
Tuberculosis screening and education
HIV risk assessment/counselling
Healthy start services

Dundalk
7700 Dunmanway 21222

Family planning
Family planning teen clinic
Prenatal
Pediatric nurse assessment
Well child
Tuberculosis screening/education
Attention deficit disorder
WIC voucher
Family centered home care
Pregnancy testing/counselling
Blood pressure screening/monitoring
HIV risk assessment/counselling
Nutritional counselling
Healthy start services

Eastern Regional
9100 Franklin Sq. Drive 21237

Prenatal clinic
Family planning clinic
Family planning nurse clinic/FPC
Child health with nurse assessment
WIC
Tuberculosis screening/education
Conservation of hearing
Cerebral palsy
Dental clinic
Cancer screening
Colposcopy clinic
Eye clinic
Family centered home care
HIV assessment/counselling
Healthy start services
Family help team
Blood pressure screening/monitoring

Essex
1548 Country Ridge Lane 21221

Child health
Pediatric nurse practitioner clinic
Nurse assessment
Family planning
Teen family planning
HIV AB anonymous testing
Sexually transmissible diseases
Attention deficit disorder
WIC
Tuberculosis screening/education
Blood pressure screening/monitoring

Pregnancy testing/counselling
Family centered home care
High risk infant services
HIV risk assessment/counselling
Nutritional counselling
Healthy start services

Hannah More Academy Center
12035 Reisterstown Road 21136

Child health
　PNP clinics
Family planning
Blood pressure screening/monitoring
Pregnancy testing/counselling
Family centered home care
High risk infant services
Dental clinic
HIV risk assessment/counselling
WIC services
Healthy start services

Liberty Family Resource Center
8737 B Liberty Road 21133

Dental clinic
Child health
　Nurse clinics
　PNP clinics
Family planning
Attention deficit disorder
Pregnancy testing/counselling
Blood pressure screening/monitoring
Family centered home care
Adolescent family planning
Sexually transmissible diseases
WIC
Tuberculosis screening/education
Chest
HIV risk assessment/counselling
Conservation of hearing
Blood pressure screening/monitoring
Family help team
Nutritional counselling
Healthy start services

Sparrows Point
4033 North Point Boulevard 21222

Family planning
Well child
Child health nurse assessment
Attention deficit disorder
WIC

FIGURE 11–3 (Continued)

Towson
8812 & 8814 Orchard Tree Lane 21204

Child health
Nurse assessment
Family planning with FP nurse clinic
Sexually transmissible diseases
HIV AB testing
WIC (certification/voucher distribution)
Tuberculosis screening & education
Pregnancy testing/counselling
Blood pressure screening/monitoring

Family centered home care
Chest clinic
HIV risk assessment/counselling
Nutritional counselling
Healthy start services

Woodlawn
1811 Woodlawn Drive 21207

Child health
Family planning

Teen family planning
Sexually transmissible diseases
HIV antibody testing
Attention deficit disorder
WIC (certification/voucher distribution)
Family centered home care
Blood pressure screening/monitoring
Pregnancy testing/counselling
HIV risk assessment/counselling
Health opportunity for teens
Healthy start services

As Figure 11–3 shows, the range of services provided by the Baltimore County Health Department is extensive. Descriptions of a selected number of those services follows. These descriptions are taken from the Department's information handbook:

• **Chest Clinic.** This clinic service is offered for the purpose of diagnosing tuberculosis. When medically indicated, services available include tuberculin testing (however, not for routine screenings), bacteriological investigation, and X-ray examinations. Anti-TB medications are also available to County residents for chemopreventive and chemotherapeutic treatment. There is no charge for any service.

• **Family Planning.** Participants are offered counselling and instruction concerning the full range of family planning methods: natural method/rhythm, intrauterine devices, contraceptive pills, foams, condoms, dia-

TABLE 11–1. Baltimore County Department of Health Professional Staff—FY 93

Statistical analyst	2	Patient care coordinator	1
Management assistant	8	Sanitarian	2
Personnel analyst	1	Coordinator, volunteer services	1
Accountant	3	Social worker	35
Financial operations supervisor	1	Social work supervisor	3
Public health educator	2	Chief, division of developmental disabilities	1
Public health investigator	5	Mental health therapy coordinator	4
Chief, administrative support	1	Psychology associate	4
School nurse	99	Psychologist	3
Occupational health nurse	2	Physician's assistant	1
Public health nurse	67	Physician	8
Nurse practitioner	5	Health planner	1
Field nursing supervisor	7	Coordinator, mental health services	3
Assistant chief, nursing services	1	Dentist	3
Chief, nursing services	1	Facilities review coordinator	1
Nutritionist	2	Deputy director, public health	1
Speech pathologist/audiologist	5	Human services program coordinator	10
Speech pathologist/audiologist supervisor	1	Total	296
School health coordinator	1		

phragms, and Norplant. Screening studies for cancer and venereal diseases are also conducted, as well as fertility counselling and referral for other diagnostic studies. Pregnancy testing and counselling is available by appointment in each health center. In some health centers there are clinics during afternoon hours for adolescents only.

- **Nursing-Home Visiting Services.** The public health nurse provides nursing care to acutely ill, chronically ill, and aged patients and their families in the home. Services are available to all ages from infancy up to and including the elderly population. The goal of the program is to help patients/families manage their health problems effectively.
- **Prenatal Clinics.** Pregnancy tests are performed in all health centers, and when pregnancy is discovered, the patient is referred to one of our prenatal clinics where regular examinations are given by an obstetrician throughout pregnancy. Patients are assisted in making arrangements for delivery at an area hospital. Nutritional advice, medical social services, and post-natal family planning are available to these patients. Tests for cancer, gonorrhea, and syphilis are given; high risk behavior is determined, and tests for the AIDS virus performed if desired.
- **Rabies Clinics.** Rabies clinics are regularly scheduled in the spring and fall. Vaccination is offered to pet dogs and cats 3 months of age and older. There is a small fee.
- **School Health.** The school health program is a joint undertaking of the Baltimore County Department of Health and the Baltimore County Public Schools. The school health program has three basic functions: delivery of health services to students and staff, implementation of an ongoing health education curriculum, [and] provision of a safe and healthful school environment. Professional school nurses from the Department of Health are assigned to every public elementary and special school and to many non-public schools. Their purpose is to identify and modify or remove students' health-related barriers to learning, prevent disease, and promote individual wellness. School health screenings include vision, hearing, and scoliosis screening.
- **Speech and Language Services.** The Division of Speech, Language, and Hearing provides complete testing and treatment for speech and language problems. We also provide consultation, family training/counselling, and referral service to County residents experiencing speech and language problems. Services are provided to a wide range of clients from infants to senior citizens. Referrals are accepted from physicians, teachers, allied health professionals, family members, or the person needing service. We evaluate and treat the following communication disorders:
  - Articulation delay/disorder
  - Language delay/disorder
  - Voice problems
  - Stuttering

Communication problems associated with:
  - Cleft palate
  - Developmental disability
  - Learning disability
  - Stroke and other neurologically based disorders

Fees are based on a sliding fee scale. Medical assistance is accepted. Detailed insurance statements are prepared if you need them. No one is denied service because they cannot pay. Each staff member is licensed and holds a Certificate of Clinical Competence. The Division is accredited by the American Speech-Language and Hearing Association. All services are by appointment only.

- **Well Child Clinics.** These clinics provide preventive care for children and adolescents from birth through 20 years of age. Routine immunization is provided for diphtheria, tetanus, whooping cough, *Hemophilus influenzae* B, polio, measles, mumps, and German measles. Screening tests for anemia, tuberculosis, PKU, lead poisoning, sickle cell anemia, and hearing, vision, speech, language, and developmental problems are performed. Health and parenting education is provided by both physicians and public health nurses.
- **WIC (Women, Infants, and Children).** The WIC program services pregnant, postpartum, and breast-feeding women and children under five years of age who are residents of Baltimore County AND meet income eligibility requirements AND have a medical/nutritional risk factor which can be helped by nutritional foods. The WIC program provides free supplemental foods such as milk, eggs, cheese, juice, dried beans, and iron-fortified cereal. Nursing mothers receive information on breast-feeding. Infants may receive iron-fortified formula. WIC also provides on-going nutrition education as well as referrals to Health and Social Services.

While public health department personal health programs and services are directed primarily toward lower-income and disadvantaged groups, some programs and services are for all people regardless of income, and as noted above, for some services a charge is made for those able to pay.

The Baltimore County Health Department does not provide any environmental health services since the county decided to place responsibility for those services with a separate agency. The inclusion of environmental services in health departments will vary from one jurisdiction to another. In adjacent Anne Arundel County, for example, environmental health services are an integral part of the county health department's work. The Anne Arundel County Health Department, based at the county seat of Annapolis, reports its environmental health functions in its "Agency Profile" as follows:

Environmental hazards to human health may cause immediate acute illness or delayed disease or disability. The Department plays a leading role in protecting the health of County residents by preventing their exposure to environmental hazards.

- Drinking water safety. In this County, 40% of all residents derive their drinking water from *private wells.* The Department regulates the site and construction of all residential wells and samples new wells for bacteria and harmful chemicals.
- Safe sewerage and solid waste disposal. The Department reviews and approves all private *residential and commercial sewage systems* and conducts thousands of *soil percolation ("perc") tests* each year. The volume of this program reflects the County's development and the fact that 40% of the County's homes have private on-site sewage systems.
- Safe food service. County residents and visitors are protected from food-borne disease by the Department's *Food Control Program.* The program annually *inspects* about 1,400 *restaurants, markets, bakeries, schools, camps, and nursing homes,* and conducts complaint *investigations and training* in safe food handling.
- Safe recreation. Bacterial contamination of waterways, streams and ponds is monitored to ensure the safety of *public and community beaches.* The County's 225 *public pools and spas* and 1,460 *lifeguards and pool operators* are licensed annually by the Department.

- License and permit inspections. As provided for under County law, the Department inspects and approves permits for about 68,000 units in *multiple dwelling housing.* Permits are also approved for *mobile home parks* and *vendors of exotic birds.*
- Investigation of community complaints. Citizens are often the first to recognize community hazards and nuisances. The Department investigates and institutes corrective action on complaints such as *hazardous waste, sewage overflows, tenant problems, noxious weeds, rodents, unsafe structures, and air pollution.*
- Liaison activities. Occasionally action on a local environmental hazard involves all levels of government: Federal, State and County. In these instances, the Department serves the County as the *liaison* or intermediary between agencies, citizens and community groups. Recent examples include Departmental leadership on indoor air and toxic waste clean-up projects.

Federal-State and State-Local Relations

Throughout the world in almost all enterprises in which a central authority has local units or branch offices, there is conflict. The branch office typically thinks the head office does not know what it is doing, and the head office reciprocates with like attitudes.

In the federal government, it is common for federal health officials to speak disparagingly of state health officers and, in state government, for officials to speak disparagingly of local health officials and distrustingly of federal officers. What the local health officers think of both, the reader can easily guess. These common attitudes stem from the fact that each level of government views the world from a different perspective and has different pressures working on it. Their respective priorities develop accordingly, and it should not be surprising that they often differ. Because the higher level of government tends to have more resources to work with and a stronger bureaucratic structure with the staying power that goes with it, the assessments by the higher government level of the next lower level tend to prevail, just as the histories written by victors in wars shape our perspectives on world history. The assessment of local and state

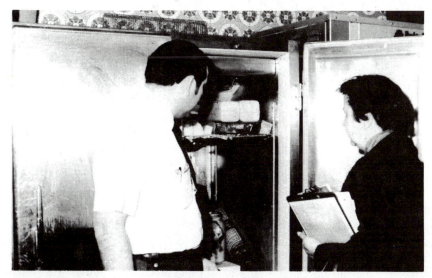

Figure 11–4. Sanitarian inspecting restaurant refrigeration equipment. Routine inspection of food-service facilities is an important part of all local health department work, serving to minimize the danger of disease from food contamination through food handling, processing, and storage. (Courtesy, Anne Arundel County Health Department.)

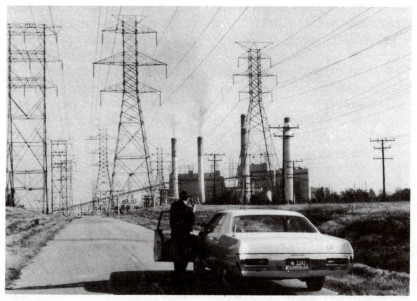

Figure 11–5. Sanitarian monitoring smokestack emissions. Air pollution control is of growing importance in our industrial society for maintenance of the public's health and the quality of the environment. (Courtesy, Anne Arundel County Health Department.)

health departments by the units of government above them should therefore be treated with caution. They may be valid assessments, but they may also be biased appraisals reflecting age-old styles of bureaucratic in-fighting.

The Federal Government and Public Health

Public health involves interplay among federal, state, and local governments. The federal government provides some direct health services, but its chief role has been that of stimulating the development of new and improved services by provision of monies to buy the action it wanted to see developed. Indeed, except in some circumscribed areas, the federal government has no constitutional authority to provide direct health services for people, this being the domain of the states and the private sector.

The Congressional Role in Health

For government to do anything requires money that must be raised by some form of taxation. The use of that money, as well as the raising of it, must have a legal base; somewhere in the U.S. Constitution there must be a clause that justifies a law and, in turn, an appropriation, for government to do what it does. This applies to all areas of government activity. The U.S. Supreme Court is arbiter when otherwise unresolvable disputes arise about whether the activity of the government is in accord with the authorities granted government by the Constitution.

The *Powers of Congress* part of the Constitution (Article I, Section 8) provides authority to raise and support armies, to provide and maintain a navy, and to make all laws "necessary and proper" for carrying out those powers. One can quickly see how this justifies the allocation of monies for military, naval, and air force hospitals and health services. It requires only a slight extension of logic to justify the Department of Veterans Affairs (VA) work in health, whether it is the building of a hospital or

clinic for treatment of veterans with service-connected disabilities or the support of medical education to ensure an adequate supply of doctors so that there will be enough to meet the staffing needs of the VA system. Similarly, one can justify the medical school for the armed forces that was recently built on the grounds of the National Naval Medical Center in Bethesda, Maryland.

The Constitution also grants to Congress the power to regulate foreign and interstate commerce. This justifies much of the federal activity regarding regulation of foods, drugs, product and occupational safety, and some environmental health activities, because they move in, or affect, interstate or foreign commerce. The power to control federal lands, along with the presidential power to make treaties (with the advice and consent of the Senate) are the sources of federal activity in providing health services for Native Americans and Alaska Natives. Other direct service activities also rely on these clauses for legitimization. By far the greatest federal influence comes from the distribution of monies to the states, local governments, and nongovernmental agencies. Sometimes these grants of money can be justified as "necessary and proper" for carrying out the specific constitutional powers already cited. An even more significant basis for grant monies derives from the power of Congress "to lay and collect taxes, duties, imports, and excises, to pay the debts and provide for the common defense and general welfare of the United States."

It is the "general welfare" clause that justifies support for medical research, Medicare, Medicaid, health employee training, and so on. The power to make monies available for certain general welfare activities also permits the writing of regulations setting out the conditions that must be met in order to get the money. The regulations are applications of the law written by the administering agencies in the executive branch and published in the *Federal Register,* a daily (Monday through Friday) official publication of the U.S. government. Since regulations have force of law, they must follow the intent of Congress. Frequently, litigation revolves around whether a regulation has followed the intent of Congress. This the courts determine, drawing not only on the law itself but also on congressional committee reports that indicate the thinking of the Senate, the House, and sometimes of the conference committee on the bill as each reports it: the House committee reports to the House of Representatives, the Senate committee reports to the Senate, and the conference committee reports to both houses of the Congress. The conference committee is an *ad hoc* group of representatives from the Senate and the House, convened to iron out or resolve different versions of similar bills, one passed by each house.

The Legislative Process

Any proposed law must begin by being introduced in the Senate or the House by one of the respective members. On introduction, it is assigned a number (e.g., HR 1 or S-9, as the case may be). To become a law, a bill must be passed in identical form by both houses of Congress and signed by the president. If the president vetoes the bill, it can become law without his signature if two thirds of both houses vote to override his veto; if the president does not sign the bill or veto it, it can still become law if, after 10 days (Sundays excepted), no such action is taken. If during these 10 days Congress adjourns, then the bill does not become law. The drafting of a bill may be done in the executive branch and be given to a member of the Senate or House for introduction, or it may be drafted within the legislative branch and be introduced by one or more members of the respective houses. Bills may also be drafted by individual citizens or groups and be given to a willing member of Congress for introduction.

On introduction, the bill is referred to an appropriate committee for study and for report to the full house. The process in the Senate is very similar to that of the House of Representatives, and each goes through the entire process in considering a bill; each, typically, holds its own hearings on a bill and writes its own report. Neither body defers to the other on such matters.

Many bills die in committee. Some die in *conference,* conference being a joint committee of the House and Senate to iron out differences on a bill that has passed each house but with different provisions or wording. More important bills typically have hearings whereby proponents and opponents to the bill may testify to give information to the committee that help or influence the committee's thinking about the bill. With the benefit of this information and advice from its professional staff, a committee can then decide what action it wishes to take on the bill. It has a report prepared on the bill, which accompanies the bill to the full House or Senate. The report explains what the bill is intended to do. Committee reports can be secured from the respective committees, as can published hearings.

The movement of a bill through the House or Senate is a complicated process, affected by the volume of business before the house as well as by political considerations of influential leaders, the administration, interest and pressure groups, and the views of individual members of the house.

There are a number of agencies of the Congress that need to be cited because of their key roles in health affairs. They are the key committees of each house, the General Accounting Office (GAO), the Congressional Budget Office (CBO), and the Office of Technology Assessment (OTA).

There are approximately 20 committees of the House of Representatives, with at least 33 subcommittees concerned with health affairs. On the Senate side there are 17 committees, with some 23 subcommittees concerned with health affairs. Some of these committees, with or without subcommittees, have major health legislative and investigative responsibilities. Some have minor or tangential concerns. The problem in part is that we can never be certain when a new committee or its chairperson will suddenly discover a need to look at some health affairs.

Bills that launch new programs or modify existing programs are substantive legislation that *authorize* the spending of money. The authorization is not, however, an *appropriation*. The appropriation of money is a separate act, and the Constitution provides that money bills must originate in the House of Representatives. The work on appropriations is done by the House Appropriations Committee, and the appropriations for health by its Subcommittee on HHS Appropriations. The House Ways and Means Committee is concerned with raising revenue by various tax measures. If a new piece of health legislation is to require new tax monies, then this committee must find the ways and means of securing new monies and then must recommend them to the full House. The committee might also be concerned with the use of monies previously raised and appropriated and might, therefore, investigate the strengths and weaknesses of what has resulted from its earlier recommendation to the House for authorization of expenditures. A national health insurance bill would undoubtedly have to clear the Ways and Means Committee at some point. To make its work more efficient, the committee has appointed a number of subcommittees that carry out the substantive work. Among its subcommittees is the Subcommittee on Health. The counterpart in the Senate to the House Ways and Means Committee is the Senate Finance Committee, which has a Subcommittee on Health. The Senate Appropriations Committee also has a subcommittee concerned with HHS appropriations.

These committees are, so to speak, the *money* committees. Most of the committees and their subcommittees are concerned more directly with substantive legislation. This may entail factfinding to enable them to ascertain what kinds of legislation are needed, or it may entail legislative oversight to examine the execution and effectiveness of existing laws. One problem in identifying the key committees and subcommittees is that the names often change. Be that as it may, on the Senate side, apart from the Senate Finance Committee and the Senate Appropriations Committee, some of the major committees and subcommittees concerned with health affairs are:

• Committee on Agriculture, Nutrition, and Forestry; Subcommittee on Nutrition and Investigation

• Committee on Armed Services; Subcommittee on Manpower and Personnel
• Committee on Commerce, Science, and Transportation; Subcommittee on Consumer Affairs
• Committee on Environment and Public Works; Subcommittee on Toxic Substances, Environmental Oversight, and Research and Development; Subcommittee on Environmental Protection
• Committee on Veterans' Affairs
• Special Committee on Aging
• Select Committee on Indian Affairs

The key Senate Committee, however, is the *Senate Labor and Human Resources Committee,* which deals most often with substantive health legislation.

On the House side one finds similar committees with sometimes similar names. Apart from the Ways and Means Committee and the Appropriations Committee, the House Energy and Commerce Committee should be noted, and in particular its Subcommittee on Health and the Environment.

General Accounting Office (GAO)

The GAO is an agency of Congress. Its job is, in part, to help Congress monitor the performance of federal agencies. It is much more than a bookkeeping operation. It conducts many studies to determine how well the intent of a law is being carried out in terms of program activites, program effectiveness, and program efficiency. As might be expected, its reports are often discomforting to agencies in the executive branch. Among its recent reports are:

• *Medicare—HCFA Needs to Take Stronger Actions Against HMOs Violating Federal Standards* (November 1991)
• *Access to Health Care—States Respond to Growing Crisis* (June 1992)
• *Long-Term Care Insurance—Risks to Consumers Should be Reduced* (December 1991)
• *Medicare—Improvements Needed in the Identification of Inappropriate Hospital Care* (December 1989)
• *Health Insurance—Vulnerable Payers Lose Billions to Fraud and Abuse* (May 1992)

• *Health Care Spending Control—The Experiences of France, Germany, and Japan* (November 1991)

GAO reports are rigorously reviewed for accuracy before release and are the closest the federal government comes to securing independent evaluation of executive branch activities.

Congressional Budget Office (CBO)

The CBO is another agency of the Congress that is assuming a critical role in fiscal affairs. Its professional staff undertakes a variety of analyses relating to fiscal policy. This, along with its studies of the budget submitted to the Congress by the president, provides Congress with an independent assessment of what is requested and where we are going in terms of fiscal policy.

Office of Technology Assessment (OTA)

New technology can be very costly. The Congress, through its OTA, now has an independent mechanism assessing the costs and benefits of technology, which can be a guide as it decides on matters relating to legislation as well as budgeting for new technology.

Health Responsibilities of the Executive Branch

There are a number of major federal agencies concerned with health services. Principal among these are the Department of Defense, with a large network of facilities to care for members of the armed forces and their dependents; the Department of Veterans Affairs, with a network of hospitals, nursing homes, and services to care for veterans of the armed forces; Department of Labor, with its Occupational Safety and Health Administration; the Environmental Protection Agency; and the Department of Health and Human Services.

Department of Health and Human Services

The Department of Health and Human Services (HHS) is the principal health agency of the federal government and has a budget second only to the Department of Defense. It is composed of five major agencies: the Public Health Service, the Health Care Financing Administration, the Office of Human Development Services, the Social Security Administration, and the Family Support Administration. The general organization of HHS is shown in Fig. 11–6. The Public Health Service and the Health Care Financing Administration are specifically related to health.

Public Health Service (PHS)

The mission of the Public Health Service (PHS) is to protect and advance the health of the American people by (7):

• Conducting and supporting biomedical, behavioral, and health services research and communicating research results to health professionals and the public.
• Helping to provide health care and related services to medically underserved populations; to Native Americans and Alaska Natives; and to other groups with special health needs, such as migrant workers and their families, the mentally ill, and persons with alcohol and drug abuse problems.
• Preventing and controlling disease, identifying health hazards in the environment and helping to correct them, and promoting healthy lifestyles for the nation's citizens.
• Ensuring that drugs and medical devices are safe and effective, that food is safe and wholesome, that cosmetics are harmless, and that electronic products do not expose users to dangerous amounts of radiation.
• Working with other nations and international agencies on global health problems and their solutions.

The PHS operates the largest public health program in the world. It is directed by the assistant secretary for health, who is appointed by the president and confirmed by the Senate. The surgeon general of the Public Health Service assists the assistant secretary in the administration of the PHS. The PHS has undergone frequent reorganizations and has an interesting history. It began in 1798 when a law was passed that provided for the relief of sick and disabled seamen, and later for the

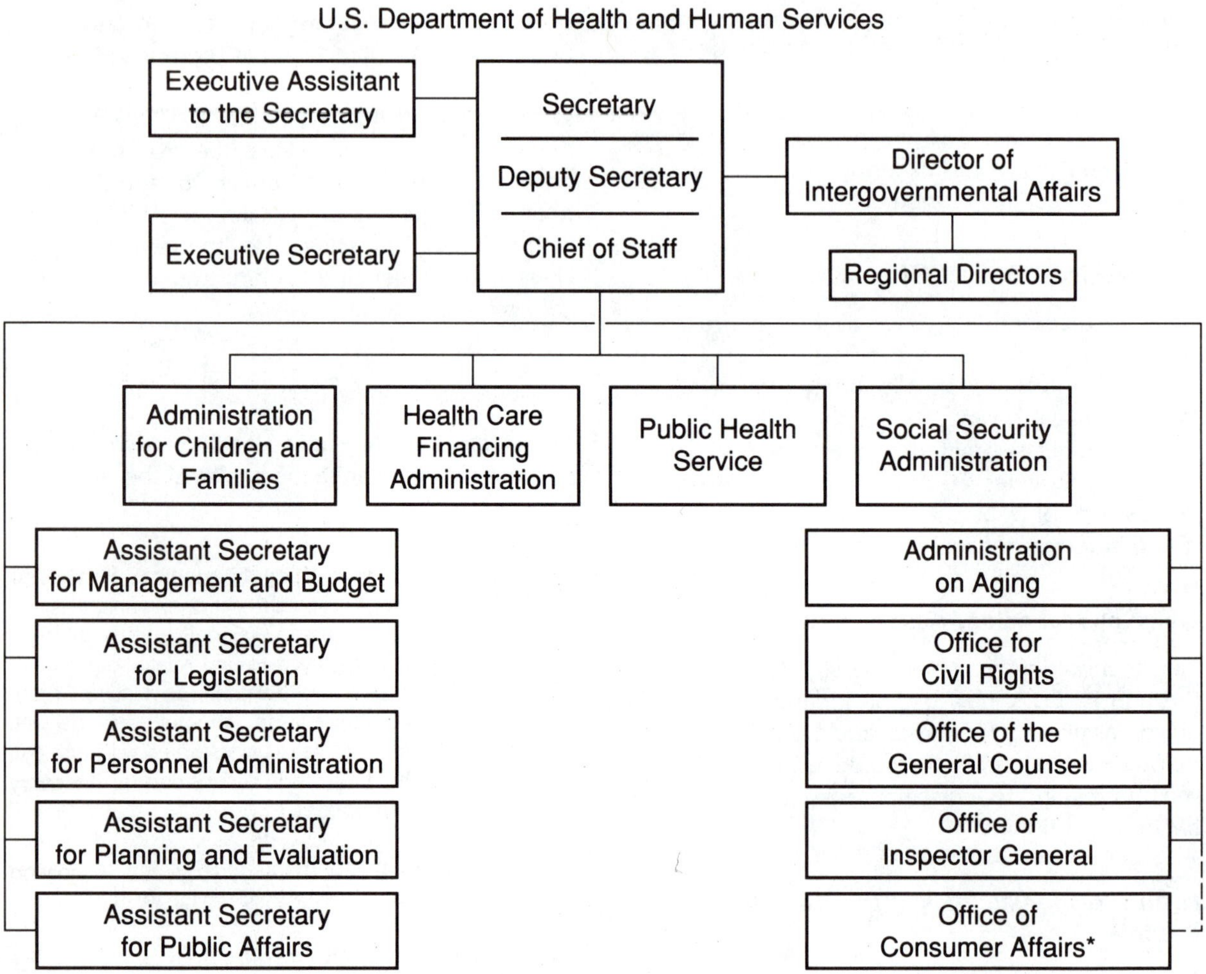

U.S. Department of Health and Human Services

Figure 11–6. U.S. Department of Health and Human Services, Organization Chart, 1992.

widows and children of seamen "who may have been killed or drowned in the course of their service as seamen." This led to the establishment, over time, of a number of marine hospitals that later became known as the Public Health Service Hospitals. It was not until 1870, however, that the hospitals were formally coordinated through a central agency initially known as the Marine Hospital Service. There were eventually eight such hospitals. For some years during this half of the twentieth century, a number of presidents sought to turn these hospitals over to the communities in which

they were located, there no longer being a need to care for American seamen and their families because of health insurance, other government medical programs, widespread availability of life insurance, and the now legal liability of American ship owners. Congress resisted for many years because the hospitals represented federal money and jobs in the states in which they were located. Finally, in the 1980s, the president succeeded, marking the end of a very significant era in the history of federal health activity.

Clearly, the hospitals fell within the constitutional

power of the Congress to pass laws regulating foreign and interstate commerce. In 1799, Congress also authorized federal officers to cooperate with state and local authorities in the enforcement of quarantine laws which were, at that time, the prerogative of the state and local governments. It took nearly a century for the Congress, inching its way forward through a series of laws, to preempt the field, making the PHS fully responsible for quarantine matters that might affect foreign and interstate commerce. The need for federal responsibility only became apparent with a number of large epidemics in the latter part of the nineteenth century.

Epidemics were serious problems, and as medical science advanced during the latter part of the nineteenth century, a one-time student of Robert Koch (discoverer of the tuberculosis and cholera bacilli) was permitted to establish a one-room laboratory at the Marine Hospital in Staten Island, New York. This event in 1887 was the beginning of what was to become the Hygienic Laboratory in 1930, and later the National Institutes of Health.

In 1902 Congress expanded the function of the Marine Hospital Service to give it responsibility for licensing and regulating the production and sale of drugs moved in interstate commerce. With this new responsibility came a new name: Public Health Service and Marine Hospital Service. Again in 1912 a new name was given, as it assumed added responsibilities for research beyond communicable diseases, with a specific authorization for water pollution research. The new name was the United States Public Health Service.

Federal activity relating to foods and drugs that typically move in interstate and foreign commerce is particularly noteworthy. *The Public Health Service Today* (8) describes the evolution of this work:

Consumers, today, can hardly imagine the conditions that prevailed in the food and drug industries at the close of the nineteenth century. People were moving from the farms to the cities, where they were no longer able to grow their own food, and, as one might expect, the food industry was expanding rapidly, with little or no

control. Such chemical preservatives as borax, formaldehyde, and salicylates were used extensively in commercial food processing; artificial colors and flavors were indiscriminately employed to enhance the attractiveness of the "embalmed" foods; the country was plagued by unsanitary conditions in meatpacking plants.

In that same era, medicines containing opium, morphine, and cocaine were sold without restriction at almost any crossroads store. Thousands of so-called patent medicines, such as "Kick-a-poo Indian Sagwa" and "Warner's Safe Cure for Diabetes," were hailed by their makers and promoters as sure cures for every known disease. Only rarely did labels list ingredients, and warnings against abuse were unheard of. What information consumers did receive came, most often, from their own bitter experience.

In 1906, public pressure for change prompted Congress to pass, and President Theodore Roosevelt to sign, the first Federal Food and Drug Act. This law was administered by the Bureau of Chemistry in the Department of Agriculture. The chief of the bureau was Dr. Harvey W. Wiley, who had worked for more than 20 years for the passage of the law.

The Wiley Act defined "adulterated" and "misbranded" foods and drugs and prohibited their shipment across state lines. Following passage of the act, Dr. Wiley and his young staff at the Bureau of Chemistry worked energetically to enforce its provisions, developing scientific methods of investigation, streamlining the legal procedures and the techniques of inspection, applying these procedures and techniques in hundreds of hard-fought court cases, and building strong precedents through administrative decisions and regulations. For their efforts, they won the respect of industry and a high degree of voluntary compliance.

The Wiley Act was a strong law for its times, but the rush of technological change outpaced it. In 1938, following a bitter, five-year debate, a new and stronger Federal Food, Drug, and Cosmetic Act was passed. This act covered therapeutic devices and cosmetics and authorized mandatory food standards. A significant provision required that new drugs be approved for safety before going on the market.

Subsequent amendments to the act of 1938 applied safety controls to a broad spectrum of pesticides, chemicals and colors used in foods, drugs, and cosmetics. With this type of industry regulation came new emphasis on scientific research and public education, it being recognized that consumers are best protected by preventing violations of the law, rather than by prosecuting violators afterward.

The Bureau of Chemistry went out of business in 1927, when the Food, Drug, and Insecticide Administration was formed in the Department of Agriculture. Four years later, in 1931, the name was shortened to the Food and Drug Administration.

In 1940, FDA was transferred to the Federal Security Agency, which became the Department of Health, Education, and Welfare in 1953. In 1968, FDA became a part of HEW's Public Health Service. [HEW is now history and the FDA, along with PHS, is part of HHS.]

The functions of the PHS became significantly broader in the mid-1930s following passage of the Social Security Act, which authorized annual grants to the states for the "investigation of disease and problems of sanitation." Though there were state health departments throughout the country and a very large number of local health departments, this legislation stimulated the development of some 175 new local departments within a year of the passage of the Social Security Act. Very quickly, the PHS began to expand and was providing technical assistance to the states in nutrition, dental hygiene, laboratory methods, and accounting. It is worth noting that these service activities to the states consisted of grants of money and technical assistance, not direct service to people.

During the 1930s we were thus beginning to witness the emergence of aggressive federal action in health affairs. Although it was confined largely to money and technical assistance, it was a federal leadership role nonetheless. Following the Second World War the federal leadership role continued to intensify for approximately 30 years. *The Public Health Service Today* describes the postwar events this way (8):

At the close of hostilities, therefore, Congress began to enact legislation that, in the years since, has significantly affected the nation's medical research and training efforts, increased health services in the states, and expanded the functions and responsibilities of the Public Health Service.

In 1946, the shortage of hospital and related medical facilities spurred the establishment of the National Hospital Survey and Construction (Hill-Burton) Program, the purpose of which was to provide federal aid to the states for the construction of hospitals and health centers. Also in 1946, the National Mental Health Act established a National Advisory Council on Mental Health and a broad program of grants for research, training, and community mental health services.

The service's research activities were strengthened in 1948 with the establishment, at the National Institute of Health, of the National Heart Institute, the National Institute of Dental Research, and the National Microbiological Institute. The National Heart Act, which authorized the creation of the Heart Institute, also changed the name of NIH to the National Institutes of Health (plural). Over the next two decades, eight more institutes were authorized by the Congress and established within NIH.

A major goal of the Public Health Service during this period of growth in the basic research area was that of putting our new knowledge to work in the nation's communities. The Community Health Services and Facilities Act of 1961 authorized the service to support community studies and demonstrations that would lead to new and improved out-of-hospital services, particularly for the chronically ill and aged.

The Mental Retardation Facilities and Community Mental Health Centers Construction Act of 1963 extended this service-development concept to the mentally ill and retarded, authorizing funds for the construction of community-based mental health centers and, generally, emphasizing treatment in the patient's community, rather than custodial care in large institutions. This construction-grant program was expanded in 1965 to include federal grant support for Community Mental Health Center staffing, as well.

In the field of infectious disease, the Vaccination Assistance Act of 1962 enabled the service to help the states and communities conduct immunization programs against poliomyelitis, tetanus, diphtheria, and whooping cough. The aim of this legislation was to eradicate these preventable diseases in the United States.

Meanwhile, another major campaign was being waged against the health hazards of the environment, from pollution of the air and water to traffic deaths and injuries, and a number of new Public Health Service divisions and laboratories were being created. The Water Pollution Control Act of 1948, for example, launched PHS programs in that field. Environmental health research and training was expanded in 1954 with the opening of the Robert A. Taft Sanitary Engineering Center in Cincinnati.

In 1958, the Division of Radiological Health was created and given the job of coordinating a national program to prevent radiological health hazards. In 1963, the Clean Air Act authorized the development of air quality criteria and limited federal abatement action in certain problem areas.

Responsibility for the health care of American Indians and Alaska Natives was transferred from the Department of the Interior to the Public Health Service in 1955. Since that time, the PHS has administered a broad program of health services for these groups. . . .

Two important steps were taken in the early 1960s to deal with the shortage of professional health manpower. The Health Professions Educational Assistance Act of 1963 authorized a new program of federal grants to help build schools of the health professions. It also provided a loan program for medical, dental, and osteopathic students. The Nurse Training Act of 1964 authorized federal aid for the construction and rehabilitation of nursing schools and established a loan fund for student nurses. It also extended the PHS traineeship program for professional nurses, which had begun in 1956, and made aid available to nursing schools for curricula improvement.

The aim of the Heart Disease, Cancer, and Stroke Amendments of 1965 was to make the most advanced techniques in the diagnosis and treatment of these "killers" available to physicians and their patients everywhere. These amendments to the Public Health Service Act authorized the service to create regional programs of cooperation (Regional Medical Programs) in research, training, and patient care across the nation.

Several programs initiated by the service in recent years have focused on the special health-care needs of communities. The National Health Service Corps, created by the Emergency Health Personnel Act of 1970, recruits and places physicians and other health professionals in areas that have critical shortages of health manpower.

The Health Maintenance Organization Service, established administratively in 1971 (and by the HMO Act of 1973), supports the development of health maintenance organizations, which provide comprehensive health care services on a prepaid basis. HMOs emphasize primary care, preventive services, and operational efficiency. The

Emergency Medical Services Systems Act, passed by the Congress in 1973, authorizes the service to provide financial support and technical assistance for the development of better emergency medical services in the nation's communities.

These are some of the key programs that evolved. There were many others, some of which are described elsewhere in the text; for example, Medicare, Medicaid, health statistics, and health services research and development. Many of the programs that developed over the years have now terminated, victims of their successes or of their failures, and some programs remain with modified, new, or diminishing responsibilities. Most health manpower monies are now gone, as are Hill-Burton construction grants and other program monies. Some programs continue to operate at significantly reduced levels of effort.

The changing federal role is caused by two major factors. The first, which transcends political parties, is the shortage of money. The nation's economy has not in recent years been able to produce enough to enable society to do all the things it would like to do. At the same time we have seen an enormous growth in federal expenditures because of Medicaid and Medicare, which command an increasing share of the monies available for health purposes. The second factor in the changing federal role is philosophical: there is a view that the federal government in the last 30 or so years has moved into fields that should have been left to the states and to the private sector. When this view is dominant, programs and growth at the federal level are generally not possible.

Let us turn now to describe the major units within the PHS and the rest of HHS, recognizing once again that they are in almost constant flux. There are eight PHS agencies: the National Institutes of Health, the Substance Abuse and Mental Health Administration, the Agency for Toxic Substance and Disease Registry, the Food and Drug Administration, the Centers for Disease Control, the Health Resources and Services Administration, the Indian Health Service, and the Agency for Health Care Policy and Research.

The National Institutes of Health

The National Institutes of Health (NIH) is perhaps the most stable and certainly one of the most professional units within the PHS. Its focus is medical research. In 1990, an estimated $12.4 billion was spent on medical research in the United States (see Table 9–5). This does not include the research and development costs of pharmaceutical companies and other manufacturers of medical equipment and supplies, which has been estimated to run well over $10 billion for the pharmaceutical manufacturers alone. Of the $12.4 billion, over 80 percent ($10 billion) was spent by the federal government, 1.2 percent by the state and local governments, and the remainder by foundations and other private sources. Some of the federal money came from the VA, Defense, and the FDA. But by far the greatest amount was provided by the NIH.

The NIH funds over 57 percent of all biomedical research in the United States, over 31 percent if one takes into account the profit-oriented research carried out by pharmaceutical companies and other medical manufacturers. The NIH's budget for 1990 was approximately $7.14 billion. Of this amount, nearly 73 percent (more than $5.2 billion) was awarded to investigators at over 1,700 institutions throughout the country, whereas only 12 percent ($875 million) was allocated to support intramural (in-house) research by NIH professional employees.

The mission of the NIH is to help improve the health of the American people "by increasing our understanding of the processes underlying human health and by acquiring new knowledge to help prevent, detect, diagnose, and treat disease." It accomplishes this by conducting basic science and clinical research in its own laboratories and clinics (which include a 470-bed research hospital, known as the Clinical Center). The major thrust of the NIH, however, is the support of research in universities, medical schools, hospitals, and other research institutions, mostly on the basis of applications submitted by scientists who seek to carry out some type of biomedical research. These applications for research grants are reviewed not only by NIH scientists for their scientific merit and appropriateness to the NIH mission, but also by advisory panels of experts who are not employees of the federal government. The monies support the time of investigators who are typically located where new physicians are being trained, where medical and other biomedical specialists are being trained, and where physicians are responsible for patient care. The interaction of investigators with these people undoubtedly contributes daily to the quality of training and to the quality of medical care. The presence of ongoing research helps create a milieu of excellence, of care, and of rigor, which infects most of those in that environment. This is not an easily measured result, but it may in fact be as significant as the research questions themselves.

Research is, of course, a never-ending process. The NIH, therefore, has a role in seeing to it that promising young research people are trained, and that there are adequate research facilities in the country. NIH monies go into these activities. Another principal activity of the NIH is to ensure access to knowledge, and to promote the dissemination of new knowledge. This effort is centered in the National Library of Medicine, a library noted not only for its collection of 4.5 million items and nearly 3,000 journals, but also for *Index Medicus* and *Medline.*

Most of NIH money for research is dispersed through its 12 constituent research institutes, the name of each indicating its central focus:

- National Cancer Institute
- National Institute on Aging
- National Institute of Child Health and Human Development
- National Institute of General Medical Sciences
- National Heart, Lung and Blood Institute
- National Institute of Allergy and Infectious Diseases
- National Institute of Dental Research
- National Institute of Neurological Disorders and Stroke

- National Institute of Arthritis and Musculoskeletal and Skin Diseases
- National Institute of Diabetes and Digestive and Kidney Diseases
- National Institute of Environmental Health Sciences
- National Eye Institute
- National Institute on Deafness and Communication Disorders

In 1992 three research institutes relating to alcoholism, substance abuse, and mental health were transferred to the NIH while keeping separate their nonresearch functions, as shall be noted shortly. These research institutes are:

- National Institute on Alcohol Abuse and Alcoholism
- National Institute on Drug Abuse
- National Institute of Mental Health

In addition to these institutes are three research centers at the NIH:

- National Center for Nursing Research
- National Center for Human Genome Research
- National Center for Research Resources

There is also the Fogarty International Center, which provides a focus for the NIH in international cooperation in all aspects of biomedical research. It serves as a base for the exchange of knowledge on biomedical research, medical education, research training, and health services through conferences and seminars, provision of postdoctoral fellowships for research in the United States and overseas, support of scientific exchanges between the United States and other countries, and sponsorship of special studies and reports that are of international significance.

The movement of the National Institute of Mental Health (NIMH) to the NIH is worthy of note. The NIMH has a long history within the PHS for its active support of research and training in the mental health area. Under its fiscal stimulus, the community mental health movement with its wide-ranging services was able to develop rapidly. In addition to support of services throughout the

country, the NIMH has financed research on the NIH campus as well as throughout the country. Historically the NIMH has been organizationally in and out of the NIH umbrella, one year an integral part of the NIH organization, another year a completely separate unit on organization par with the NIH. The 1992 reorganization split its functions, placing the research component under the NIH and placing the training and services functions in a newly created Substance Abuse and Mental Health Services Administration.

Most NIH activities are located on the 310-acre campuslike setting in Bethesda, Maryland, a suburb of Washington (Fig. 11–7). Located here are the bulk of its laboratories, its research hospital (the Clinical Center), and offices. All but one of the institutes are on this campus. The National Institute of Environment Health Sciences is located at Research Triangle Park in North Carolina, and a relatively small number of other NIH installations are in other locations. All told, the NIH had, in 1992, approximately 13,000 employees; nearly 23 percent (3,600) held doctoral degrees. Over the years, the NIH has supported the work of 82 scientists who were later awarded the Nobel Prize, four of whom have been NIH intramural scientists.

Substance Abuse and Mental Health Services Administration

The Substance Abuse and Mental Health Services Administration (SAMHSA) is the principal federal agency addressing the problems of alcoholism, drug abuse, and mental health. It provides technical assistance to states and communities that operate health service programs in these clinical areas by providing program support grants to assist them and by disseminating information.

Agency for Toxic Substances and Disease Registry

The Agency for Toxic Substances and Disease Registry (ATSDR) assesses data and information on the effects of hazardous substances that are

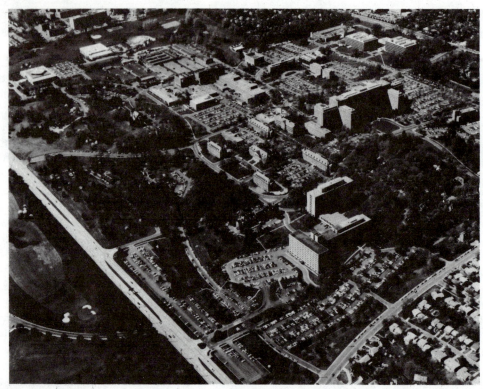

Figure 11–7. The National Institutes of Health in Bethesda, Maryland. (Courtesy, the National Institutes of Health, Bethesda, MD.)

released into the environment, and as appropriate issues advisories and information to the public. It also inspects hazardous waste sites that are on the National Priorities List as well as in response to complaints filed with the agency. In addition to maintenance of registries of persons exposed to, and ill from, hazardous substances, the agency stands ready to assist state and local governments, and others, in emergency situations involving exposure to hazardous substances.

Food and Drug Administration

The Food and Drug Administration (FDA) is a regulatory agency ensuring the safety of foods and radiologic devices, as well as drugs and other biologic products that move in interstate commerce. It is without a doubt the nation's largest and oldest consumer protection agency. It inspects food processing plants. It tests foods and food additives in its laboratories to make certain they are safe for public consumption. Its inspectors check for false and misleading labeling of foods and for deceptive packaging.

Perhaps its best-known role is that relating to drugs. Before any new drug can be marketed, the manufacturer must provide the FDA with evidence of its safety and effectiveness. The agency in its laboratories also tests on a regular basis every batch of most antibiotics and all insulin before they go on sale. In addition, the FDA has a variety of other functions and authorities relating, for example, to blood banks, biological products other than those mentioned, cosmetics, and radiation devices.

Its standards relating to pharmaceuticals have,

from time to time, been subject to criticism from the manufacturers because of what they feel are the sometimes inordinate delays in securing FDA approval. They point to the frequent availability of many drugs on the European markets (where regulations are also rigorous) long before the FDA grants approval. Not all agree with the industry's complaint in this regard. The FDA's role has been most prominent in recent years as it has worked with the pharmaceutical industry on problems that have developed with drugs previously certified as safe.

Centers for Disease Control

The Centers for Disease Control (CDC) programs seek to prevent and control infectious and chronic diseases; to prevent disease, disability, and death associated with environmental and workplace hazards; and to reduce health risks through education and information. Currently the prevention and control of AIDS is a high priority.

The CDC is based in Atlanta, Georgia, although its personnel and some of its units are found in different parts of the country, and some of its personnel are even overseas. It maintains laboratories for the study of infectious and communicable diseases, and it provides training and technical assistance for state and local public health officials (Fig. 11–8). Its personnel go out to the states whenever requested to help in tracking down the cause(s) of infections and communicable diseases. Historically, its work with the states in connection with sexually transmitted disease control (often referred to as VD control), tuberculosis control, and immunization programs has been particularly significant.

Within the CDC is the National Institute of Occupational Safety and Health, whose personnel conduct laboratory research and epidemiologic studies relating to hazards in the workplace. It advises the Department of Labor on exposure limits for toxic substances, and it has a program directed toward coal miners for the early detection and treatment of black lung disease.

As the name suggests, the CDC's activities can range far and wide, depending on the kinds of problems that arise. Those activities cited are only a brief sample of the breadth of its work. Like the NIH and the FDA, it is a very professional organization within the PHS.

The National Center for Health Statistics

The NCHS is the nation's focal point for national health statistical data. Based in the Washington, D.C. metropolitan area, it is presently a unit within the CDC. Working closely with state and local health departments, which are the sources for much of its data, but also generating significant amounts on its own initiative, its reports on morbidity and mortality (including the causes), published regularly in its *Monthly Vital Statistics Report,* are indispensable sources for health care investigators, and its other reports are also invaluable sources of data on the health of the American people. Of particular note are the data that flow from the National Health Interview Survey. Its data are secured from a continuing sample of households in the nation. Using a questionnaire, it gathers information on such items as utilization of professional personnel, perceived illnesses, injuries, impairments, and chronic conditions. It also gathers data on family size, educational levels, and income. Its findings are usually reported in the *Vital and Health Statistics* publication series.

Health Resources and Services Administration

The Health Resources and Services Administration (HRSA) is assigned the task of helping to improve the nation's health delivery system by providing grant support for a variety of educational and health service activities. A major focus has been on trying to improve basic health services in underserved areas. It has done this by supporting community health centers in both urban and rural areas, and special services for an estimated 500,000 migrant and seasonal farm workers and their families. It also provides monies for programs to assist in care

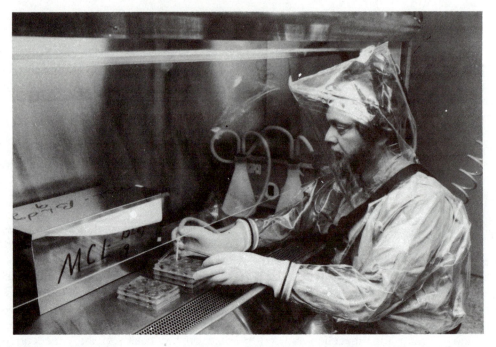

Figure 11—8. A scientist removing fluid from cell cultures under the laminar flow cabinet in the CDC's Suit Lab, Maximum Containment Lab. (Courtesy, Centers for Disease Control, Atlanta, GA.)

of the homeless, for substance abuse programs, and for a wide range of AIDS treatment and prevention programs. The grants are awarded mainly to state and local health departments, community service agencies, hospitals, and medical schools.

One of the most important grant programs for the PHS, administered through the HRSA, is the maternal and child health block grant to states to improve services for both mothers and children. Grants are also made for special projects such as those directed toward genetic disease screening, hemophilia, and pediatric emergency medical services. As new problems arise in the nation, and as the Congress appropriates monies to deal with these new problems, the HRSA is usually asked to administer the grants. As a consequence, the HRSA from year to year has programmatic money for new activities, and no money for activities that have taken on a lesser national priority. It continues to administer a direct service program for persons afflicted with Hansen's disease (leprosy). It also

continues to monitor health facility compliance with obligations incurred when they received monies under the former Hill-Burton legislation. The chief objective of this monitoring process is to make certain that the facilities provide a certain amount of free care each year.

A recent responsibility assigned to the HSRA is that of administering the National Practitioner Data Bank, which is a national registry of actions taken against medical practitioners by disciplinary agencies and of medical malpractice payments made as a result of lawsuits. Historically, the HRSA has been a major source of funds for medical, dental, nursing, health administration, and other health professional academic programs, though support for many of these has from time to time declined because of national budget crises. Currently, a high priority for funding are programs to increase the supply of primary care practitioners and for improving the number of minorities and other disadvantaged persons in health career educational programs. The agency also provides technical assistance for modernizing or replacing health care facilities, and provides leadership in the education, training, supply, and quality of the nation's health personnel. It also administers the National Health Service Corps, which assigns recent medical school graduates and other health professionals to rural and inner-city primary care centers, centers which are mostly community (not government) sponsored. Many of these assignees provide service in lieu of repayment for government educational loans.

The HSRA has perhaps experienced the most tumultuous changes in recent years. Because most of its activities in grant support have been on the socioeconomic side of health care, it has been subject to the changing winds of the political climate. In the budget reductions and in the program eliminations of the 1980s, this organization within the PHS has probably suffered the most.

Indian Health Service

The Indian Health Service (IHS) runs a comprehensive medical care system throughout the 50 states, serving the needs of the more than one million Native Americans and Alaska Natives. The services for these peoples are considered a federal responsibility as a result of early treaties between the federal government and the numerous Native American tribes. Scattered in strategic places throughout the country are 7 hospitals, 134 service units, 153 health centers, 118 health stations, 8 school health centers, and 173 Alaskan Village clinics (Figs. 11–9, 11–10). Most of these services are administered through tribes and tribal organizations. Federal personnel run the hospitals, increasingly less and less of the other services.

Agency for Health Care Policy and Research

This relatively new agency was formed in 1989 by merging the National Center for Health Services Research with the office of Health Care Technology Assessment. It has three principle functions: funding demonstration projects on new ways to orga-

nize, finance, and administer health services that aim to improve access to care and to measure the effectiveness of services; to assist in the development of practice guidelines for use by health professionals as guides to providing quality care; and to assess new technologies to determine their effectiveness and the appropriateness of their being paid for by Medicare and Medicaid.

The Public Health Service—the Commissioned Corps and the Decline of Professionalism

In most developed countries, health professional and administrative leadership rests with a career civil service. There is political accountability and control through an elected or politically appointed official (e.g., minister of Health, secretary of HHS), but the health service is granted considerable autonomy. It is an area generally thought of as the domain of the health professionals, mostly physicians, with minimal political interference and political control limited largely to budget and to major policy directions such as the institution of a national health service or a national health insurance program.

In the United States, the professional elite at the federal level was in the Commissioned Corps, which was almost synonymous with the PHS. The corps was a quasi-military organization headed by a surgeon general (as in the army), with associate surgeon generals and assistant surgeon generals with other ranks below this. The corps had its uniforms, which were worn at many official functions, as well as on duty in some PHS installations. In recent years, the wearing of uniforms has sharply declined. Over the years, the composition of the corps changed with the admission of many health workers who joined the ranks with physicians, dentists, and nurses. But alongside the corps' personnel was a large number—and a growing number in the years after World War II—of civil servants who did not have the benefits of the corps or its kind of military personnel system. But until the 1960s, the corps held the key leadership positions. The surgeon general was appointed by the presi-

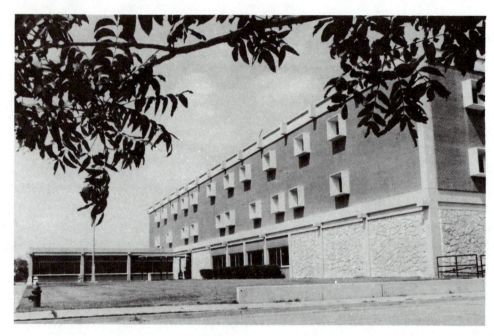

Figure 11–9. The U.S. Public Health Service Indian Hospital in Lawton, Oklahoma. (Courtesy, Indian Health Service, U.S. Public Health Service.)

dent for a four-year term, but he was normally from the ranks of the corps.

The control of key positions by the corps, as in the army, allowed the development of a highly professional service with people committed to a lifelong career in the PHS. Presidents would come and go, as would secretaries and assistant secretaries of HEW, and currently HHS, but the PHS, the corps—like the country—would carry on. This kind of stability tends to build an even-keeled organization. Some would see this as leaning to the conservative side; others might see it as liberal. But the corps certainly recognized the political constraints under which it operated; although political winds of change might blow, the Constitution and the federal system of government would go on. Corps leaders understood the federal system and the constitutional limits on the PHS insofar as what constituted federal authority and what properly belonged to the states. Many in the corps rotated for limited periods

of service to state and local health departments.

Since the end of the Second World War, the expansion of federal programs has caused a rapid expansion in the numbers of people needed to run them at the federal level. Corps personnel increased in numbers, but the greatest increase came in the U.S. Civil Service, with physicians, dentists, nurses, health administrators, and others. The corps occupied the key positions. This caused some resentment, and the resentment played into the hands of elected and appointed officials (some of the latter being health professionals from outside the corps), who held bold new ideas and wanted them put into operation. They found the corps resisting, not so much as *corps* but as professionals who would be around long after the political people had gone off to greener, or at least to other, pastures. This was no small problem, for the Civil Service system is very open. One can enter at senior levels without previous government experi-

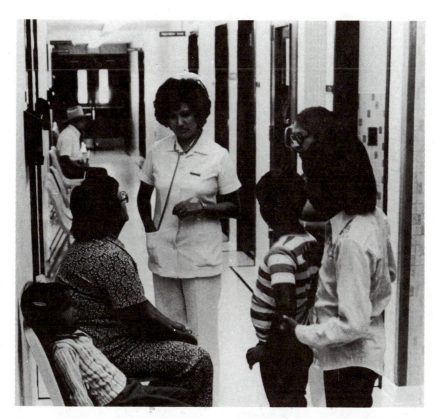

Figure 11—10. A nurse discussing a case with a Native American family at the Indian Health Service Clinic at Claremore, Oklahoma. (Courtesy, Indian Health Service, U.S. Public Health Service.)

ence, let alone federal experience. But because of the ease of entry and because of American high employee mobility, particularly in positions of responsibility, many entered the Civil Service and worked in the PHS and then moved on to other government agencies (federal, state, and local), to medical schools and other university units, to private industry, to professional commissions and associations, and to hospitals. The corps was, however, a stabilizing force, for it was there to keep the service on a steady course after "the best and the brightest" left.

In the late 1960s, the pressures on corps personnel were considerable. There were strong political pressures that proved destabilizing: an enormous number of new programs, aggressive political drives that were altering the very nature of our

federal system, whereby the states were becoming increasingly dependent on the federal authority, and agitation by the new people who perceived the corps as stodgy and unprogressive and too conservative. The various pressures, including the upheavals of frequent major reorganizations, prompted many in the corps to leave. Many simply waited until they could take, as in the military, a 20-year retirement. Key offices were increasingly filled by noncorps people, people who appeared more responsive to the political winds of change, and an increasing number who had to pass political screening, that is, political party identification, in order to get their jobs. For several years in the 1970s, there was no surgeon general, only one who was acting and who represented our government in the international arena. But during most of the 1970s the surgeon general had no significant operational responsibility for the PHS, this responsibility being assigned to the Assistant Secretary for Health. With the administration of President Carter the Assistant Secretary of Health also became the surgeon general. He was not only from outside the Commissioned Corps but also from outside the federal Civil Service. During the Reagan administration the Surgeon General was again placed under the Assistant Secretary for Health and given little, if any, operational responsibility, and this continued during the Bush administration. Some see in all this the emergence of new opportunities for aggressive federal initiatives or tighter political control, as the case may be. Others see in this a deprofessionalization of the PHS and the loss of experienced career personnel.

Health Care Financing Administration (HCFA)

The Health Care Financing Administration (HCFA) was established in 1977, bringing together the Office of Long-Term Care, the Bureau of Quality Assurance, and Medicare and Medicaid. The Office of Long-Term Care was concerned primarily with the development of standards for nursing homes and ensuring their enforcement. The Bureau of Quality Assurance was responsible for administering the End-Stage Renal Disease Program, which paid for the care of nearly all persons with end-stage renal disease, renal dialysis, and renal transplants. The bureau was also responsible for developing the Professional Standards Review Organization program. The functions of the Office of Long-Term Care and the Bureau of Quality Assurance have now been integrated within HCFA.

Medicare was moved to HCFA from the Social Security Administration. Medicaid was transferred from the PHS. Both programs were launched in 1966, each funded differently and each designed mostly for different clientele. Both programs are dealt with in Chapter 10. The HCFA is the federal focal point for administering these two programs. It is the agency that issues the regulations, oversees the administration of these programs, and deals

with the Congress regarding them. Though it is a part of HHS, it is not part of the PHS.

Health Care Financing Review is a quarterly journal published by HCFA and is important for the analytical studies and statistical data that it reports relating to national health expenditures, health costs, health insurance, and Medicare and Medicaid. Periodically the agency also issues special reports on Medicare and Medicaid and on factors that affect these programs.

Department of Veterans Affairs

Our government has, over the years, provided a variety of benefits for those who served in the armed forces, and among these is a wide range of health services administered by the Veterans Administration, elevated in 1988 to a cabinet level department and renamed the Department of Veterans Affairs (VA). Veterans who have some health problems connected with their service in the armed forces are clearly entitled to be cared for by the government for those problems. The emphasis here is *service connected* and *not* war or combat connected. Other veterans are entitled to government health care also, specifically veterans with nonservice-connected disabilities who cannot afford private care. The Civilian Health and Medical Care Program of the VA (CHAMPVA) provides for medical care to the spouse and child of a veteran who is totally and permanently disabled from a service-connected injury or illness or who died as a result of such disability. Their care is provided for mostly by contract with nongovernment providers.

Congress has been sensitive to the government's moral obligation to meet the health care needs of those who served, and it has also been responsive to the veterans' lobby. As a result it has liberalized, over the years, veteran and veteran family entitlements to VA care. The importance of the VA system is that it is a *total* system as well as a large one that interacts and affects the civilian sector. Moreover, the liberalization by the Congress over the years as to the persons who might have programs was designed to facilitate an integrated and coordinated attack on the environmental problems of air, water, pollution, solid-waste management, pesticides, radiation, and noise. The EPA is a regulatory agency, setting and enforcing standards in the areas mandated. It works through regional offices and through state and local governments. In some instances, state or local governments enforce EPA standards. In other instances, the EPA inspects and enforces. As with the OSHA, the EPA is having a significant impact, both positive and negative. On the positive side, it is orchestrating an effort to improve the quality and safety of the environment in which we live and work. On the negative side, its regulations are forcing businesses and industries to incur costs that either make the enterprises unprofitable (resulting in loss of jobs and taxes) or make the enterprises pass on the costs to the consumer.

Controversy surrounded the agency in the 1980s and early 1990s concerning the political direction of its activities, which exposed the population to health risks. This would not have been the case had the agency had more independence and had professional standards been applied more vigorously.

Federal Trade Commission

The Federal Trade Commission (FTC) was established to protect the public against anticompetitive behavior and against unfair and deceptive business practices. Its rulings affect such things as advertising practices (no deceptive advertising) and warranties and consumer rights for refunds.

In recent years, it has moved against what it perceived to be anticompetitive forces in the health field. These included the AMA's role in medical school accreditation through the Liaison Committee on Medical Education, the AMA's Code of Ethics, which the FTC ruled, in late 1978, created an unfair practice because it effectively banned advertising and patient solicitation, and the restrictive practices of the American Society of Plastic and Reconstructive Surgeons in allowing, among

other things, only board-certified specialists into the society and setting standards for notices and advertisements in its journal. The efforts of the FTC in these and other cases have been troublesome to the medical profession and others. In the health field, in the absence of meaningful public regulation, it was only through ethical codes, accreditation processes, and professional control and certification of specialty training that the public's health and safety were protected, as was brought out in Chapter 1.

But the efforts of the FTC seemed to undermine many of the profession's positive initiatives without an adequate substitute, and the costs of fighting the FTC were causing serious financial problems for the organizations that felt compelled to resist what they saw as FTC intrusion into areas where it did not belong. The editor-in-chief of *Medical World News* put it this way: "This isn't to argue that medicine should be immune to antitrust laws. It is arguing that in applying those laws to medicine, the FTC should use more discrimination, precision, and judgment. The FTC's charter does not include the remaking of medicine to satisfy the perceptions of a handful of anti-elitist government attorneys nor does it call for the undermining of the quality of medical care" (9).

Because of cost considerations, some groups caved in to the FTC. Foreseeing more trouble from the FTC, the AMA has sought to defuse the situation by modifying the language in its ethical code to minimize the risk that the language would become the vehicle for FTC action claiming restraint of trade. In addition, the AMA has raised the question with the Joint Committee for Accreditation of Healthcare Organizations (JCAHO) about changing the references to *medical staff* in JCAHO criteria to some more innocuous phrase so as to preclude FTC action, as well as legal action by other professions, over hospital privileges. *Medical staff,* the AMA felt, could too easily be interpreted as physician staff. It is not that the AMA or its members want to see every clinical psychologist, chiropractor, nurse-midwife, and so on get hospital privileges, but they do not want the AMA or JCAHO access to VA care makes the VA system a potentially more pervasive force on the health care scene.

The VA currently has 171 hospitals with approximately 67,000 beds, and it cares for over one million patients. Outpatient visits have soared to 13 million annually. These outpatient visits are provided through its 171 hospitals and over 300 clinics. The VA also has 127 nursing homes with nearly 14,000 beds, caring for more than 29,000 patients. The agency has, in addition, 35 domiciliary facilities that provide medical and other professional care to nearly 18,000 patients. To cope with the need for nursing home care, the VA also finances care for over 50,000 veterans in more than 3,100 community nursing homes. This is just a short summary of the extent of the agency's activities in health, though it might be added that the VA also provides a variety of other services, including home care.

What makes the VA system unique is that it is a total system of care under the direction of a single agency. Another critical element is the fact that there are 30 million veterans in the nation today who, particularly as they age, will force some major public policy decisions.

Presently, about 29 percent of the veterans are over 65 years of age. By the year 2000 the percentage is expected to jump to 37 percent, although the total number of veterans by then will have dropped from 27 to 24.1 million. One VA source put the issue in these words: "Even if over-65 users of our system remain at about the 25 percent level, it is evident that [the VA] would be experiencing overall demands for care that would far exceed all current ideas about 'adequate' resources. In fact, however, it seems likely that the percentage of users will increase as both Medicare and Medicaid find ways to limit the costs of their programs, making the VA health care system more attractive." In other words, to the extent that Medicare is deficient in terms of the hospital costs that must be borne by the patient, the limitation of benefits in both hospitals and nursing homes, and the unpredictability about how much of the physician's fee will have to be paid by the patient, it is

anticipated that the demand for VA servi[increase. For VA care, there are no deducti[co-insurance charges to be made.

Occupational Safety and Health Administr[

The Occupational Safety and Health Act o[was designed "to assure as far as possible[working man and woman in the nation sa[healthful working conditions and to preser[human resources" (Public Law 91-596). [this, the law (act) provided that each em["shall furnish to each of his employees en[ment and a place of employment which ar[from recognized hazards that are causing [likely to cause death or serious physical ha[his employees." To carry out the mandates [legislation, the Occupational Safety and Healt[ministration (OSHA) is required to issue l[enforceable standards and regulations that[govern the work environment and the work[tices to be employed. The OSHA is also res[sible for enforcing the standards and regulat[to do this, it carries out periodic inspectior[establishments covered by the legislation. The [is in the Department of Labor.

It is generally acknowledged that the OSH[play an increasingly important role in health a[and in the nation's economy, the former bec[of the growing body of knowledge we have a[hazardous substances, practices, and machi[in the work environment, and the latter bec[many of the changes may seriously affect[financial standing of the firms, which, in so[cases, may force businesses to close, or in ot[instances, may cause a rise in the cost of[products produced.

Environmental Protection Agency

The Environmental Protection Agency (EPA) w[also established in 1970. Before its establishme[by presidential order, there were 15 environmen[control programs in various federal agencies, i[cluding many within HHS. Consolidation of th[

to be sued over the issue. Better let each hospital board do what it believes is best.

The AMA also went a political route vis-à-vis the FTC. Being too costly to resist the FTC demands, it sought to clip the FTC's power over the professions by seeking relief from the Congress. Congress, however, was unwilling to go along. Subsequently the AMA and the FTC reached an agreement on the ground rules that would govern FTC actions. The agreement provided that the FTC would not involve itself in bona fide professional matters or in matters governed by state law, but it would retain authority to monitor and take action over business/economic matters. There would still seem to be considerable ambiguity, and only time will tell whether the medical profession has won the relief it sought.

Office of Management and Budget

The Office of Management and Budget (OMB) is technically part of the Executive Branch. Its job is to pull together the budget requests of the various federal agencies and to propose to the president a consolidated budget that falls within presidential policy guidelines. In recent years, the OMB has assumed an increasingly influential role. Its choices about which programs to fund and at what levels have a profound effect on health policy. When the OMB proposes a cut, the agency can appeal to the president; increasingly, however, presidents have been relying on OBM choices as the only viable way to control the growing burden on government of health care expenditures. Particularly irksome to HHS has been the tendency for the OMB to make the policy choices rather than to let HHS make the choices when budgets must be cut. HHS's view has been that it, and not OMB, should be the principal adviser to the president on health policy, and if a budget cut is necessary, it (HHS) is in a better position to give the president sound advice about what programs to cut.

There is, here, a basic conflict between the professionals and the president. The former seek to strengthen the health services as they perceive the need and to persuade the president to adopt their advice. The president, on the other hand, knows well that the agency's advice is frequently self-serving and may not, in fact, represent what is best for the country in terms of health or in terms of the relationship of health to the total economy. Hence, the tendency to rely on a more independent body: the OMB. This, in turn, prompts the professionals in HHS to employ a variety of strategies to force the president's hand. Among these strategies are the unleashing of outside interest groups to pressure the president and Congress, as well as the outright appeal to congressional committees and individual congressmen, through the subtleties of testimony while "supporting" the president's decision to the "behind-the-scenes" persuasion of key members of Congress.

How Federal Money Is Disbursed

Federal monies to the states, to local governments, and to nongovernmental agencies are distributed by grant or by contract. *Contracts* are usually thought of as government buying the effort for someone to do specifically what the government wants done. By contrast, a *grant* is usually viewed as getting money from government to do what the recipient wants to do but which also is in the government's area of interest. The recipient of grant money generally has greater freedom of action. There are different kinds of grants, but they fall, essentially, within two basic groups: formula grants and project grants.

A *formula grant* is money distributed to a class of entitled agencies (e.g., state or local governments, universities). All members of the class are entitled to receive a portion of the total sum appropriated as long as they meet the conditions governing entitlement to the money. The money is distributed on approval of the application on the basis of some mathematical formula, which, with state government, typically is weighted according to population and per capita income. Other elements may also be factors. With universities, the formula may weigh different factors such as the number of graduates and length of curriculum. The amount distributed to each entitled agency is thus objectively obtained. *Capitation grants* to universities were one kind of formula grant. *Block grants* are also a kind of formula grant given to cover a wide range of activities, usually with considerable discretion left to the recipient.

Project grants are not entitlements. These are grants awarded on a competitive basis. The applicant develops a plan or proposal stating what is to be done if money is awarded. The applications are reviewed competitively, though, in fact, the government is sensitive to the need to spread the awards around. Some grant programs have delegated the review and approval process, and the money, to HHS regional offices. Others are handled centrally with comments from the regions. The extent to which the 10 regional offices of HHS are involved varies from time to time (Fig. 11–11). Still others, particularly NIH research grants, are reviewed without regional comments.

Some grants, both formula and project, require the applicant to match the requested government grant. In other words, the government expects the applicant to contribute some of the agency's funds to the effort. Some *matching grants* have a fixed ratio governing applicant contribution or match; other grants are flexible.

Project grants, whether for research, training, demonstration, or another purpose, have typically been reviewed by outside, peer review committees, which make recommendations to the granting authority that the granting authority usually accepts. These outside committees of experts, who are usually peers of the applicant, have been a vehicle for ensuring that grant proposals are of high quality and that they merit support. These committees have also helped government agencies to withstand political pressures to approve certain grants. The bureaucrat can say to anyone applying pressure: This expert committee said that the proposal did not merit support; you would not want us to

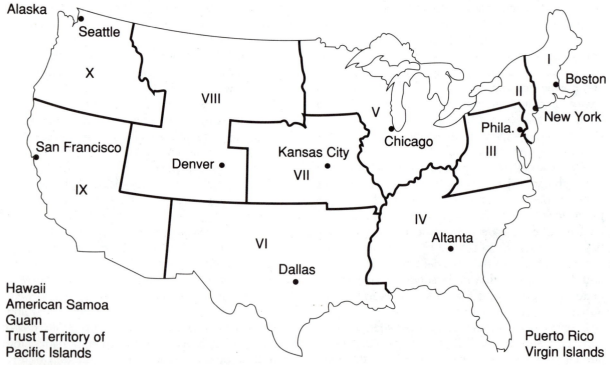

Figure 11–11. HHS regions and regional offices, 1990.

spend public money for something that is without merit, would you? This is not to say that political pressures do not exist but that they are less because of the peer review process.

Typically, what happens is that a grant proposal is reviewed by agency staff first. From there, it goes to a peer review committee. The recommendation to the agency head from the committee may be to disapprove, approve, or approve with certain conditions. The agency head then decides what to do. As indicated, the agency usually accepts the advice, for if it does not, it would not be long before the committee would not take care in rendering advice because it is usually ignored. Not all projects that are recommended for approval are, in fact, funded. Many are approved but not funded because there is insufficient money available.

The committees are drawn mainly from universities, research institutions, and health agencies from around the country. Expenses and a modest honorarium are paid each member.

In recent years, there has been pressure on HHS to reduce its dependence on outside committees, to do in-house reviews only. The argument has been that the committees are costly and that the agency probably has or should have enough expertise to do the job. This is very reasonable, though one can appreciate why some agencies, and particularly NIH, have resisted this, for it would open the door wide to the worst of political influence.

With the inflationary period following the Vietnam War, there has been a sharp reduction in the availability of grant funds in many categories. This has proved a problem for agencies and universities that had grown to depend on federal grant monies for their operations. Grant money, from government or foundations, is considered *soft money*, as distinct from *hard money*. Soft money is short-term money, for fixed project periods—often up to five years. The project period may cover several years, but the money is usually awarded year by year and thus is not assured. By contrast, hard money is money that is fairly secure. Legislative annual appropriations to a university and student tuition are fairly reliable sources of funding; hence,

the money is hard, albeit not always assured, for a legislature can cut budgets (but not likely the entire budget), and student enrollment can decline (but not likely to zero).

The review process for grants can take a year, and sometimes longer. If an investigator or an agency has a brilliant idea and it captures the imagination of the granting agency, the agency can sometimes go the contract route rather than the grant route. Getting a contract through the bureaucratic machinery can take less time. To use a contract as a substitute for a grant is, of course, expedient, and some agencies have a mechanism for peer review of contracts. But the contract mechanism is also subject to abuse since the money can flow for weak proposals. The government has sought to curb the worst abuses in contract work by requiring that most be awarded on a competitive basis. When this is done, the agency lists the proposed contract in the Commerce Department's *Commerce Business Daily*, a publication that is scanned by many who seek government business. Usually, there is a short description of the proposed contract and an agency contact for more information. The listing in the *Commerce Business Daily* is a call for an *RFP*, which is *request for proposal*, by the agency that would issue the contract. Not all RFPs are in good faith. Sometimes the agency knows the group that it wants to get the contract and is only advertising to meet the legal requirement to do so. Sometimes, too, the agency has no intention of issuing a contract, but it advertises in order to get some information about a particular subject.

SUMMARY

Society as we know it could not have developed without organized public health programs at the local and state levels. Through a variety of preventive measures, health departments have assured the population of safe drinking water, milk, and other perishable food products and an environment relatively free of harmful substances and elements. They initiated environmental health and personal prevention programs to deal with a variety of communicable and infectious diseases. Early on they addressed the prevention of problems affecting the poor at points of their greatest vulnerability, that is, in the areas of maternal and child health and school health.

The record of state and local health departments is, on the whole, worthy of praise in most of our states. There are things yet to be done, and old problems sometimes rise again, resisting even the best of efforts. This is not necessarily a reflection on public health departments, but more often is a result of the inability of public health officials to control all of the variables by the very nature of the variables—the citizens of the areas who are free people, and the advance of knowledge and technology that often causes new problems as well as providing new ways to deal with old problems.

The track record of public health agencies in providing treatment and care services for the mentally ill, mentally retarded, and the poor is not nearly the success record that it is for old-line public health activities. There are, to be sure, state and local governments that have performed well, but all too often the efforts of government in these treatment and care areas have been compromised by the inability and unwillingness to provide the environment within which excellence can emerge in terms of facilities, salary structures, support staff, reimbursement levels for purchased treatment and care services, and bureaucratic rules, regulations, and paper work.

The differences in performances between traditional public health (in the areas of *environmental* and *personal prevention services*) and public health's *treatment* and *care services* may result from society's perception that in prevention "there but for the grace of God go I," and, therefore, it is for government to do what has to be done, but that in the treatment and care areas the public as a whole will not, or cannot, project itself into the position of those needing publicly financed or provided services.

States can determine how they organize public health activities at the state level. Historically, in most states there was a state health department and separate departments for mental health (in-

cluding mental retardation), welfare, and education. In almost all cases, the health department had a board of health that supervised, set policies, or advised the department. The historical pattern of organization has changed considerably. Many states are switching to a cabinet system of government, making the board of health advisory only. In some states, umbrella agencies are being created incorporating a variety of state human service functions in departments of human resources including (and this varies from state to state) health, mental health, mental retardation, welfare, education, and corrections. Some states are merging health and mental health. Other states are creating separate departments of mental retardation. Still others are removing environmental health activities from the health department and placing them in special environmental protection agencies.

There is, of course, no single *right* way to organize for the public's health. Each state adopts a model that it believes will achieve the objectives of that state. History and personalities, as well as idealized models, all play a role in determining how a state sets up its agencies.

Some public health services are administered directly by the state, but an objective of most states is to encourage the development of local health departments to deliver the services under state standards. One thus finds a mix throughout the country in terms of what services are delivered by what level of government. The tendency is for licensure, vendor payments under Medicaid and other programs, state hospitals, and laboratories to be administered at the state level with standard setting for deliverance of local services through clinics, screening programs, public health nurses, and sanitary inspections. But again, the pattern varies from state to state. Typically, local (city or county) health services are partially state subsidized.

Although the federal government provides some direct health services, its principal role has been that of stimulating the development of new and improved services by the provision of monies to buy the action it wanted to see developed. Except in some circumscribed areas, the federal government has no authority to provide direct health services for people, this being the domain of the states and the private sector.

The Congress plays a key role in all federal activity, not only in the adoption of laws and a budget, but also in its investigative and information gathering roles which are expressed through the work of its key committees and subcommittees. The GAO is an important agency of the Congress in that it is an independent program-auditing body that assesses the performance of executive agencies in carrying out congressional mandates. Of growing importance also are the Congress' Congressional Budget Office and Office of Technology Assessment.

Although there are a large number of federal executive agencies concerned with health affairs, for example, Defense, Labor with its OSHA unit, the VA, and the EPA, by far the most important is the Department of Health and Human Services.

The principal unit within HHS is the Public Health Service, which has eight basic units.

In addition to PHS, there is the Health Care Financing Administration (HCFA), which is the agency responsible for administering Medicare and Medicaid, including the formulation of the federal standards that apply to both programs.

Each of the other federal agencies with health responsibilities, particularly the OSHA, EPA, FTC, and VA, have important roles to play. The VA, however, is particularly significant in terms of its potential impact on the overall organization of health services in the nation, owing to the rapidly aging veteran population who might shift to VA care because of the shortcomings of Medicare and Medicaid.

The president's OMB has been a key factor in all health policy considerations: though the secretary of HHS may be a key advisor on health to the president, it is the director of OMB who figuratively sits in the Oval Office and has, in recent years, been able to be more influential on selected health policy matters than the secretary. This, in turn, has only strengthened the resolve of the HHS bureaucracy, if not the secretary also, to secure assistance for their programs from outside interest groups.

It is important to understand how federal money is disbursed, and the advantages and disadvantages of each mechanism. Essentially, the money goes out by *contract, formula grant,* and *project grant.* To minimize the influence of political considerations and thus ensure that grant and contract recipients have proposals of merit and quality and are qualified to perform, HHS has used outside peer groups to advise it, particularly for grants. The extent to which peer groups have been used has been questioned in recent years by some in the executive branch of government, ostensibly because of the costs involved, but undoubtedly also because the peer review mechanism inhibits the award of grants to favored groups and individuals.

DISCUSSION QUESTIONS

1. Should the NIH decrease the influence of its outside consultants in grant review by relying less on peer review committees?
2. In what ways and areas would you favor expansion of federal health activities?
3. To what extent should there be political direction and political control over federal health activities?
4. How are the health responsibilities in your state government organized? How effective is the organizational structure? What changes should be made, and why?
5. Does the mechanism for financing local health services in your state encourage the development of strong local health departments?
6. How effective are the local health departments in your state? Account for their effectiveness, or lack thereof.
7. To what extent can the state legislature, the mental health association, and medical societies be positive or effective forces in helping your state meet its public health responsibilities?
8. If you had the choice of being paid under a federal contract, formula grant, or project grant, which mechanism for salary support would you prefer, and why?

REFERENCES

1. Gossert, D.J., Miller, C.A.: State Boards of Health, Their Members and Commitments. *Am J Public Health,* Vol. 83, 1973.

2. Miller, C.A., Brooks, E.F., DeFriese, G.H., Gilbert, B., Jain, S.C., and Kavaler, S.: A Survey of Local Public Health Departments and Their Directors. *Am J Public Health,* Vol. 67, 1977.

3. Hanlon, J.J.: *Public Health Administration and Practice.* 6th ed. St. Louis, Mosby, 1974.

4. Miller, C.A., et al.: Statutory authorizations for the work of local health departments. *Am J Public Health,* Vol. 67, 1977.

5. Becker, A., Schulberg, H.C.: Phasing Out State Hospitals—A Psychiatric Dilemma. *N Engl J Med,* Vol. 294, 1976.

6. National Association of County Health Officials: *National Profile of Local Health Departments.* Washington, D.C., July 1990.

7. U.S. Department of Health and Human Services: *Public Health Service Fact Sheet.* Washington, D.C.

8. U.S. Department of Health, Education, and Welfare: *The Public Health Service Today.* Washington, D.C., 1976.

9. *Medical World News,* January 8, 1979.

Chapter 12

Health Care Reform: Lessons From Abroad

More than 35 million Americans are estimated to be without health insurance and few of these have the means to pay for their hospital care, nor to pay a physician except for the most routine care. Countless other millions are inadequately insured and will face burdensome costs should they become seriously ill, and they may also face cancellation of their health insurance policies. At the same time the costs of care are skyrocketing, fueled by an increasing array of technological developments—new drugs and new equipment—that enable physicians to treat people more effectively and in many cases to treat successfully what was previously untreatable. Total expenditures are also rising as a result of an aging population, people who require more health care because the conditions that afflict the elderly tend to require more frequent and longer hospital treatment. All of these increased costs are borne primarily by employers and government, but ultimately they are passed on to the public through increased taxes and the increased cost of services and manufactured goods.

Employers complain about the increasing cost burden of health care because it affects adversely their competitive position in the marketplace. Government resists raising taxes because to do so is unpopular and limits other government programs.

The uninsured pose a special problem. While most who need hospital care get it—though not always in the most timely fashion—the costs of their care are borne by the hospital, which tries to shift those costs to patients who are insured or who are covered by government programs. Employers resist this and are increasingly self-insuring their employees and negotiating hospital charges. Medicare has also sought to control this situation by instituting the diagnosis related group (DRG) system of payment for hospital care, and many state governments have followed suit in the Medicare program. States have also coped by not paying hospitals for the actual cost of care for Medicaid enrollees. As a consequence, the hospital is frequently placed in a precarious financial position, and the uninsured and Medicaid patients may encounter some difficulties in obtaining both hospital and physician care.

Financing the health system has thus become a major problem. Government, insurers, and employers are unhappy with the present situation. A growing number of citizens who are uninsured would like to secure health insurance but find it too expensive. Hospitals and nursing homes are unhappy about inadequate payments, and about the growing number of people without any means to pay for their care. Physicians are unhappy about the increasing criticism of their incomes and the increased amount of regulation imposed by insurers and government, and they fear that reform efforts may affect adversely their freedom to treat patients and how they are paid.

Government, employers, physician groups, and others have been proposing different types of reform of the health care field, seeking to control costs and yet ensure access for all to needed health services of high quality. Some of the proposals are self-serving, designed to address the problems while protecting the interests of the group making the proposal. Proposals have come forth but most, though appealing to the proposing group, are not acceptable to other groups, which have their own perspectives. There are no simple solutions to the problems we face, for if there were, there would be general agreement on what to do. Increasingly health policy makers have been studying the experiences of other countries that have faced the problems of access and cost to see if they can provide some insights for solving our problems. As noted in Chapter 10, the German and Canadian systems are viewed favorably by a number of these people.

Most industrialized countries ensure universal access to needed medical services. No one is denied treatment by a physician or denied admission to a hospital because they cannot pay. Available data suggest that in comparison with Americans those populations are as healthy and live as long or longer. Although a health system is a product of the country's history and culture, and is not readily transportable to another country,

there are similarities sufficient to merit their study. The health systems of those countries from which we have much to learn are described below. Each is a democratic nation and their peoples have as much freedom as Americans. The countries are affluent and, as a consequence, their peoples have a high standard of living. Their physicians are well trained, and the hospitals are comparable to ours except that the more sophisticated, costly equipment is strategically placed in a restricted number of hospitals. Most noteworthy is the fact that the life expectancy and health of their populations, as evidenced by morbidity and mortality data, is roughly comparable to that of the United States and their infant mortality rates are considerably lower (Table 12–1). An important difference is that, unlike the United States, everyone in these countries has access to whatever health services are needed. One system that is being studied by U.S. policy analysts is that of the Federal Republic of Germany.

Federal Republic of Germany*

Germany relies on a decentralized insurance mechanism to finance health care (1–3). While nonprofit insurance companies dominate the system for paying both hospitals and physicians, there remains a significant role for private insurance. Patients have free choice of physician for ambulatory care, and these physicians are paid on a fee-for-service basis. There are therefore some marked similarities to the traditional American way of doing things.

Ninety-eight percent of the German population is insured for medical care. About 90 percent are protected by federally mandated legislation that requires that insurance premiums be paid, half by the employer and half by the employee, to one of more than 1,100 nonprofit, public "sickness funds." The premiums employees pay are based on a

*All references and data to Germany refer to the area of what was West Germany. With reunification, the health system for the area of what was once East Germany is in a transitional stage, but the principles of the West German health care system are being extended to the former East German sector.

TABLE 12–1. 1989 Comparative Health Data

Country	Total Expenditure on Health (% of GDP)	Life Expectancy at Birth (in Years)		Infant Mortality (Deaths/100 Births)
		Females	Males	
United States	11.7*	78.5	71.8	0.97
Denmark	6.4	77.7	72.0	0.75
Sweden	8.7	80.6	74.8	0.57
Germany	8.2	79.0	72.6	0.75
Netherlands	8.1	79.9	73.7	0.68
Canada	8.7	79.7†	73.0†	0.79†

SOURCE: Organization for Economic Cooperation and Development (OECD) Health Data. August 1991, and OECD Health Care Reform Project—Canada. June 1992.
*Gross national product.
†1986.

percentage of their salary, so that those with a higher salary pay more, thus making the insurance more affordable for those in the lower income categories. Those in the higher income brackets can either be covered through the sickness fund arranged for through their place of employment or elect to take out a private insurance policy that may provide certain extra benefits such as a private hospital room and freedom to choose the hospital doctor. An estimated 8 percent of the German population is privately insured in this manner. The remaining 2 percent are uninsured and are primarily the very well-to-do who can afford to pay out-of-pocket. Those who are unemployed have their sickness fund insurance paid for by the government. The sickness funds and private insurance companies pay for virtually all costs relating to hospital care and for most ambulatory care. Physicians in hospitals are salaried, and most do not practice outside of the hospital. In fact, except in very few cases, hospital physicians may not practice outside of the hospital. The salaries of hospital physicians are set by negotiations between an association of the hospital physicians and the appropriate regional hospital association. Those salaries are considered a part of hospital costs and are included in the per diem reimbursement by the sickness funds. Until recently hospitals were paid on a per diem basis but, as a result of legislation

adopted in December 1992, a DRG system of payments will be instituted as a means of controlling costs, some of which were generated by keeping patients in hospitals longer than necessary and by a variety of inefficiencies. Hospital expenditures are further controlled by separating the operating costs (financed by the sickness funds) and capital costs (financed by state and local governments). This type of arrangement controls new construction and the acquisition of expensive high tech equipment. Because capital expenditures are financed by the government, this has proved a more effective cost control mechanism than the certificate of need process in the United States, which relies mostly on private sector funding.

Ambulatory care is paid for on a fee-for-service basis. The fee schedules are negotiated between the sickness funds and associations of ambulatory care physicians that represent general practitioners and those specialists who restrict their practices to ambulatory care. Ambulatory care payments cover the full charge for each patient visit—in other words, there is no out-of-pocket cost for the patient. Fees paid for services provided to privately insured patients are typically much higher than those paid by the sickness funds, and thus the privately insured patient is a valued patient. Because ambulatory physicians are not allowed to practice in hospitals, a significant number of them have acquired sophisticated medical equipment and perform many procedures in their offices, which augments their incomes significantly. Germany, it might be noted, uses a relative value scale for paying for ambulatory care services. The relative values are negotiated nationally but the conversion factor—that is, how much each relative point is worth in German currency—is set by negotiations between the local sickness fund and regional physician association.

A unique and important feature of the German system is that each sickness fund turns over the money budgeted for physicians' ambulatory care services to the regional association of physicians for the association to pay out. Ambulatory physicians have legal status for negotiating and this encourages social responsibility in the fee-setting process.

Government works collaboratively with the sickness funds and with hospital and physician representatives, and others, seeking through semiannual conferences to build a consensus on major public policy issues relating to health. Called the "Concerted Action Conference for Health," this group focuses in part on health cost issues and agrees on global guidelines for payments to hospitals, ambulatory physicians, and dentists, and for pharmaceuticals. These recommendations become negotiating guidelines for the sickness funds as they negotiate with hospitals over payments and with regional physician associations over the relative value scale conversion factor—the factor that gives a monetary value to the service.

Negotiating guidelines may mean little for control of health care costs unless there is some limit. The German Parliament sets limits by adopting legislation mandating that health insurance premiums could not rise more rapidly than wages generally. Iglehart notes that this has affected "providers through tighter control on physicians' fees and hospital budgets and on pharmaceutical manufacturers by forcing them in essence to reduce the prices of their brand-name drugs" (3). This legislation essentially establishes a cap on health expenditures for the coming year. For ambulatory physicians this has major significance: since the

total monies available from a given sickness fund are limited (capped) for the year, physicians who significantly increase their services, and thus their incomes, deplete the available pool of money for all physicians for that year. To prevent running out of money, Iglehart reports that when the regional physician association finds that "physicians' bills in the aggregate exceed the negotiated global budget in any given quarter, the conversion factor [on the relative value scale] for all claims is reduced slightly, to keep the final annual tally within the fixed budget" (3). This means that each physician receives a lower payment for each office visit. Legislation in December 1992 applied the formula which controls sickness fund premium increases—i.e., limited to increases in overall wage rates—to increases in physician and hospital payments. Thus, in negotiating with the sickness funds, ambulatory care physicians and hospitals can only try to secure payment increases in line with increases in overall wage rates.

Glaser notes that Germany has relatively few nursing homes and that such care is not paid for by the sickness funds since the homes are considered part of the social sector and not the health sector (1). If a patient goes into a nursing home, the patient must pay for the full cost unless covered by private insurance or, if poor, by some social welfare program. Glaser points out that health insurance "may be used only if a physician certifies that the patient is sick. Then the patient is treated by a doctor and placed in an acute-care hospital." As a consequence, many of the patients in American nursing homes would, in Germany, be found in the German acute care hospitals. This would account in part for the long average length of stay in German hospitals.

While health care costs continue to rise in Germany as elsewhere, the rate of increase in Germany has been less than in the United States.

The German approach provides some ideas for American health care reform. They have adopted, to begin with, a fairly rational means for controlling the rise in health costs by not allowing sickness fund premiums to rise faster than overall wage rates. This forces providers to think carefully about what they do, rather than just charging ahead and incurring costs, figuring that the system will somehow pay them. The control with regard to primary care physicians is particularly noteworthy in light of the proliferation of diagnostic equipment in their offices and their being paid a fee for service. Their professional associations negotiated both the global budget for ambulatory care and the conversion factors, and their regional professional association is the body that pays them. If they try to maximize their incomes by generating more services that is alright, but if those extra services threaten the overall budget allocation for the year, then the conversion factor for their services will be downgraded so that their association does not run out of money. Since ambulatory physicians must belong to a regional association in order to receive payments for care, this means in a very real sense that the profession has collective responsibility and accountability for the success of the insurance system.

A somewhat similar practice existed in the United States with the founding of the Blue Shield movement. Blue Shield was commonly referred to as "the doctors' plan" because the organizations were sponsored by the medical societies and their boards of directors were dominated by physicians. Unlike Germany, however, physicians did not have to be a participating physician with a Blue Shield plan to be paid, and there was no effective mechanism for controlling physician charges or Blue Shield premiums.

The German system suggests some practices we might consider in the United States. First, the Germans have retained the fee-for-service principle for ambulatory care but have implemented a mechanism to control the temptation for a physician to overservice in order to maximize income. While there are critics of the fee-for-service principle, the fact remains that the payment of a fee gives greater assurance that the patient will get the services needed and not be denied a service, which may occur under other payment mechanisms. Second, the Germans encourage professional group

solidarity and the negotiation of fees between the sickness funds and the physician associations. The hand of government is there in the Concerted Action meetings but is only one among many. Government's main control is in ensuring that premiums, and payments to ambulatory care physicians and to hospitals, do not go up faster than wages. This stands in sharp contrast to current American practices under both Medicare and Medicaid, where government listens to the professions but does not negotiate meaningfully. The idea of the payer negotiating fees with the providers has merit. Given the ambivalence of U.S. citizens over the role of government, the idea of mandating health insurance for all, turning the monies over to the equivalent of sickness funds (i.e., insurance companies), and allowing the professions and hospitals to negotiate with those funds may be an interesting approach for the United States to consider. The U.S. government could then enter into a partnership with the hospitals, professions, and the insurance companies, and allow its heavy hand to be restricted to setting some type of limit on premium rate and payment increases. Additionally, the German experience also provides some ideas on who should make the payments to hospitals and to physicians. Currently in the United States payments come from a variety of sources—state governments, federal government through fiscal intermediaries (Medicare), Blue Cross and Blue Shield and other nonprofit programs like Kaiser-Permanente and HIP, private insurance carriers, self-insuring employers, and patients. The Germans have simplified the process of payments by working mostly through a variety of nonprofit sickness funds that pay the hospitals and allocate to regional physician associations money for the associations to pay ambulatory physicians. The savings for the United States in administrative costs could be enormous if it simplified its payment mechanisms.

In summary, the Germans have universal access to health care, financed by compulsory health insurance to which both the employer and employee contribute. Insurance premiums vary according to the employee's salary to make the insurance more affordable to all. Physicians are more socially responsible because they have a legal role in determining what society's health costs will be by virtue of their negotiating fees (within wage increase limits) and their administration of the payments. The German health administration system is more simple and much less costly than the U.S. system, and the separating of capital costs from operating costs makes it easier to control unnecessary construction and the proliferation of unneeded high technology.

The Netherlands

The Dutch health care system has many similarities to the German system: like Germany there is universal access to care by physicians and for care in hospital; care is financed principally by sickness funds and private insurance (4, 5, 6). Over 60 percent of the population is covered by 62 sickness funds, coverage that is mandated by law for people below a certain income. These people pay no out-of-pocket costs for either physician or hospital services. Those above a specified income, and the self-employed, are encouraged to take out private health insurance, and approximately 32 percent of the population has done so. These private insurance policies cover most of the costs of care, but the patient may have to pay a nominal amount for physician services and some portion for in-hospital amenities such as a private room, as well as for treatment by a particular physician. The remaining population (e.g., civil servants, police) are covered by the government on a basis comparable to the sickness fund coverage.

Primary care physicians in The Netherlands are paid on a capitation basis for each sickness fund patient on the physician's list. This payment is made whether the patient sees the physician or not. No additional charge is made by the physician regardless of the number of times the patient visits. For privately insured patients the primary care physician is paid a fee for service, an amount that is regulated. Specialists are also paid a fee for

service both by the sickness funds and private insurers, unless the specialist is salaried. While the sickness fund patient does not have to pay out-of-pocket, the privately insured patient may have to pay a portion of the fee for both general practitioner and specialist services. Hospitals are paid on a per diem basis.

The Dutch health care system is undergoing significant change in terms of finance. Following a report from an independent, government-appointed commission, the government proposed to eliminate the distinction between the sickness funds and private insurers, and to require all insuring bodies to accept all who apply for coverage. While the insuring bodies might have different premiums based on the services covered, they would not be able either to select their risks or to charge different rates for different risks. The insuring bodies would get their money from two sources—a fixed premium paid by the person who is to be insured, and a sum given them by government. Government would collect its monies through the tax system on an income-related basis. The premium monies collected through the tax system would cover an estimated 75 percent of the total premium cost, and the insured person would be responsible for the balance, which would be paid directly to the insuring body. The insured person would be able to select the insuring body depending on the benefits offered and the premium charged. This new financing system is designed to introduce an element of competition among insuring bodies, leading to increased efficiency and, one hopes, some cost control. When the government appointed the study commission in 1986, the Dutch were spending 10 percent of their gross national product (GNP) on health care, and that percentage rose to 10.3 percent in 1987, the year in which the study commission's report was published. Since then, Dutch expenditures as a percentage of the GNP have declined even though the report's recommendations had not been implemented.

Each of the old sickness funds was limited to a specific geographic area. Under the new system, all sickness funds would be able to market their policies throughout the country, and would have to compete for their share of the market. Hospitals would have to compete with each other to convince the sickness funds to use their services. This will give the sickness funds leverage in negotiating low hospital payments. Patients would continue to have the same benefits as before, though there may be more out-of-pocket payments for drugs and the first specialist consultation.

The Netherlands has also developed the Exceptional Medical Expenses Act, which pays the costs of care in nursing homes, institutions for the handicapped, and long-term care in hospital, as well as a variety of long-term care community services. Financed by a payroll tax on employers and a government subsidy, this program is administered through the sickness funds. It is the only country to provide complete coverage of long-term care on an insurance basis. As we shall see, Denmark also provides such benefits, but Denmark does not work on an insurance basis.

The Dutch system is also of interest because it contains many elements of the U.S. system, such as its retention of fee-for-service payments to in-hospital specialists except for certain hospital specialists who are salaried. Payment for physician services in hospitals is thus partly comparable to the U.S. experience. We say "partly" because in the United States whenever a salaried physician in a hospital provides care, a charge is made to the insurance company and a fee is paid even when the fee is retained by the hospital. The Dutch system of paying primary care physicians a capitation payment, while not comparable to the mainstream of U.S. medicine, does find an American parallel in health maintenance organizations (HMOs), where the HMO is typically paid a capitation payment for the complete care of enrolled patients. How much an individual HMO primary care physician is paid in the United States is an amount negotiated between the physician and the HMO.

What is significantly different from the U.S. tradition is the mechanism used by the Dutch for paying for primary care. The capitation system may not be acceptable to a majority of American primary care physicians. The Germans, by contrast, have retained fee-for-service payments for all primary care services, but in doing so have created a situation whereby ambulatory care specialists have generated significant incomes by acquiring a large amount of equipment in their offices for procedures that when done in other countries are done in hospital outpatient departments. This leads to the concern that tests in Germany might be done to generate income instead of done for patient need. This is, of course, a concern in the United States as well. The Germans attempt to control an increase in volume by turning physician payment monies over to physician associations for disbursement and capping the total amount available for the year so that physician excesses can be monitored and controlled by the physician's own professional body. This may be better than having an outside group, the sickness fund, or the government control physician utilization and payments. It may well be that some combination of the German and Dutch systems will lend themselves to reform in the United States. One can envision a combination that would interfere least with traditional U.S. practices. The easiest reform comes when there is the least amount of adjusting required by those affected by the reform.

The Netherlands, like the United States, has nonprofit and for-profit insurance companies but, unlike the United States, proposes to level the playing field so that they can compete in a fair manner. Unlike the United States, however, the Netherlands system has solved the problem of providing long-term care coverage by paying all long-term care costs.

Denmark

Denmark is an interesting country because of its method for paying physicians, its waiting lists, and its financing of long-term care. Like most countries of Scandinavia, Denmark has a strong tradition of decentralized government. With the exception of one national hospital in Copenhagen, the provision of health care is the responsibility of county and municipal governments (7, 8). Hospitals and all medical care services are a county responsibility. Nursing homes, home care services, and school health services are a municipal responsibility.

Most of the money necessary for these services is raised through county and municipal taxation, and is supplemented by block grants from the central government. The central government, in addition to block grant support, sets overall national policy through legislation, and through its National Board of Health sets national guidelines for the operation of the health system. The Board controls where primary care physicians may practice if they want to be paid by the public system. Since most of the money comes from local sources, there is considerable flexibility in the health care system. The national government may set national spending limits, but if a county wishes to expand in a given area and can find the money, it is difficult for the national government to stop it. Parliament did decree a few years ago that counties could not increase their taxes beyond a certain amount in an effort to control national health expenditures, but this had only limited impact because for many counties and municipalities additional tax revenue was created through inflation and business successes without having to raise taxes.

In Denmark the physician is paid by a combination of a capitation payment for each person on his or her list and a fee for service for each patient visit. No charge is made to the patient. The amounts paid to the physician are negotiated between the General Practitioners Union and the Association of County Councils. Their agreement must, however, be approved by the Minister of Health. Efforts to control the growth in national health expenditures by having the general practitioners charge patients for some part of each visit have been opposed by the general practitioners. This issue arose several years ago when the central government refused to ratify the agreement negotiated between the union and the county association: the primary doctors went on strike, continuing to see patients but billing them directly for services, which they had the right

to do in the absence of an agreement. Public reaction to the physicians' move was negative and forced the general practitioners to reach a new agreement acceptable to the Minister.

Patients needing hospitalization are referred by the general practitioner to one of the county hospitals, where care is provided without charge to the patient by salaried specialists. On discharge the patient is once again cared for by the general practitioner. If home care or nursing home care is required, the municipality becomes responsible for providing the necessary services. Persons who become permanent residents of nursing homes must turn over their pensions to help pay for the care, a small amount of which is returned to the patient for purchase of personal items.

As in most European countries, patients sometimes have to wait for nonemergency surgery. Emergency cases are always admitted without delay. The nonemergency cases tend to be in orthopedics, ophthalmology, and cardiac surgery, problems most commonly present in the elderly. In Britain, where surgical waiting lists are also common, and are a bone of contention in both Parliament and the press, some assert that part of the problem stems from manipulation of the waiting list by specialists who want to increase the number of patients they can treat in private hospital, thereby increasing their incomes. Data to prove this are generally lacking. In Denmark, however, this explanation for the waiting lists does not hold since the private sector is infinitesimal. The Danish system is thus instructive with regard to the explanations advanced in some countries for the existence of nonemergency surgical waiting lists. Governments in Britain and in New Zealand have at times blamed the professions in part for the waiting lists when in fact the problem may be as much or mostly insufficient investment in the health sector.

A significant number of beds in Danish acute care hospitals are occupied by chronically disabled elderly. Since hospital care is financed by the county, and nursing home care by the municipality, the cost of discharging a patient to a nursing home shifts the cost of care from one government level to another. This has led to the backup of patients in the acute care hospitals because of an inadequate supply of municipality services.

Movement of patients from a county-financed facility to a municipally financed facility or service illustrates a common problem that occurs when there is an absence of health service integration and no focal point for seeing to it that the needed services are provided uninhibited by roadblocks, which in this case is financial responsibility falling upon different authorities. One Danish county is reported to be charging the municipality for hospital care it is providing to patients who should be in a municipality-run nursing home or at home with municipality-run home health services. According to Holst, "The experience from this experiment has been so positive that it will likely be put into effect nationally" (8). Sweden, it might be noted, recently moved its nursing home administration from counties to municipalities, making it comparable to the longstanding Danish practice, and requiring the municipality to pay for hospital care whenever their patients have to stay there because of insufficient municipality services.

The Danish system is instructive on several points. First, the problem between the counties and the municipalities over the transfer of patients demonstrates the kinds of problems that can occur when there is divided financial responsibility in payment for services. One solution is being adopted in Denmark and in Sweden. Another possible solution, proposed some years ago in the State of Maryland (but not adopted), is to put all funds for state government-financed health services at the local level and have the local level be responsible for provision of local services and the purchase of other services as needed, thereby creating an incentive for the local government to develop an optimal range of local services to prevent unnecessary and more costly institutional services. A somewhat similar approach is currently being adopted in Britain, where large group practices are being permitted to manage funds and purchase services from the sources that best provide for

their patients' needs—in terms of cost and quality. The danger here is that the holder of the money, if also a provider of service, may seek to conserve resources and not use expensive services even when they would be appropriate. Separating the provider from the payer, as in an insurance system, tends to overcome this danger.

Another point to note about the Danish system is the reason for the Danish abandonment of capitation payments for primary care in Copenhagen and Fredriksberg. Years back Denmark paid general practitioners in these two large cities only a capitation payment for care of patients on their lists, whereas general practitioners in other parts of the country were paid a smaller capitation payment plus a fee for service for care provided. Denmark abandoned the capitation-only method of payment because general practitioners were referring their patients more frequently to hospital outpatient departments even though the general practitioners were well able to treat them. As Krasnik et al. note, general practitioners had no incentive to provide an optimal range of services because they were not paid for them, but that after fee-for-service payments were introduced "the general practitioners seemed to have taken the opportunity to undertake some services previously provided by the hospitals and specialists" (9). The problem faced by the Danes found a clear parallel in Maryland before the advent of Medicaid, when the state paid general practitioners a capitation fee for care of inner-city poor patients. This attracted physicians to the inner city of Baltimore, but it was later found that the general practitioners did not provide as broad a range of service as they could, and instead referred an unexpectedly large number of patients to hospital outpatient departments.

Finally, it is worth noting that the Danish primary care physicians feared a policy that would require them to make the patient pay even a part of the cost of a patient care visit. Their fear apparently was that such a practice would be so objectionable to the public that they could end up in a worse situation than before. This led them to be more amenable to agreement at the bargaining table.

Unreasonable resistance by the medical profession in the United States to needed reforms could conceivably follow a similar course, whereby public indignation in light of extraordinarily high incomes could work to the profession's disadvantage.

Canada

For many years the Canadian health system paralleled that of the United States. Medical schools, hospitals, and medical practice were virtually identical to those south of their border. While most similarities remain, Canada began to shift its system of finance in the mid-1960s, and today its health system stands as a model that many Americans believe should be adopted here (10, 11).

As in the other countries, Canadians have equal access to high-quality medical care and pay no bills for the services provided. The Canadian system is financed in all but two provinces through progressive federal and provincial taxes, and is administered by the provincial government. Two of the provinces mandate monthly premiums rather than general provincial taxes. The federal government grants monies to each province, a sum tied each year to growth in the GNP. Because of rising health care costs that have outstripped percentage growth in the GNP, the provinces have been forced to pick up an increasing share of health expenditures.

Canadians have a free choice of physician. Physicians in all provinces typically have private, office-based, fee-for-service practices. As in the United States, physicians in ambulatory care may treat their patients in hospital if they have admitting privileges. The fee levels for both primary care physicians and specialists are negotiated between each provincial government and the provincial medical association. Federal law provides that if a province allows physicians to bill patients over and above the amount paid by the provincial insurance system, the federal grant to the province will be reduced. The practical effect is that Canadian patients do not have to pay the physician. Private

practice is permitted but a physician cannot treat private patients and also be paid under the provincial insurance scheme. As a consequence, medical practice outside of the insurance system is almost nonexistent. There is a concern that fee-for-service medicine encourages physicians to provide additional services to maximize their incomes. As we have noted, the Germans and Dutch, while retaining fee-for-service medicine, have instituted procedures to prevent an excessive increase in the volume of services. The Canadians have done so as well. Each province monitors what fee-for-service physicians do. If a physician's billings to the health insurance system exceed a certain amount, future payments are paid at only 25 percent of the scheduled fee.

Iglehart notes that Canada is unique among Western democracies in prohibiting private insurance for services covered by the provincial insurance systems (11). Evans and his colleagues note that this serves to prevent a private insurer from skimming off the good risks, and that it also ensures that there will not develop a two-class system, whereby some get better service than others (12).

Hospitals negotiate individually a global yearly operating budget with their provincial government. Included in this budget are the salaries of hospital-based physicians. As with most countries, capital budgets are separate, and typically subject to government advance approval. This has led to a more restricted dispersion of technology, though technology in Canada is generally more widespread than it is in European countries.

While the federal government originally transferred to each province about 50 percent of the total costs of care, by 1990 the federal government's share, for reasons noted above, was reduced to about 35 percent. This often happens in countries where one level of government transfers monies to another level for the provision of certain services. The central government typically grants money as an incentive for the other level to develop a certain type of service. Over time the central government's contribution drops, either because, as in Canada, the federal share is tied to growth in the GNP while costs rise faster, or because the federal government, having seeded the development, chooses to withdraw its contributions. State governments in the United States are well familiar with this practice. Local governments in the United States are also aware of this practice when it comes to state government grants to local authorities.

The Canadian system is attractive on a number of accounts. First, it provides universal, free access to needed health services. Everyone is treated alike. Second, since there is only one payer—the provincial government—the cost of administration is much less than in the United States. Not only is a single claim form used, as against a multitude of different forms required by the different insurance companies in the United States, but in Canada there are no acquisition costs, no need to advertise for enrollees, no need to generate a profit—whether to pay the stockholders or to cover losses from unpaid bills—and no need to compete for business since there is only one carrier per province. Evans and his colleagues suggest that "the costs of running the American payment system itself, independent of the costs of patient care, may account for more than half the difference in cost between the Canadian and the U.S. systems" (12).

As attractive as the Canadian system is, there is one major shortcoming, one that is common to virtually all other countries, and that is the presence of nonemergency waiting lists for certain tests and for certain surgical procedures. This has to be kept in balance, however. Waiting lists exist in the United States as well, though they are not typically as long as one finds in the other countries. Waits of six to eight weeks in the United States are not uncommon. These waits are for conditions that are not emergencies—no need to rush. Reports of Canadian patient frustrations over lengthy nonemergency waiting periods, and reports of their crossing the border for care in the United States are numerous, but the extent to which this occurs is not well documented. A telephone survey of major U.S. hospitals along the U.S.-Canadian border by the

authors found few Canadian cases. Some cross-border flow, however, undoubtedly occurs. Some people are impatient and do not want to wait, and so, as they say in Britain, they "pay to avoid waiting while others wait to avoid paying." Some cross-border flow is done on a contract basis, whereby a Canadian hospital arranges to pay a U.S. hospital for certain services, usually because the Canadian hospital is unable to handle that case, either because of its critical nature and a backup of cases in the Canadian hospital or because the American hospital has pioneered a particular technology that is not yet commonly available in Canada. The bottom line, however, is that the quality of care in Canada—by every available index—is as high as in the United States, and that the system is extremely popular with virtually all Canadians.

The Canadian system, like those of Europe, provides many suggestions for ways we might develop. Unlike Germany and The Netherlands, the Canadians use a single payer—the province. Their costs of administration are thus significantly less than those of the United States, and probably also less than those of Germany and The Netherlands. Because of the cultural similarities nourished by an enormous cross-border flow of information, people, and goods, and because their system developed along parallel lines to the U.S. system, there would likely be an easier and more successful transfer of methods. There is, however, a major factor that militates against a complete transfer of the Canadian system, and that relates to their reliance upon government administration. Trust in government in the United States is much less than in Canada. As one Canadian has noted: "We did not rebel." Their traditional reliance on government differs from the U.S. experience. Notwithstanding, the similarities are enormous, and perhaps the Canadian system would be possible if, instead of government administration of the financial mechanisms, we used an intermediary such as the Dutch and Germans use. Whether that intermediary would be a single agency in each state or region (as in Canada) or multiple agencies (as in Germany and The Netherlands) would be points for discussion.

Insights for Reform

The countries whose health systems have been briefly summarized have dealt more or less successfully with two of the most pressing health care problems faced by the United States—access and cost. Access has been achieved by compulsory health insurance financed either by general taxes or by insurance programs in which the employers and employees contribute. The growth in health care costs have been slowed by capping operating expenditures, controlling capital costs, negotiating hospital global budgets or per diem charges, and negotiating physician fees and salaries.

In a democratic society, if everyone is in favor of a given course of action, that course will be taken. The greater the opposition to a course of action, the more difficult it is for a democratic society to decide what it should do. Good government and good public policy thus require a harmonization of interests to as great an extent as possible, and securing of support for a given course of action by as many as possible.

When it comes to health care reform, the importance of this principle should be clear. People agree that they want all to have access to care of the highest quality possible at a reasonable price. Their concerns are shared by government, by employers, by the health professions and hospitals, by Blue Cross and Blue Shield and other nonprofit insurance programs, and by the private insurance companies. All agree on the goal, but each has its own perspective on how best to attain the goal, perspectives that often serve to protect their interests and their traditional ways of doing things, and that would cause them the least amount of adjustment. To attain unanimity of approach may well be impossible but to secure overwhelming support for one course of action may be possible. Let us examine some possibilities.

Retention of the fee-for-service principle is a near-sacred issue for the majority of physicians in

the United States, notwithstanding the fact that there is a trend toward salaried practice in hospitals and medical groups. The Canadians, Dutch, and Germans have also maintained fee-for-service payments. The Danes, having used capitation payments for primary care in their two largest cities, abandoned that form of payment and introduced fee-for-service payments as was used in the rest of the country. As we have noted, however, the objection to fee-for-service payments is that they are an inducement to overservice, but the Canadians and Germans have dealt with this by reducing physicians payments per service if the physicians greatly exceed their past frequency of service. Monitoring physician practices in the United States would be simple since most large insurance companies and Blue Shield plans already have profiles on each physician's practice, profiles developed from claims they have submitted. Some physicians might object to having their payments reduced for excessive services, but this might be dealt with by having independent physician appeal boards, which have been common among Blue Shield plans. One could also envision adopting the German practice of turning the annual allocation for physician fees over to a physician association to disburse.

Critical to reforming the physician payment system is the creation of a mechanism through which physicians could have some say in how much they are to be paid. This is where it becomes important for physician organizations (state medical associations, state speciality societies, etc.) to have the right to negotiate the amounts they will be paid. At this writing the Federal Trade Commission (FTC) has ruled that such negotiations would be tantamount to restraint of trade and therefore illegal. Importantly, however, the AMA has asked the FTC to look again at its ruling on this matter and to reverse it. Thus, organized medicine seems to have reached the point where it would like the freedom to negotiate their payments, which is common in all of the countries noted above.

The problem with fee negotiations, however, is that the playing field is not altogether level. The physicians have enormous power, power emanating from their possession of unique training, knowledge, and skill, and their ability to withhold their services. Physician strikes do occur in many industrialized countries, though never to the point of withholding acute, emergency medical treatment. Medical services, however, are vital to a nation and therefore the right to strike may have to be subject to some restraint such as compulsory arbitration. Even so, to slow the growth of health care costs it may be necessary to adopt what the Canadians, Germans, and Dutch have done in tying growth in monies available for physicians services to growth in the GDP, inflation, or some such factor.

Capping the money available for health services, as the countries described above have done, is probably necessary given the growth in technology. Just imagine what the national health cost picture would look like if a successful, small, artificial heart were developed! But capping monies would be subject to the whim of politicians unless the politicians adopted some rational, objective standard to control growth in national health expenditures. Here again, all of the above countries have set a standard that controls the growth of health expenditures.

The notion of paying hospitals on a retrospective basis is rapidly disappearing in the United States. More and more a DRG type of payment system is being adopted. The problem this creates in the United States is that of "gaming," trying to get the best possible (i.e., highest-paying) diagnosis per admission. In addition, hospitals, in order to maintain solvency because of the costs in caring for the uninsured and of underpayments by Medicaid, seek to maximize their income through a variety of cost-shifting strategies (admission of discretionary well-insured patients, extra tests, etc.). Given all the computer data we now have about individual hospitals, we might begin to think about the Canadian, Danish, and Swedish systems of global hospital budgeting, simplifying the process for paying a hospital and giving hospitals more flexibility in management. Hospitals could negotiate their yearly

allocation with the insurer under some agreed upon guidelines.

Few policy experts in the United States believe that a federal or state goverment-administered system is politically feasible. In a few states, tradition may make such possible, but in the main the antipathy toward government is so pronounced that the interest groups that oppose a mandated government system would stall health care reform. Stability would seem to dictate that the health system be insulated from mometary political passions and crises. The Dutch and Germans have done this by the use of fiscal intermediaries (the sickness funds). The Canadians do not use fiscal intermediaries but their traditions with government are different, and for this reason this element of the Canadian system is probably not politically acceptable in the United States. Adopting the German approach—nonprofit insuring agents comparable to Blue Cross, Blue Shield, HIP, and Kaiser-Permanente—would be one alternative. Another alternative would be what the Dutch are planning to do, allowing both for-profit and nonprofit companies to compete, requiring that all comers be accepted and that a community rating system apply. Whether a quasi-Canadian-type approach of using a single nongovernment payer per state or region would be preferable is certainly an option that merits consideration, though it would undoubtedly generate widespread opposition from many health insurance companies, both for-profit and nonprofit.

Finally, a word on long-term care. The Danes, Swedes, and Dutch have all provided for long-term care in nursing homes and in the community without requiring depletion of all of the patient's resources. What is particularly significant is that these countries have provided a standard for these nursing homes that is matched in the United States only by our most expensive homes, which few of our citizens can afford.

Perhaps the most important factor that contributes to the success of the German, Dutch, Danish, and Canadian systems is the societal view that health care is a social right and that government has a responsibility to make certain that services are available for all. This does not mean that the government must provide the services, finance the services, or control all aspects of their provision. It does mean that government must be certain that those services are accessible for all whether provided by government, nonprofit entities, the for-profit sector, or some combination thereof. Until the United States accepts the principle that ensuring health care for all is a social responsibility, there may never be the political will to achieve meaningful health care reform in the United States.

DISCUSSION QUESTIONS

1. What advantages do you see to having the U.S. health system financed through taxes? Disadvantages?
2. What advantages do you see to having the U.S. health system financed on an insurance basis? Disadvantages?
3. If we were to continue financing health care on an insurance basis, should insurance be voluntary or compulsory?
4. What role should be played by the U.S. federal government in administering whatever health care reforms occur? State governments? For-profit and nonprofit health insurance companies?
5. Should we set a spending limit or goal for national health expenditures as in other countries? If desirable, how could this be done?
6. If we were to cap health care expenditures, what structural and financial changes in our health system would that require?

REFERENCES

1. Glaser, W.A.: *Health Insurance in Practice.* San Francisco, Jossey-Bass, 1991.
2. Eichhorn, S.: Health Services in the Federal Republic of Germany, in Raffel, M.W., ed.: *Comparative Health Systems.* University Park, The Pennsylvania State University Press, 1984.
3. Iglehart, J.K.: Germany's Health Care System, *N Engl J Med,* Vol. 324, No. 7, February 14, 1991, and Vol. 324, No. 24, June 13, 1991.
4. Tiddens, H.A., Heesters, J., and van de Zande, J.: Health Services in The Netherlands, in Raffel, M.W., ed.: *Comparative Health Systems.* University Park, The Pennsylvania State University Press, 1984.
5. Janssen, R.: *Costs and Financing of the Dutch Health Care.* Maastricht, University of Limburg, 1990 (mimeo).
6. Schoyvers, A.J.P.: The Netherlands Introduces Some Competition into the Health Services. *JAMA,* Vol. 266, No. 16, October 23/30, 1991.
7. Sondergarrd, W., Krasnik, A.: Health Services in Denmark, in Raffel, M.W., ed.: *Comparative Health Systems.* University Park, The Pennsylvania State University Press, 1984.
8. Holst, E.: *The Danish Healthcare System.* Copenhagen, University of Copenhagen, 1992 (mimeo).
9. Krasnik, A., Groenewegen, P.P., Pedersen, P.A., Scholten, P.V., Mooney, G., Gottschau, A., Flierman, H.A., and Damsgaard, M.T.: Changing Remuneration Systems: Effects on Activity in General Practice. *Br Med J,* June 30, 1990.
10. Hatcher, G.H., Hatcher, P.R., and Hatcher, E.C.: Health Services in Canada, in Raffel, M.W., ed.: *Comparative Health Systems.* University Park, The Pennsylvania State University Press, 1984.
11. Iglehart, J.K.: Canada's Health Care System Faces Its Problems, *N Engl J Med,* Vol. 322, No. 8, February 22, 1990.
12. Evans, R.G., Loomas, J., Barer, M.L., Labelle, R.J., Fooks, C., Stoddart, G.L., Anderson, G.M., Feeny, D., Gafni, A., Torrance, G.W., et al.: Controlling Health Expenditures—The Canadian Reality. *N Engl J Med,* Vol. 320, No. 9, March 2, 1989.

Appendix: Acronyms in Common Use

AAFP American Academy of Family Physicians

AAFPRS American Academy of Facial Plastic and Reconstructive Surgery

AAGP American Academy of General Practice

AAMC Association of American Medical Colleges

ABMS American Board of Medical Specialties

ACCME Accreditation Council for Continuing Medical Education

ACP American College of Physicians

ACS American College of Surgeons

ADA American Dental Association; American Dietetic Association; American Diabetes Association

AFDC Aid to Families with Dependent Children

AHA American Hospital Association

AHCPR Agency for Health Care Policy and Research

AHEC Area Health Education Center

AHME Association of Hospital Medical Education

AHPA American Health Planning Association

AID Agency for International Development

AIP Annual Implementation Plan

AJPH American Journal of Public Health

AMA American Medical Association

ANA American Nurses Association

AOA American Osteopathic Association

APHA American Public Health Association

APhA American Pharmaceutical Association

ARC Appalachian Regional Commission

ASPRS American Society of Plastic and Reconstructive Surgeons

ASTHO Association of State and Territorial Health Officers

ATSDR Agency for Toxic Substances and Disease Registry

AUPHA Association of University Programs in Health Administration

BC Blue Cross

BCHS Bureau of Community Health Services

BHM Bureau of Health Manpower

BMS Bureau of Medical Services

BS Blue Shield
BSN Bachelor of Science in Nursing

CAHEA Committee on Allied Health Education and Accreditation
CAT Computerized Axial Tomography; See CT
CBO Congressional Budget Office
CCFMG Cooperating Committee on Foreign Medical Graduates
CCME Coordinating Council on Medical Education
CDC Centers for Disease Control (formerly, Communicable Disease Center)
CETA Comprehensive Education and Training Act
CHAMPUS Civilian Health and Medical Program of the Uniformed Services
CHAMPVA Civilian Health and Medical Program of the Veterans Administration
CHP Comprehensive Health Planning
CME Council on Medical Education; Continuing Medical Education
CMIT Current Medical Information and Terminology
CMP Competitive Medical Plan
CMSS Council of Medical Specialty Societies
CON Certificate of Need
COPA Council on Postsecondary Accreditation
COTRANS Coordinated Transfer Application System
CPHA Commission on Professional and Hospital Activities
CPR Cardiac Pulmonary Resuscitation
CPT Current Procedural Terminology
CT Computed Tomography

DC Doctor of Chiropractic
DDS Doctor of Dental Surgery
DHEW Department of Health, Education, and Welfare; succeeded by the DHHS
DHHS Department of Health and Human Services
DMD Doctor of Dental Medicine
DO Doctor of Osteopathy
DPM Doctor of Podiatric Medicine

DRG Division of Research Grants
DRG(s) Diagnosis Related Group(s)

ECFMG Educational Commission on Foreign Medical Graduates (formerly, Educational Council for Foreign Medical Graduates)
EENT Eye, Ear, Nose, and Throat
EMS Emergency Medical Services
ENT Ear, Nose, and Throat
EPA Environmental Protection Agency
EPSDT Early and Periodic Screening Diagnosis and Treatment
ESP Economic Stabilization Program

FAH Federation of American Hospitals
FDA Food and Drug Administration
FHA Federal Housing Authority
FIC Fogarty International Center
FLEX Federation Licensing Examination
FMG(s) Foreign Medical Graduate(s)
FMGEMS Foreign Medical Graduate Examination in Medical Sciences
FSMB Federation of State Medical Boards
FTC Federal Trade Commission
FY Fiscal Year

GAO General Accounting Office
GDP Gross Domestic Product
GHA Group Health Association
GNP Gross National Product
GP General Practitioner
GYN Gynecology

H-B Hill-Burton Act
HCFA Health Care Financing Administration
HEW Health, Education, and Welfare; Succeeded by HHS
HHS Health and Human Services
HIAA Health Insurance Association of America
HII Health Insurance Institute
HIO Health Insuring Organization
HIP Health Insurance Plan of New York
HMO Health Maintenance Organization
HRA Health Resources Administration
HSA Health Services Administration

HSP   Health Systems Plan
HUP   Hospital Utilization Project
HURA   Health Underserved Rural Areas

ICF   Intermediate Care Facility
IHS   Indian Health Service
IMG   International Medical Graduate
IPA   Individual Practice Association

JAMA   The Journal of the American Medical Association
JCAH   Joint Commission on Accreditation of Hospitals; Succeeded by JCAHO
JCAHO   Joint Commission on Accreditation of Healthcare Organizations
JME   The Journal of Medical Education

LCCME   Liaison Committee on Continuing Medical Education
LCGME   Liaison Committee on Graduate Medical Education
LCME   Liaison Committee on Medical Education
LCSB   Liaison Committee for Specialty Boards
LPN   Licensed Practical Nurse
LVN   Licensed Vocational Nurse

MAP   Medical Audit Program
MCAT   Medical College Admission Test
MCH   Maternal and Child Health
MD   Doctor of Medicine
Med   Medicine
MEDLARS   Medical Literature and Analysis Retrieval System
MH   Mental Hygiene; Mental Health
MPP   Medicare Participating Physician
MR   Mental Retardation
MRI   Magnetic Resonance Imaging
MSKP   Medical Sciences Knowledge Profile

NBME   National Board of Medical Examiners
NABPLEX   National Association of Boards of Pharmacy Licensing Examination
NCHS   National Center for Health Statistics
NCI   National Cancer Institute
NEI   National Eye Institute

NEJM   The New England Journal of Medicine
NHC   Neighborhood Health Center
NHI   National Health Insurance
NHIS   National Health Interview Survey
NHLBI   National Heart, Lung, and Blood Institute
NHSC   National Health Service Corps
NIA   National Institute on Aging
NIAAA   National Institute on Alcohol Abuse and Alcoholic
NIAID   National Institute of Allergy and Infectious Diseases
NIAMSD   National Institute of Arthritis, and Musculoskeletal and Skin Diseases
NICHD   National Institute of Child Health and Human Development
NIDA   National Institute on Drug Abuse
NIDDKD   National Institute of Diabetes and Digestive and Kidney Diseases
NIDR   National Institute of Dental Research
NIEHS   National Institute of Environmental Health Sciences
NIGMS   National Institute of General Medical Sciences
NIH   National Institutes of Health
NIMH   National Institute of Mental Health
NINDS   National Institute of Neurological Disorders and Stroke
NIOSH   National Institute of Occupational Safety and Health
NIRMP   National Intern and Resident Matching Program
NJPC   National Joint Practice Commission
NLM   National Library of Medicine
NLN   National League of Nursing
NLRB   National Labor Relations Board
NMA   National Medical Association
NMR   Nuclear Magnetic Resonance; See MRI
NRMP   National Residency Matching Program

OB   Obstetrics
OD   Doctor of Optometry
OEO   Office of Economic Opportunity
OIH   Office of International Health
OMB   Office of Management and Budget

OR   Operating Room
OSHA   Occupational Safety and Health Administration
OTA   Office of Technology Assessment

PA   Physician Assistant
PAHO   Pan American Health Organization
PAS   Professional Activity Study
PHR   Public Health Reports
PHS   Public Health Service
PHSA   Pennsylvania Hospital Services Association
PL   Public Law
PMA   Pharmaceutical Manufacturers Association
PNHA   Physicians National Housestaff Association
PP   Preferred Provider; Participating Physician
PPO   Preferred Provider Organization
PPS   Prospective Payment or Pricing System
PRO   Professional Review Organization
PSRO   Professional Standards Review Organization

RFP   Request for Proposal
RHI   Rural Health Initiative
RMP   Regional Medical Program
RN   Registered Nurse

SAMHSA   Substance Abuse and Mental Health Services Administration

SHCC   State Health Coordinating Council
SHMO   Social Health Maintenance Organization
SHPDA   State Health Planning and Development Agency
SHUR   System for Hospital Uniform Reporting
SMI   Supplementary Medical Insurance
SMSA   Standard Metropolitan Statistical Area
SNF   Skilled Nursing Facility
SSA   Social Security Administration
SSI   Supplementary Security Income
STD   Sexually Transmitted Disease

TB   Tuberculosis

UCR   Usual, Customary, and Reasonable
UR   Utilization Review
USFMG   U.S. Foreign Medical Graduate
USMG   United States Medical Graduate
USMLE   United States Medical Licensing Examination

VA   Veterans Affairs
VD   Venereal Disease
VE   Voluntary Effort
VNA   Visiting Nurse Association
VQE   Visa Qualifying Examination

WHO   World Health Organization
WIC   Women, Infants, and Children

About the Authors

Marshall W. Raffel is Professor of Health Policy and Administration at The Pennsylvania State University. He has had extensive experience in the health field, first as a corpsman in naval hospitals during the Second World War, later with Blue Cross and Blue Shield in New York City, then in industrial health and safety programming for the Baltimore and Ohio Railroad, followed by four years as the principal health planner for the Maryland State Planning Commission. After teaching political science in New Zealand and doing research on the health services of that country, he returned to the United States to serve on the U.S. Surgeon General's staff as Chief for Program Research and Development in the Office of Comprehensive Health Planning. At Penn State he pioneered in developing the baccalaureate program in Health Planning and Administration, and continued his research interests in New Zealand health services (to which he returns periodically for field research) and in health manpower education. In 1973, he served as a consultant to the World Health Organization in India and Nepal, and in 1978 he was a World Health Organization travel fellow, studying the health services of England, Denmark, Sweden, and Czechoslovakia. Under sponsorship of the United States and former Yugoslav governments, he also spent time studying the health services of Yugoslavia. He has visited and studied the health services of Hungary, Poland, Romania, and the former Soviet Union (with study visits to Russia, Estonia, Georgia, Uzbechistan, and Yalta). In addition to authoring papers in professional journals, he is editor and co-author of a text, *Comparative Health Systems.* He is also co-editor with Norma K. Raffel of *Perspectives on Health Policy: Australia, New Zealand, United States.* A graduate in philosophy from the University of Illinois, Dr. Raffel holds a Ph.D. in political science from the Victoria University of Wellington, New Zealand.

Norma K. Raffel received a Master of Science and a Doctor of Philosophy from the University of Maryland. After completing her studies, she was on the faculty in the Department of Medicine at the University of Maryland School of Medicine. She has taught biological sciences at Goucher College and The Pennsylvania State University, and at Penn State, a course on the U.S. health system, and has served as a consultant to state education agencies and universities on educational policy. Her international activities include professional travel in the People's Republic of China, the Middle East, Latin America, eastern and western Europe, and the Soviet Union, studying the health services and the position of women. Her published works include articles on the health systems of New Zealand, Denmark, the Soviet Union, Hungary, Czechoslovakia, and the United States. In 1987 she co-edited with Marshall W. Raffel the book, *Perspectives on Health Policy: Australia, New Zealand, United States.*

Index

Numerals in *italic* indicate a figure; "t" following a page number indicates a table.